Neurological Classics
in Modern Translation

Neurological Classics in Modern Translation

Edited by
David A. Rottenberg, M.D.
and
Fred H. Hochberg, M.D.

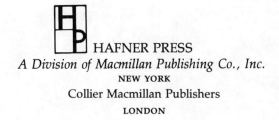

HAFNER PRESS
A Division of Macmillan Publishing Co., Inc.
NEW YORK
Collier Macmillan Publishers
LONDON

Hafner Press
A Division of Macmillan Publishing Co., Inc.
866 Third Avenue, New York, N. Y. 10022

Collier Macmillan Canada, Ltd.

Library of Congress Catalog Card Number: 77-74853

Printed in the United States of America

printing number
1 2 3 4 5 6 7 8 9 10

Library of Congress Cataloging in Publication Data

Main entry under title:

Neurological classics in modern translation.

    Includes index.
    1. Nervous system--Diseases--Addresses, essays, lectures. I. Rottenberg, David A. II. Hochberg, Fred. H. [DNLM: 1. Neurology--Collected works.
O4NLM / WL5 N494]
RC346.N39   616.8'08   77-74853
ISBN 0-02-851180-8

CONTENTS

LIST OF TRANSLATORS

Walter H.O. Bohne
Associate Professor of Surgery
Cornell University Medical College

Steven L. Fish
Washington, D.C.

Carol N. Hochberg
Instructor in Medicine
Peter Bent Brigham Associated Hospitals

Fred H. Hochberg
Instructor in Neurology
Harvard Medical School

Kate Liepmann
London, England

E.P. Richardson, Jr.
Professor of Neuropathology
Harvard Medical School

David A. Rottenberg
Assistant Professor of Neurology
Cornell University Medical College

William C. Schoene
Associate Professor of Pathology
Harvard Medical School

Claude G. Wasterlain
Associate Professor of Neurology
University of California at Los Angeles

PREFACE

Neurological Classics in Modern Translation represents a concerted attempt on the part of the editors and translators to provide English-speaking medical students, general physicians, neurologists, and neurosurgeons with ready access to some of the most significant—and, in several instances, most controversial—contributions of nineteenth and twentieth century European neurology. Most of the papers in this volume have never before been translated into English. Some have appeared in specialty journals in condensed or in grossly abbreviated form; others have been so awkwardly or imprecisely rendered as to demand retranslation.

We have decided to translate each original article in its entirety (including figures, illustrations, and tables) in order to allow the reader to interpret the author's conclusions in the light of the latter's declared prejudices, clinical observations, and pathological correlations. The selection of articles for inclusion in this volume has been based almost exclusively upon their relevance to the themes and controversies of contemporary neurology; though often quoted, their inaccessibility to most English-speaking readers has led inevitably to misunderstanding and misinterpretation. Several inclusions were prompted by our desire to interject unfamiliar and thought-provoking contributions into the English neurological literature.

We hope that our neurologist translators have succeeded in accurately conveying the spirit as well as the erudition of their European predecessors.

MORPHOLOGY

Introduction

Sanford L. Palay, M.D.
Bullard Professor of Neuroanatomy
Harvard Medical School

SANTIAGO RAMÓN Y CAJAL (1852–1934) began his epochal investigations of the nervous system in 1887. During the next two years he made the essential revolutionary discoveries that resulted in our present conception of the nervous system. Before the work of Ramón y Cajal the prevailing conception of the nervous system was that enunciated by Gerlach in 1858 and subsequently. According to this idea the processes of nerve cells were all indiscriminately united in a continuous reticulum, in which the nerve cell bodies appeared here and there as swollen nodal points. The incoming nerve fibers of the sensory roots joined this reticulum by means of their terminal branches, and the fibers of the motor roots originated from it. Since Gerlach's conception did not at first recognize any differences between the processes of nerve cells, it had to be slightly modified when Deiters (1865) showed that there are two kinds of processes—dendrites (protoplasmic expansions) and axons (axis cylinders, neural processes)—and that the axons of anterior horn cells could be traced into the ventral roots. This new piece of information, however, suggested no essential change in the reticular theory. When Golgi (1873) invented his method for staining (impregnating) individual whole nerve cells in their natural places within the brain, an adequate method had at last become available for analyzing the morphological organization of the nervous system. But although Golgi (1885) saw that dendrites were independent of the pervasive reticulum, he concluded that they ended freely about blood vessels, and although the discovered the recurrent collaterals of axons, he thought that they joined the reticulum. He relegated dendrites to a nutritive role. Golgi was too conservative to discard the prevailing point of view. The modern reader should not underestimate the enormous difficulty of discovering the three-dimensional form and interrelationships of nerve cells. Even with an adequate technique it was difficult to read new signals. Neurohistologists had no reason to suspect that nerve cells were discrete and independent since animal cells lacked distinct walls. In any case, the Golgi method hardly altered any fundamental concepts before 1890, since it was, to quote Ramón y Cajal, "un peu capricieux et aléatoire."

By 1888 Ramón y Cajal had seen enough Golgi preparations to convince

3

himself of the marvelous utility of the method, and he set himself the task of making it reliable. He started from two premises: (1) since nerve cells are very large in large animals like man, it is desirable to use small animals like mice in which whole nerve cells might be visualized in a single preparation; and (2) since the central nervous system is complicated in large adult animals, it should be advantageous to study the immature, simple nervous system of very young animals, which is not only small but, also, less complicated. In addition, he was already keenly aware of the still unexplained inhibition of the Golgi impregnation by the presence of myelin. Immature small animals have little or no myelin in their central nervous system. Acting on these premises, Ramón y Cajal succeeded so brilliantly that within a few years he had explored the entire nervous system not only in mammals, but also in birds, reptiles, amphibians and fishes, and in many invertebrates as well. The range of his discoveries was enormous, and the accuracy of his observations continues to astound each succeeding generation of neuroscientists.

But in 1888 and 1889, when he published his first results, he was alarmed and disappointed, as he recounts in his autobiography, by the calm with which the scientific world greeted his discoveries. Those to whom he sent reprints of his papers responded with silence, and the few citations of his work that appeared in the foreign literature suggested to him that the authors had not even read his papers, especially in view of his provocative opinions. Ramón y Cajal determined to have a hearing. This he managed first by having French translations of his papers (often with significant emendations and additions) published in the most prestigious German journals and second by attending the next Congress of Anatomists in Berlin (1889). Although several of his papers on the nervous system had appeared in a language everyone could understand by the time he arrived in Berlin, he was received with skepticism and disdain by most of those who deigned to examine his demonstration of original preparations. But several of the great histologists of the time—His, Schwalbe, Retzius, Waldeyer, van Gehuchten, and Kölliker—carefully studied his slides and pronounced themselves convinced. Especially significant was the conversion of Kölliker, the most important personality in German biology, who acclaimed Cajal as his own greatest discovery. The success of Ramón y Cajal from this point onward was assured. In 1906 he and Golgi shared the Nobel Prize for their discoveries in the structure of the nervous system.

The paper chosen for the present collection is the first English translation of a segment of Ramón y Cajal's earliest comprehensive description of the nervous system. The paper was originally one of a series of lectures delivered at the Academy of Medical Sciences of Barcelona and published in Spanish in the Revista de Ciencias Médicas de Barcelona in 1892. The whole series was amplified by the author and then translated into German by Hans Held at the request of Wilhelm His and published in Archiv für Anatomie und Physiologie, Anatomische Abteilung, for 1893 (pp. 319–428) as "Neue Darstellung vom histologischen Bau des Centralnervensystems." The same texts, somewhat enlarged, were translated from the Spanish into

French by Ramón y Cajal's friend, L. Azoulay, and published in 1894 with a preface by the great French histologist Mathias Duval under the title "Les Nouvelles Idées sur la Fine Anatomie des Centres Nerveux." In his annotated list of his most memorable publications, Ramón y Cajal wrote that in these lectures all the new facts about the morphology of the vertebrate central nervous system were brought together for the first time, as well as the physiological implications he had deduced from them.

In this paper Ramón y Cajal first summarizes his approach to the most important questions of cortical structure and then goes into a rather sketchy histological description of the cerebral cortex. Although regional differences in the physiology of the cerebral hemispheres had already been noted (Fritsch and Hitzig; Ferrier), Ramón y Cajal does not identify the region of the cortex that he studied, even in the figure legends. This work was done long before the rise of cortical cytoarchitectonics, and his intention was clearly to establish the general cellular characteristics of the layers distinguishable in Golgi preparations. In this paper he recognizes only four layers; later he would distinguish nine. The present mode of recognizing six layers with many subdivisions of the deeper four did not become established until a dozen years later, after the work of Brodmann and Campbell (1905).

The description of cells and fibers in the cortex is concerned with two major questions: (1) the classification of the principal neuronal types according to their morphology and (2) the discovery of connections between the nerve fibers and the nerve cells. On the basis of his observations Ramón y Cajal tried to construct probable circuits involving not only the incoming fibers but also the axons and recurrent collaterals of the cells located within the cortex. The audacity of this attempt is unlikely to impress the modern neurologist, who regards the central nervous system as obviously an immensely complicated network of cells and is accustomed to thinking in terms of pathways and connections. But it was Ramón y Cajal who made this conception obvious. He recognized that since axons and recurrent collaterals impinge on the dendrites and cell bodies of nerve cells in the cortex, the nerve impulse must be transmitted from the axon of one cell to the dendrites and cell body of another. A few years later, Sherrington (1897) would apply a new name, the synapse, to the microscopic site where the nerve impulse passes from one cell to another. He recognized that the impulse was transmitted at this site and started a new impulse in the receiving cell. But Ramón y Cajal in 1892 speaks only of connections between axons and dendrites. His observations showed him first that the connected cells are related only by contact, not by protoplasmic continuity, and second that the direction taken by the "nervous current" in the nerve cell proceeded from dendrites to cell body to axon, whence it was transmitted to another cell through the axonal terminals impinging on the dendrites of the second cell. The first observation later became codified in the Neuron Doctrine and the second became the law of dynamic polarity, which Ramón y Cajal enunciated in the present paper. The importance of this law lies not in its intrinsic correctness (it has had to be modified in order to allow direct synaptic interaction between dendrites and between axons and for electrotonic coupling between nerve cells), but in its rationalization of the form of all nerve cells and, thus, of the link between the morphological organization of the nervous system and its function.

A New Concept of the Histology of the Central Nervous System

S. RAMÓN Y CAJAL

THE STRUCTURE of the mammalian cerebral cortex has always intrigued neurologists, among whose number Gerlach, Wagner, Schultze, Deiters, Stieda, Krause, Kölliker, Exner, Meynert, Edinger, Betz, Golgi, Martinotti, Flechsig, and Retzius should be cited for their outstanding contributions to our knowledge in this area.

Prior to the publication of Golgi's famous book, _Sulla fina anatomia degli organi centrali del sistema nervoso_ (1885), all that was known about the structure of the cortical gray matter could be summarized as follows:

1. The gray matter contained pyramidal cells with branched protoplasmic sprouts (dendrites) directed toward the cortical surface and descending axis cylinders, which were thought to be unbranched. The presence of neural expansions (axon collaterals) had been established only for the largest cells.

2. Several cortical layers were distinguished, each of which seemed to contain a distinct neuronal population. The following layers were described by Meynert, whose authority was accepted blindly by Hugenin and many others: (from outside inward) I, composed of neuroglia, nerve fibers, and a few small fusiform or triangular ganglion cells; II, containing small pyramidal cells; III, Ammon's formation, composed of large pyramidal cells similar to those seen in Ammon's horn; IV, the layer of small spherical and triangular cells; and V, the layer of fusiform cells.

NOTE: Translated by D. A. Rottenberg from: Ramón y Cajal, S., "El Nuevo Concepto de la Histología de los Centros Nerviosos," _Revista de Ciencias Médicas de Barcelona_ 18 (1892), 457–76.

Aside from the shape of the cell body and its thickest protoplasmic expansions (largest dendrites), nothing at all was known about the neurons which populated these layers; absolutely nothing was known about the arrangement of their finest dendritic branches, and there was little information regarding the existence and course of the majority of their axons. Gerlach's theory of protoplasmic networks was invoked to explain the dynamic interaction of cortical neurons.

3. It was known that myelinated fibers were irregularly disposed within the intermediate cortical layers, giving rise to plexiform structures, and that they formed convergent fascicles within the deeper cortical layers. These myelinated fibers were continuous above with the axis cylinders or basilar expansions of pyramidal cells, and below they constituted the myelinated fibers of the corona radiata.

Such was the state of our knowledge of the fine structure of the cerebral cortex when Golgi appeared on the scene, armed with a powerful method for staining nerve cells. Golgi's work firmly established the following:

1. the arborization of the protoplasmic processes of pyramidal cells and the absence of anastomoses;
2. that the vast majority of pyramidal cells possess descending axis cylinders which give off branched collaterals;
3. the existence in gray matter of two cell types based on axon morphology: cells whose axons lose their identity after multiple branchings (sensory cells) and cells whose axons, in spite of sprouting numerous collaterals, retain their identity and join up with nerve fibers in the white matter (motor cells);
4. the morphology of the neuroglia, relating the interweaving (without anastomoses) of the innumerable fibrillary expansions which radiate from astrocytes* to the background matrix of the nervous system.

Except for his speculations in the realm of physiology, such as the abovementioned distinction between motor and sensory neurons, Golgi's findings have been confirmed in all of their essentials by Tartuferi, Mondino, Fusari, Nansen, Kölliker, Todlt and Kahler, Obersteiner, Edinger, Retzius, and Cajal.

Since the publication of Golgi's important book six years ago, our knowledge of cerebral histology has hardly advanced at all. However, we should not neglect the contributions of Flechsig, who by means of a special staining technique succeeded in demonstrating the presence of myelin in the collaterals of cortical nerve fibers (1890), and Martinotti, who recently (1891) demonstrated that some of the fibers in the first

---

*"Spider cells (Dieters' cells)" in the original—EDS.

cortical layer derive from certain pyramidal cells with ascending axis cylinders.

In spite of the unremitting efforts of many investigators and of the recent advances in analytical methodology the problems awaiting solution, as regards the structure and function of the cerebral cortex, are as numerous as they are extraordinary.

What are the properties of the nerve cells in the first cortical layer? Do axon collaterals form a network, or do they terminate freely like those in the white matter of the spinal cord? What cells give rise to the fibers of the corpus callosum? Do the cells of origin of the association, projection, and commissural fibers lie within different cortical layers, or are they intermingled, as is the case in the spinal cord? Where within the pyramidal cell does the nervous impulse originate, and what is the significance of that singular tuft (apical dendrite) which, in all vertebrates, the pyramidal cell directs toward the cortical surface? Are there motor and sensory cells in the cerebral cortex? Do protoplasmic-neural (axodendritic) contacts mediate the interaction of cortical neurons in conformity with the law of cellular interconnection that obtains in the cerebellum, spinal cord, olfactory bulb, etc.?

Although a number of rather ingenious solutions to these problems have been proposed by anatomists and physiologists during the past two decades, these solutions are based on flawed observations or on data obtained from pathological material susceptible of various interpretations—thus the need for a thoroughgoing reappraisal of the subject, a calm and impartial study of the cerebral cortex employing those analytical methods that have so vastly increased our knowledge of the spinal cord and cerebellum.

The study of the cerebral cortex is an extremely difficult undertaking, perhaps the most difficult that has ever confronted any anatomist. The supreme dignity which surrounds the brain and the awesome complexity of its workings presuppose the existence of an extremely complicated warp, sure to ensnare those who imagine that nature unfolds multifarious exalted phenomena according to schematic formulae or by means of simple mechanisms, whose threads can be partially unravelled by only the most sagacious investigators. But it should also be recognized that the approach adopted by Golgi and his disciples, however excellent for demonstrating certain fine points of cellular morphology, is not the approach best suited to demonstrate the connections between cortical neurons. Golgi and his co-workers, and nearly all those who have tackled this problem using modern histological methods, have preferred to study the human cerebrum and the brains of large mammals. Because of the enormous extent, the intricacy, and the labyrinthine quality of the warp, it is almost impossible to follow a single mammalian axon or axon collateral from its origin to its termination.

On the other hand, if one elects to study small mammals (mouse, rat, bat, guinea pig, etc.), preferably neonates or even embryos, the cortical layers become more compact, the distances shorter and the staining of nerve fibers more constant; it becomes possible to specify the origin, course, and termination of some nerve fibers. I have proceeded in this fashion and, consequently, have made several discoveries which, though they do not resolve all of the outstanding problems (an impossible task, especially for me, given the scope of the undertaking), may by furthering our knowledge contribute to the early solution of these problems.

The results obtained using this approach can be confidently generalized to higher mammals and to man since all mammalian brains are fundamentally similar, differing only in macroscopic form and in the relative size of their constituent parts.

Let us move on now to consider the cerebral cortex, concentrating on those structural arrangements which are observed in all mammalian species, and which, therefore, represent the essential features of cortical organization.

Four cortical layers may be distinguished: I, the *molecular layer*; II, the *layer of small pyramidal cells*; III, the *layer of large pyramidal cells*; IV, the *layer of polymorphic cells*. Layers I and IV are well defined, but such is not the case with Layers II and III, which gradually merge one into the other (Fig. 1).*

MOLECULAR LAYER

In sections stained with carmine or with aniline dyes this layer has a finely granular or reticular appearance. Here and there one encounters small neuroglial nuclei; these are especially numerous near the pial-cortical junction. Other larger nuclei surrounded by triangular or fusiform protoplasmic bodies are exceedingly rarely encountered and probably correspond to nerve cells.

In the most superficial region of the molecular layer Kölliker described a zone of horizontally oriented myelinated fibers; his results were subsequently confirmed by Exner, using an osmic acid-ammonia method, and by Edinger, Obersteiner, Todlt, Martinotti, etc., who employed the more definitive technique of Weigert and Pal (Fig. 3A).

Little or nothing was known about the origin of these fibers, some of which appear to descend to deeper cortical layers, until two years ago when Martinotti, using Golgi's method, made two important observations: (1) that some of these fibers change direction, becoming vertically oriented, and merge with the ascending axis cylinders of certain pyram-

---

*Figures 1–7 in this translation were numbered 7–13 in the original article—EDS.

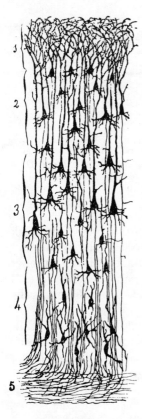

Figure 1. Vertical section through the gray matter of a cerebral convolution: 1, molecular layer; 2, small pyramidal cell layer; 3, large pyramidal cell layer; 4, polymorphic cell layer.

idal cells; and (2) that the majority of the horizontally oriented fibers in the molecular layer branch repeatedly, as if they were the terminal arborizations of axis cylinders.

But the origin of most of these fibers remains to be determined. Recognizing that the molecular layer contains autochthonous myelinated fibers which are thicker and more numerous than the fibers that descend to subjacent cortical layers, I suspected that perhaps all of the thicker fibers and a substantial number of the thinner ones derive from the autochthonous cells of the molecular layer. The existence of these cells is still not widely recognized; many workers who were unable to demonstrate them in Golgi preparations tended to regard them as neuroglia. But my suspicions were confirmed by studies in small young mammals, which revealed the existence of four distinct cell types:

1. Polygonal cells. These are medium-sized cells (Fig. 2C); four to six slender, irregular, highly branched, more or less divergent protoplasmic processes originate from the angles of the cell body. Some of these processes descend as far as the small pyramidal layer. The thin axis

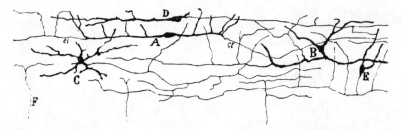

Figure 2.   Nerve cells in the first cortical layer: A, fusiform cell with two horizontal axis cylinders; B, triangular cell; C, polygonal cell with a single axis cylinder; D, fusiform cell with a horizontal axis cylinder; E, small cell with a bifurcate axis cylinder.

cylinder usually emerges from the cell body or from one of its thick protoplasmic processes. Directed obliquely or horizontally it ramifies throughout the molecular layer, ultimately resolving itself into a number of tortuous twig-like prolongations which course parallel to the cortical surface. Unlike pyramidal cell axons, the axis cylinders of polygonal cells never descend into the white matter.

2. *Fusiform cells.*   These are markedly elongated, slender ovoid cells with smooth contours (Fig. 2A). Thick characteristically rectilinear protoplasmic expansions take origin from the two poles of the cell body; after pursuing a long horizontal course they change direction and terminate near the cortical surface. The collaterals of these sprouts are directed upward and terminate freely.

Two, sometimes three axons are associated with a single polygonal cell, a truly unique state of affairs, not observed elsewhere in the mammalian nervous system. When two axons are present they emerge from the polar protoplasmic expansions precisely where the latter change direction (see above), and, coursing horizontally in opposite directions through the molecular layer, they give off a multitude of collateral and terminal branches (Fig. 2ci).

3. *Triangular cells.*   These cells (Fig. 2B) represent a morphological variant of the preceding type, from which they can be distinguished by their greater bulk and by the presence of three divergent, infrequently branching expansions, one of which ordinarily ascends obliquely toward the cortical surface. Sometimes the multiple axons arise from the cell body, sometimes from its various protoplasmic expansions; each axon courses more or less horizontally within the molecular layer, terminating in extensive tortuous arborizations which, in common with the terminal arborizations of the other cells in this layer, appear to make contact with the peripheral sprouts of pyramidal cells.

4. *Unipolar fusiform cells* (Fig. 2D). Elongated, spindle-shaped, more or less uniform cells are frequently observed in the cortex of embryonic and newborn animals (rat, cat, dog). Each horizontally oriented cell body is prolonged at one end into a thick horizontal protoplasmic expansion which ramifies without delay. A long horizontal nerve fiber arises from the opposite pole; after sprouting collaterals at right angles it ends in extensive horizontal arborizations.

I shall ignore for the present the question as to whether or not these cells, which to date have only been observed in newborn mammals or in full-term fetuses, represent a stage in the evolution of the abovementioned fusiform cells, or whether they persist into adulthood as a distinct cell type.

The assembled autochthonous nerve fibers together with the ascending fibers from subjacent layers form a compact plexus in the molecular layer. The terminal branches of ascending pyramidal cell tufts penetrate this meshwork (Fig. 3A). One cannot but consider this singular arrangement, which is certainly common to all vertebrates, as an important example of contact-mediated neurotransmission, comparable to

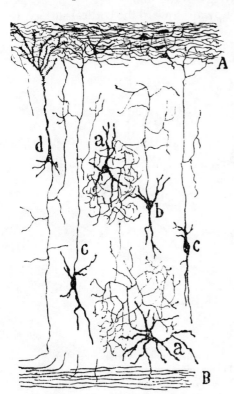

Figure 3. Section of the cortical gray matter: A, molecular layer; B, white matter; a, cells with short, extensively ramified axis cylinders; b, cell with ascending axis cylinder that does not reach the molecular layer; c, cells with ascending axis cylinders that ramify in the molecular layer; d, small pyramid.

that which occurs in the cerebellum between parallel fibrils and the protoplasmic arborizations of Purkinje cells. As these contacts are oblique or transverse the terminal branches of pyramidal cells are provided with collateral spines; the finest unmyelinated nerve fibrils appear to fit snugly into the clefts between spines.

SMALL PYRAMIDAL CELL LAYER

The layer consists of many small to medium-sized (10–12 micra) polyhedral or pyramidal cells.

All pyramidal cells, whether they belong to Layer II or to another cortical layer, possess certain general morphologic features which should be mentioned briefly before proceeding to a description of the individual cell layers. The cell body is conical or pyramidal, and the axis cylinder always arises from its basal surface. The protoplasmic processes are extremely numerous and should be distinguished according to their origin: *ascending sprout* or *primordial expansion, sprout collaterals* and *basilar expansions arising from the cell body* (Figs. 1 and 4D).

The *sprout* is thick and directed upward toward the cortical surface; it

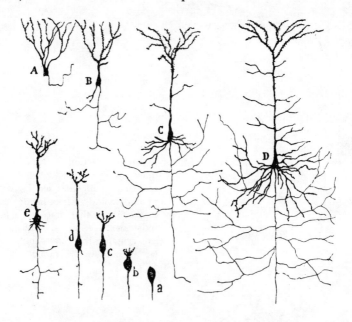

Figure 4. Upper series—the psychic cell in various vertebrates: A, frog; B, newt; C, mouse; D, man. Lower series—stages in the development of the psychic (pyramidal) cell: a, neuroblast without protoplasmic sprout; d, appearance of axon collaterals; e, formation of protoplasmic expansions of the cell body and sprout.

parallels the sprouts of adjacent pyramidal cells, and on reaching the molecular layer it terminates in a splended tuft of protoplasmic branches which end freely among the nerve fibrils of this layer. The assemblage of peripheral tufts gives rise to a dense protoplasmic plexus, which accounts for the finely reticulated appearance of this cortical region in routine carmine preparations.

According to Golgi and Martinotti these protoplasmic processes are associated with blood vessels or neuroglial cells; but, in fact, such preferential associations are not observed, and these processes are distributed (and terminate) throughout the molecular layer, that is to say, wherever terminal arborizations occur. Retzius has confirmed this arrangement in human fetuses.

I have referred to the sprouts as primordial because they appear earlier during the development of the nerve cell than any of the other protoplasmic rami, as is apparent from the evolutionary scheme in Figure 4.

Lateral expansions of the sprout (sprout collaterals) arise at focal dilatations, forming acute or right angles; they course laterally and end freely after several bifurcations.

Basilar expansions leave the cell body and proceed laterally or inferiorly, branching repeatedly and disappearing into the surrounding neuropil.

As noted above, the *axis cylinders* of pyramidal cells arise either from the base of the cell body or from a basilar protoplasmic expansion; they course downward, traverse all of the cortical layers, and end in the white matter, where they become associated with nerve fibers. It was previously thought that this continuation was always accomplished by means of an axonal bend, but I have demonstrated that it is often effected by means of a bifurcation, with the result that two nerve fibers are initiated in the white matter. During its progress through the gray matter the axis cylinder emits six to ten fine collaterals which branch off at right angles and, proceeding horizontally and at times obliquely, terminate in two or three extremely delicate fibrils.

So much for the structure of the mammalian pyramidal cell. By virtue of its unique morphology and its exclusive occurrence in the cerebral cortex, the substrate of higher nervous function, the pyramidal cell may be considered as a truly *psychic cell*.

In lower vertebrates the *psychic corpuscle* is morphologically less well developed, being correspondingly shorter and less voluminous.

In *Batrachia* (Fig. 4A) all of the protoplasmic expansions are reduced to the terminal tuft, which ramifies in a well-developed molecular layer. Sprout collaterals and basilar expansions are lacking.

The peripheral sprout has made its appearance in *Reptilia* (Fig. 4B), but collaterals have not yet developed; the basilar expansions of mammalian cells are represented by a variably branched descending prolongation of the cell body.

Now that the general features of pyramidal cells have been described, there is little more to add about the pyramids of the second cortical layer (Fig. 1). They increase in size from above downward, and their peripheral sprouts become progressively longer. The sprout, which gives off numerous collaterals near its cell body, terminates in a generous tuft; the latter occupies nearly the entire thickness of the molecular layer and interdigitates with the tufts of neighboring cells. Basilar expansions are quite numerous and highly branched.

Suffice it to say that the axis cylinder is extremely fine, that it descends, and that at a certain distance from the cell body it gives off four or five fine collaterals which dichotomize once or twice. On occasion I have observed the highest collaterals of these axons to ascend as far as the molecular layer (Fig. 3d).

How do the collaterals terminate? Golgi, who discovered them, supposed that after several branchings they anastomose among themselves, contributing to the formation of a continuous interstitial network in the gray matter.

This is one of many problems whose resolution depends upon embryological and comparative anatomical observations. The axon collaterals in man and in large mammals are extraordinarily long, and no single section, however thick, enables one to examine the entire length of a single fiber.

In embryonic and newborn mammals, however, the collaterals are extremely short, and it is readily apparent that they end in varicosities without terminal arborizations. By studying sufficiently young fetuses it is possible to observe the growth of collaterals from their first appearance as warty appendages on the axis cylinder to their development of terminal bifurcations (Fig. 4d and e).

Although the distances are much greater it is possible to confirm the existence of a similar arrangement in small adult mammals such as the mouse, bat, and white rat (Fig. 4C).

LARGE PYRAMIDAL LAYER (Meynert's Ammonic layer)

Only the larger size of its cells (20–30 micra) and the greater length and thickness of their peripheral sprouts distinguish this layer from the one immediately above it. Above, this layer merges imperceptibly (as regards cell size) into Layer II; it is better delimited below, though pyramids are often scattered among the polymorphic cells of the subjacent layer [Fig. 1 (3)].

The axis cylinder is very thick; it courses almost directly downward to the white matter, where it usually continues as a projection fiber. It occasionally bifurcates or emits a thick collateral to the corpus callosum (Fig. 7B).

During their progress through the gray matter these axis cylinders give off six to eight horizontal or oblique collaterals, which dichotomize two or three times. The terminal twigs end freely in nodular swellings.

The ascending sprout, the basilar expansions, etc. are similar to their counterparts in the small pyramidal cell layer.

POLYMORPHIC CELL LAYER [Fig. 1(4) and 7D]

A few pyramidal cells are found in this layer—some giant, some medium-sized; their peripheral sprouts are directed toward the molecular layer. But the majority of the cells in this layer are ovoid, fusiform, triangular or polygonal. Two characteristics of their peripheral sprouts are noteworthy: (1) that they lack a definite orientation (there are exceptions), and (2) that they never reach the molecular level, where the pyramidal cell tufts are concentrated. The sprout is occasionally absent, being represented by two or more short oblique processes, and it is not unusual to find a cell with three thick protoplasmic expansions, two of which descend to the white matter.

The thin descending axis cylinder emits three or four branched collaterals, makes a sharp bend or a T bifurcation and becomes associated with one or two myelinated nerve fibers in the white matter (Fig. 7G).

Cells with short axis cylinders (Fig.3). Mixed in among the cells of Layers II, III, and IV, though present in limited numbers, are two types of cells, unique in that their axis cylinders arborize within the gray matter. These are Golgi's *sensory cells* and Martinotti's *cells with ascending axons.*

The *former* tend to be large polygonal cells which send out protoplasmic processes in all directions. The axis cylinder arises from the superior, inferior, or lateral aspect of the cell body, pursues a short variable course and ends freely in a tortuous arborization; the terminal twigs envelop neighboring cell bodies.

Golgi, who discovered these cells, concluded that they were sensory cells because of their atypical axons. As I shall indicate below, there is no basis in fact for this supposition. We are dealing with cells whose short axons would appear to interconnect several neighboring cells. It is impossible to surmise anything about the nature of their physiologic function (Fig. 3a).

Cells with ascending axons. These were first described by Martinotti (Fig. 3C). I have studied these cells in the brains of small mammals and have found them in the three deeper cortical layers, especially in the polymorphic cell layer. They are sometimes fusiform, sometimes triangular, with ascending and descending protoplasmic expansions. The axis cylinders, which often arise from an ascending sprout, pass directly upward to reach the molecular layer, where they divide into two or three thick branches; these branches spread out and ramify, forming extensive terminal arborizations. Occasionally, the terminal arborization is observed within the small pyramidal cell layer.

WHITE MATTER

The white matter is composed of four types of nerve fibers: *projection fibers, callosal* or *commissural fibers, association fibers,* and *centripetal* or *terminal fibers.* These fiber types are intermingled in the white matter of large mammals (dog, sheep, cow, man, etc.), and it is impossible by direct observation to determine their origins or terminations. Fortunately, the technical problems are less formidable when the mammals are smaller, and it becomes feasible to follow many of these fibers for a considerable distance.

Projection fibers (Fig. 6a). These fibers originate from all regions of the cerebral cortex and converge within the corpora striata to enter the cerebral peduncles. In small mammals they contribute thick collaterals to the corpus callosum and descend in small bundles separated by gray-matter partitions, to which they supply delicate collaterals. Some projection fibers do not contribute to the corpus callosum, remaining intact and unbranched throughout the entire thickness of the corpus striatum.

From what cells do projection fibers originate? Certain authors, Monakow among them, maintain that these fibers represent the continuations of giant pyramidal cell axons whereas association and callosal fibers originate from small pyramidal cells.

In this regard my observations, though far from comprehensive, would seem to establish beyond any reasonable doubt that projection fibers arise from both large and small pyramids and even from some polymorphic cells. The fact that projection fibers originate from cells of different sizes might explain why the fascicles of these fibers which descend through the corpus striatum contain a mixture of thick and thin axis cylinders.

As regards the distal synapses of these fibers, histological observations have so far failed to provide a definitive answer. But pathological anatomy and Flechsig's method have taught us that many projection fibers contribute to the *pyramidal tract,* the descending pathway for voluntary motor impulses.

Association fibers (Fig. 5). These fibers probably originate from cells in the small and large pyramidal cell layers and in the polymorphic cell layer, but to date I have only succeeded in confirming their origin from polymorphic cells and from the odd giant pyramidal cell, which may

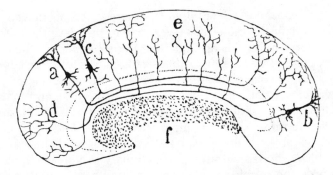

Figure 5. Diagrammatic representation of a sagittal section of the brain illustrating the arrangement of association fibers in the anterior and posterior lobes: a, medium-sized pyramid; d, terminal arborization; e, ascending arborizations of axon collaterals; f, corpus callosum in cross section.

merely reflect the relative ease of following the axons of cells that lie adjacent to the white matter.

In general these axons join association fiber bundles by making a sharp bend; T branchings with equal or unequal limbs are also encountered (Fig. 5c). In the latter case the internal limb may insinuate itself between callosal fibers. At all events, it should be noted that many association fibers, as a result of the course and connections of the two branches of a bifurcation, connect one cell in a given cortical region with many other cells in different regions (and perhaps even in different lobes) of the same cerebral hemisphere.

The number of association fibers is proportional to the gray-matter mass. Therefore, in man and in large mammals, where the gray matter is folded into convolutions, association fibers are so abundant that they constitute the largest proportion of the white-matter mass. In consequence of the quantity and extraordinary length of these fibers and their commingling with projection and callosal fibers it is totally impossible to follow the course of a single association fiber in histological preparations. Thus, it becomes absolutely necessary to study small brains (mouse, bat, rat, etc.), not only because the distances are relatively shorter, but also because the various fiber systems (association, commissural, projection) are individually distinct in certain cortical regions.

Association fiber collaterals.   The application of Golgi's method to the study of neonates and small mammals has enabled me to make a discovery of some consequence: that extremely fine ascending association fiber collaterals ramify in various layers of the superficial cortical gray matter (Fig. 5e). An examination of certain favorable cortical regions—for example, the medial surface of the hemispheres—reveals that some collaterals even attain the molecular layer, where they terminate freely in extensive arborizations; this arrangement is also evident in the cerebral cortex of reptiles. In addition to these radially disposed collaterals to gray matter, other collaterals appear to end in the white matter or near the gray-white junction; their orientation is less regular, and they seem destined to synapse with the numerous descending protoplasmic expansions that terminate in the white matter. These *white-matter* collaterals are comparable to the peripheral collaterals of batrachians and reptiles, which arborize within a perimedullary protoplasmic plexus.

As regards the termination of association fibers, these fibers, like those in the white matter of the spinal cord, end freely in extensive varicose arborizations which occupy almost the entire thickness of the cortex, including the molecular layer (Fig. 5a).

Callosal fibers (Fig. 6A).   These fibers course underneath the association fibers, and in small mammals they form a well-defined transverse plane that serves as a roof for the lateral ventricles. In adequately stained sections of the corpus callosum one is immediately struck by the extreme delicacy of its constituent fibers, which resemble axon collaterals; their myelin sheaths also appear extremely thin in Weigert-Pal preparations. Callosal fibers originate from the cortex of one hemisphere and project to the cortex of the opposite hemisphere. All cortical regions receive and project callosal fibers except the sphenoidal cortex, where the commissural fibers cross in the anterior commissure (Fig. 6B).

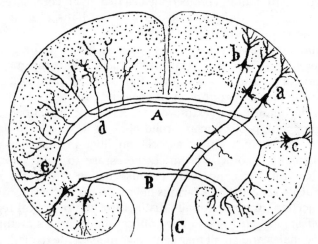

Figure 6.   Diagrammatic representation of a transverse section of the brain illustrating the probable arrangement of commissural and projection fibers: A, corpus callosum; B, anterior commissure; C, pyramidal tract formed by projection fibers.

Transverse sections of neonatal mouse brain in which the callosal fibers have been preferentially stained with silver carbonate reveal that many of these fibers, especially in certain areas, give off fine collaterals and that these collaterals behave in the same manner as association fiber collaterals. In general, each callosal fiber supplies two or at most three such filaments, which, ascending at nearly right angles, disappear within the overlying gray matter where they end freely. Branchings resembling true bifurcations are observed: the commissural fiber divides into one branch which continues to course horizontally and another which penetrates the gray matter (Fig. 6d).

Where do callosal fibers originate? Do they represent the continuations of axis cylinders, or do they correspond to white-matter collaterals? Could it be that the corpus callosum, like the anterior commissure of the spinal cord, contains axis cylinders and white-matter collaterals?

This latter view is most consistent with my own observations. Indeed, throughout the white matter certain axons (association fibers, projections fibers) give off fine collaterals that enter the corpus callosum. At times, rather than being a collateral branch, the fiber bound for the corpus callosum appears to be one limb of an axonal bifurcation.

On the other hand, one frequently observes that fibers deriving from various cortical layers, especially from the small pyramidal cell layer, descend to the level of the corpus callosum and, changing direction, continue on with the callosal fibers. Granted, similar fibers, which resemble axis cylinders, may represent the direct continuations of functional expansions of small cortical cells. I might hasten to add, however, that I have not yet been able to verify this supposition by direct observation.

How do callosal fibers terminate? This is an extremely difficult problem, and my unremitting efforts to resolve it have so far met with little success. On occasion I have observed certain callosal fibers ascending through and ramifying within the gray matter; but, unfortunately, I have been unable to follow their arborizations or to determine the connections of their terminal branches (Fig. 6e). This matter, then, requires further study.

To summarize: the callosal fibers, in my view, do not represent mere interconnections between symmetrical regions of the two hemispheres (as was formerly believed) but rather a complex transverse association system; a fiber arising, for example, at a given point in one hemisphere may make contact not only with symmetrically situated cells in the opposite hemisphere but also with many other cells (by means of collaterals) in different cortical regions and in different cortical layers.

Fibers arborizing in the gray matter (Fig. 7E).   I have already stated that association fibers originating from more or less distant regions of the same hemisphere penetrate the cortical gray and arborize extensively.

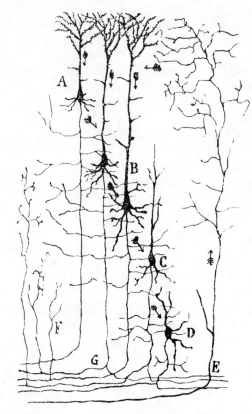

Figure 7. Diagrammatic representation of the neural-protoplasmic
connections between cortical cells
and of the probable flow of nerve impulse traffic: A, small pyramid; B,
giant pyramid; C and D, polymorphic cells; E, terminal nerve fiber
arriving from other centers; F, collaterals from the white matter; G, axis
cylinder bifurcating in the white
matter.

But, in addition, there exist other much thicker fibers emanating
perhaps from the spinal cord, cerebellum, etc.; these fibers generally
course horizontally or obliquely in the gray matter, ramifying extensively throughout its entire thickness including the molecular layer. The
terminal rami form tortuous arborizations, which seem to preferentially
envelop small pyramidal cells. Do these fibers represent the cerebral
terminations of sensory nerves or, perhaps, of axis cylinders projected
by cells in contact with the terminal twigs of sensory axons? Probably,
but one cannot be certain. These fibers are easily stained in reptiles,
where their peripheral arborizations ramify within the molecular layer.

Having disposed of the fundamental features of the histology of the
cerebral cortex, let us now consider the connections of cortical neurons.

CONNECTIONS OF THE FIRST CORTICAL LAYER

I have already established that all pyramidal cells project protoplasmic tufts to the molecular layer, where an infinite number of terminal
nerve fibers converge. By virtue of this assemblage of axons and

dendrites—which must be of great importance as it is present in all vertebrates—each pyramidal cell can be excited by a multitude of other cells. Let me state at the outset that in my opinion these connections are effected by contacts between terminal arborizations and axon collaterals, on the one hand, and cell bodies and protoplasmic expansions on the other. The direction of the impulse traffic is *cellulofugal* in the axis cylinder and *cellulopetal* in the cell body and protoplasmic expansions (Cajal, van Gehuchten), or, in other words, the protoplasmic expansions and cell bodies receive impulses transmitted by the terminal ramifications of axis cylinders and their collateral rami.

With these concepts in mind we shall proceed to a description of the connections of the first cortical layer. At this level the pyramidal cell tufts receive impulses from: (1) autochthonous cells in the molecular layer (via their neural ramifications); (2) vertically oriented fusiform cells (via the superior arborizations of their axis cylinders); (3) pyramidal association cells in distant cortical regions (via their ascending collaterals and the terminal arborizations of their axis cylinders); (4) ? cells in the spinal cord, cerebellar cells, etc. (via the extensive arborizations produced by certain thick fibers that emerge from the subjacent white matter); (5) ? cells of the opposite hemisphere (via the terminal branches of callosal fibers).

Connections at the level of the pyramidal and polymorphic cell layers. These connections are enormously complicated; they involve cell bodies, sprouts, and protoplasmic expansions on the one hand and five types of nerve fibers on the other: collaterals from the white matter, collaterals from the corpus callosum, terminal interlobar and peripheral association fibers, arborizations of Golgi (sensory) cells, and an infinite number of collateral fibrils given off during the intracortical progress of the axis cylinders of cells within the three deepest cortical layers. The plexus which is formed around pyramidal (and polymorphic) cells by so many filaments is of such intricacy that it would be foolhardy to attempt to describe the connections of a single pyramid.

I might add, under the heading of conjecture, that this plexus enables the pyramids to receive impulses from: (1) cells with short axons (Golgi cells) in the same cell layers; (2) association cells in different lobes of the same hemisphere; (3) cells in the opposite hemisphere (via callosal fibers or via the anterior commissure); (4) sensory neurons; and (5) cells in the overlying layers of the same cortical region (Fig. 7).

The last-mentioned circuit is surely one of the most important, and it appears to depend upon the axon collaterals of superposed pyramids and the bodies, sprouts* and basilar expansions of pyramids in subjacent layers. By virtue of its great length, its ramifications and its more or

*Here "sprout" = main-stem dendrite, shaft or apical dendrite—EDS.

less horizontal course, each axon collateral can make transverse contact with the bodies and sprouts of hundreds of cells, with the result that a single small pyramidal cell can modulate the activity of a multitude of subjacent small and medium-sized pyramids. And, in turn, each large pyramidal cell, in consequence of the considerable surface area available for contacts presented by its sprouts, its protoplasmic collaterals, and its descending basilar expansions, can receive impulses from a large number of overlying pyramids (Fig. 7A-D).

In the above-mentioned hypothesis of the dynamic polarity of cellular expansions, nerve impulses in the cortical gray travel from small pyramids to large pyramids and thence to polymorphic cells. The arrows in Figure 7 indicate the direction of impulse transmission.

If we knew more about the terminations of sensory nerve fibers arriving from the spinal cord or from more proximal relay stations, it might be possible to establish with some degree of certainty the site within projection cells where the impulses mediating voluntary movement arise. In spite of our ignorance in this regard there are sufficient data to formulate a hypothesis. Thus, for example, special sensory afferents, which are more or less comparable to peripheral sensory fibers, always terminate freely by arborizing within the cortical molecular layer (or the equivalent layer of other nerve centers, e.g. the cortical layer of the avian optic lobe), making contact with the peripheral protoplasmic tufts of elongated cells. This arrangement is readily demostrable within the mammalian olfactory lobe, where a significant proportion of the fibers arriving from the olfactory bulb project collaterals and terminal rami to a superficial layer which includes the tufts of pyramidal cells and is, therefore, an exact replica of the molecular layer of the cerebral cortex. In the cerebral cortex of reptiles not only olfactory fibers but all subcortical axis cylinders (some of which are probably sensory fibers from the spinal cord) arborize preferentially in the superficial molecular layer.

For these and other reasons I am inclined to believe that voluntary movement is initiated in the pyramidal cell tufts within the molecular layer. This formulation would explain why physiologists have produced movement in specific muscle groups by mechanical, chemical, and electrical stimulation of the cerebral cortex: the excitation, spreading through the molecular layer, acts preferentially on the pyramidal tufts directly, or indirectly on the nerve fibrils intimately associated with them; thus, the stimulus would act at the same locus as the will of the experimental animal.

MORPHOLOGIC TYPES OF CEREBRAL CELLS

Anatomists have always been fascinated by the possibility of deducing the function of a nerve cell from its morphological characteristics.

Thus, Golgi postulated that the nervous system contains two different classes of cells: cells whose axis cylinders lose their identity immediately upon ramifying (Type I) and cells whose axis cylinders retain their identity as far as the white matter, having previously supplied collaterals to the gray matter (Type II). He assumed that Type I cells were sensory cells, inasmuch as the branches of their axis cylinders make contact with the terminal networks of centripetal fibrils, and that Type II cells were motor cells, since their axons are continuous with motor roots.

Golgi's classification is unsatisfactory (as Kölliker, His, Waldeyer, van Gehuchten, etc. have recognized) both morphologically and physiologically.

Morphologically, Type I (sensory) cells differ from Type II (motor) cells only in respect of the length of their axons. The axons of Type I cells are short and do not pass out of the gray matter, where they end freely in proximal arborizations. In Type II cells the functional expansion is long; it enters the white matter and projects terminal arborizations to other neural centers or to peripheral organs. In view of the above, I have designated Golgi's two cell types as *cells with short axons* and *cells with long axons*, a nomenclature which, because it lacks physiological overtones, has gained acceptance by various authors.

Moreover, Golgi's two cell types cannot be distinguished physiologically because: (1) sensory organs such as the retina, the olfactory bulb, the olfactory mucosa, etc. contain large numbers of cells with long axons (Golgi's motor cells); and (2) motor organs such as the cerebellum and the psychomotor cortex contain large numbers of cells with short axons.

In point of fact, there are three morphological types of cortical neurons: (1) *cells with short axons* (Golgi's sensory cells, polygonal cells, and some fusiform cells in the first cortical layer); (2) *cells with long axons* (pyramids, polymorphic cells, etc.); and (3) *cells with multiple axons* (the bipolar and triangular cells in the second cortical layer). Cells with multiple axons also exist in batrachians and reptiles; curiously, all of their expansions, which are somewhat thick initially, gradually acquire the appearance of nerve fibers as they ramify. If it were possible to demonstrate in mammals that all of the protoplasmic expansions of fusiform and triangular cells in the first cortical layer terminate in fine filaments similar in appearance to nerve twigs (something which I have not yet succeeded in doing), then the brain could be likened to the retina and the olfactory bulb, which, in addition to the two principal cell types, contain a third cell type characterized by its lack of differentiated neural and protoplasmic expansions.

To summarize: it is not yet possible to assign a specific function (sensory, motor, special sensory, commissural, associative, etc.) to a given nerve cell on the basis of its morphology. And this same conclusion seems to apply, with certain restrictions, to the cortical layers; that is to say, commissural, association, and projection cells are not segregated in specific cortical layers but appear to be inextricably intermingled in all of the cortical layers. This arrangement would seem to explain the extreme rarity of intellectual impairment limited to one sphere of activity as well as the preservation of higher integrative functions in patients with severe focal cerebral lesions.

ANATOMICAL-PHYSIOLOGICAL CONCLUSIONS

After this lengthy anatomical excursion through the central nervous system it is high time to pause—before your patience and kind attention are exhausted—and consider some physio-psychological conclusions which follow directly from what I have said regarding the arrangement of psychic cells.

1. Neither the external morphology of psychic cells nor the manner in which they are interconnected can explain, in the light of current knowledge, the supreme dignity of the intellect. Their morphology, which represents only a slight departure from that of the common neuron, reflects the vast number of contacts that each psychic cell must make. In fact, each nerve cell, whatever its functional category, appears to be constructed according to the same model and to possess the same texture and chemical composition. The motor cells of the anterior horn of the spinal cord, the ganglion cells of the retina, the cells of the sympathetic chain all possess the same axis cylinder and the same protoplasmic expansions and employ the same methods of establishing contacts and transmitting impulses—the essential characteristics of the psychic cell to which, nevertheless, we attribute the most exalted of life's activities (association of ideas, memory, intelligence, etc.). As regards the complexity of its connections and the variety of its cell types, the cerebral cortex cannot compete with the marvelous fabric of the cerebellum or of the retina, whose functions, though important, are menial offices when compared to those of the cerebral cortex. Science, then, in order not to become discouraged in its perpetual, stubborn attempt to defend the mechanistic explanation of intellection must assume (1) that the internal structure and chemical composition of the cortical cell, rather than its external form, distinguish it from the medullary or ganglionic cell; and (2) that the mechanical phenomena which occur within the protoplasmic matrix of the psychic cell are not of the same order (far from it) as those which occur within the protoplasm of cells of a lesser category.

2. Another conclusion to be drawn from the anatomical-physiological study of the cerebral cortex, a conclusion which many anatomists have reached and which Letamendi has defended brilliantly, is that the brain does not contain a center for receiving sensory inputs, nor is there a single source of all motor impulses. Instead, the entire

cortex may be regarded as a series of centers, each of which receives one class of sensory or special sensory fibers and activates a specific class of motor fibers. These centers are interconnected by the association and commissural fiber systems for the performance of mental (as well as sensory-motor, conscious, and unconscious) associations. They do not exhibit any structural peculiarities which might explain their functional specialization; rather, as Golgi has observed, their functional specialization derives from the unique peripheral connections of their afferent and efferent fibers (with sense organs, muscles, etc.).

3. It is fair to say (with some reservations) that in the animal kingdom higher integrative functions are related to the presence of pyramidal (psychic) cells. In fishes, where the anterior cerebral vesicle lacks true pyramids, intellectual activity as such does not exist, as Edinger recently noted.

The pyramidal cell, or psychic corpuscle, exhibits certain constant morphologic features in batrachians, reptiles, and mammals (see Fig. 4): a sprout and protoplasmic tuft directed toward the cortical surface and protoplasmic rami bearing collateral spines; in the molecular layer these structures make contact with a dense plexus of terminal nerve fibers.

4. The elongation of the pyramidal cell and the diversity of its (protoplasmic) expansions enable a single pyramid to receive nervous impulses from a large number of other cells. Just as the cerebellar Purkinje cell attains a high degree of development, each of its several parts (body, principal sprout, and protoplasmic expansions) synapsing with various kinds of nerve fibers, so, too, the pyramidal cell becomes extensively elongated in order to receive afferent impulses on its body, basilar expansions, sprout, and terminal tuft. The number of synapses which a given cell can make is determined by the size and complexity of its protoplasmic arborizations.

4. [sic] Since the psychic cell enlarges as one ascends within the animal kingdom, it is natural to relate increasing functional capacity to progressive morphological complexity. However, this progression may determine the form and extent of psychical activity rather than its essence.

It would appear that the greater the number of protoplasmic, somatic, and collateral expansions and the greater the number and length of axon collaterals, and the more extensive their ramifications, the more efficient and effective is psychic cell function. The extent to which a neuron has evolved is sometimes related to its size, but this is often not the case. In general, cell size appears to vary with the size of the animal. Thus, the hen and the lizard have larger pyramidal cells than the sparrow and the newt, respectively, but the former are not better differentiated, and consequently are not capable of generating superior intellectual activity.

5. The pyschic cell begins its ontogenetic development as a simple neuroblast, that is to say, as a pyriform cell with a single (protoplasmic) expansion, the axis cylinder. Next, it puts forth a sprout, or primordial expansion, and in time the lateral branches of the sprout, cell body, and axis cylinder appear.

6. The thesis which I have just expounded relating the functional capacity of cells to their complement of collaterals may serve to rationalize two observations which are not adequately explained by the generally accepted hypothesis that intelligence is directly proportional to the number of cerebral cells (whether these are regarded as a mere instrument of the soul or as the morphological substrate of psychic acts). These two observations are: (1) the remarkable intellectual growth that accrues from habitual profound mental exertion and (2) the existence of talent and even of genius in men with medium-sized brains or brains that are smaller or weigh less than normal.

With respect to the first observation, one might suppose that intellectual activity, since it cannot lead to the production of new cells (nerve cells, unlike muscle cells, do not proliferate), promotes the further development of protoplasmic expansions and nerve collaterals, fostering the establishment of new and more extensive intercortical connections. In order to explain the maintenance of a constant cerebral volume one must postulate that this process involves either a concomitant decrease in the size of nerve cell bodies or a concomitant rarefaction of the neuroglial meshwork.

Apropos of the second observation, there is no reason not to believe that certain brains, whether owing to the inheritance of prior adaptations or to other factors, compensate for their decreased cellularity by a remarkable development of all manner of collaterals.

These arguments are based on a rational hypothesis concerning the function of nerve cells and their protoplasmic prolongations. It would seem that each psychic cell, once activated, contains—in some mysterious vibratory [sic] or chemical form—a simulacrum of each sense impression received from the external world or from the viscera (muscle sense).

Therefore, whatever the nature of this superior activity which associates, passes judgment, compares, etc., its workings cannot but be mediated by cellular, neural, and protoplasmic expansions.

If to understand is, as Bain would have it, to perceive similarities and differences, then the excellence and scope of our judgment will be the greater, the more numerous the acquisitions or images that serve as its subject matter and the more extensive the interconnections that can be established by the neuronal substrate of the brain.

The above considerations refer only to some aspects of psychic activity, not to its essential nature, which no current hypothesis can elucidate. Neither materialism nor spiritualism can explain how a nervous impulse arriving in the first cortical layer is converted there into something as tangible as a conscious act.

As regards the interconnection and continuity of the sensory–special sensory and motor spheres both constructs provide a relatively satisfactory explanation. According to spiritualist doctrine, the soul acts as a receptor in one region of the brain and as an effector in another region, functioning something like a telegrapher who, located at a central station, is capable of sending and receiving messages on all of the converging wires. The physical interaction between motor and sensory pathways would only account for automatic behavior; conscious behavior would require the interposition of the soul.

The materialist hypothesis proposes much the same thing, except that the conscious link between centripetal and centrifugal excitations, instead of being represented by an immaterial substance which generates and destroys movement, is represented by a special mechanism that transforms sensory inputs and produces motor excitations. No interruption of the impulse traffic between the two ends of the conscious arc would result; the arc would be reestablished by different means. The nature, the extent, and the complexity of the motor reaction elicited by a sensory impulse, as well as the registration of this impulse as an engram or an idea, would depend upon the anatomical configuration of the receptive cortical region. Each such region would contain a group of cells associated for the retention of impressions and a subordinate system of projection and excito-motor cells.

PRESENILE DEMENTIA

Introduction

H. Richard Tyler, M.D.
Professor of Neurology
Harvard Medical School

THE TERM DEMENTIA was first used by Pinel in relation to the progressive mental changes seen in some idiots. This term was popularized by Rush in 1812 in his classic "Medical Inquiries and Observations upon the Diseases of the Mind." In the first half of the nineteenth century the specific neuropathological entity *general paralysis of the insane* was described by Boyle, Calmeil, and Esquirol. Webster made observations on the pathology of the brain in patients with intellectual deterioration.

A great deal of controversy existed relating to the classifications of mental illness, psychosis, and organic brain disease. It was clear that general paresis of the insane was associated with a diffuse organic pathology, and it was widely accepted that this was the explanation for the mental changes observed in this illness.

Wernicke strongly felt that all mental disorders had an organic basis. Attempts to find the pathology of the other psychotic states, memory, speech, and intellectual disorders were actively pursued with great enthusiasm. Huntington's description of a familial organic disorder accompanied by memory failure gave impetus to this search.

The editors have chosen three papers of historic interest to translate. These complement others that are available elsewhere.

Pick's paper relates to the proposition that was prevalent at the time that only syphilis (general paralysis of the insane) could have focal clinical findings yet have a diffuse nonfocal pathology. It was the only form of mental disease known with focal features. Pick described a patient with senile dementia and a focal aphasic disorder who did not have a focal lesion at post mortem to account for the clinically predicted lesion (although in his case the atrophic process was more marked in the appropriate area). He noted that focal findings could be seen in other diffuse brain disorders

33

besides syphilis. The pathological and technical details in this paper are scanty, and in light of the patient's history of sudden onset of speech difficulty and "right facial deficit" one wonders if focal pathology could have been overlooked. The disorder *Pick's Disease,* named after him, followed the description of a specific pathology and a specific cell change nineteen years later by Alzheimer.

About the time of Pick's paper (1892) there were significant contributions by Blocq and Marinescu (1892), who described scattered silver staining plaques in the cortex; Binswanger (1894), who described a subcortical encephalopathy due to arteriosclerosis; and Alzheimer (1895, 1898), who described cortical changes of atrophy and focal cell changes in relation to arteriosclerosis and blood vessel thickening. Alzheimer did not feel these changes could account for senile changes and separated arteriosclerotic dementia from other cases. It is in this setting that we should read the simple, direct, and clear paper of Alzheimer, which clearly recognizes a unique pathology and puts the changes into their appropriate perspective. This paper was given at a clinical meeting in 1906 and published in 1907. It is clear that Alzheimer knew he was describing something specific which should be separated from other cases. The subsequent paper by Bonfiglio contributes little except for its excellent discussion and confirmation of Alzheimer's findings. That this was not purely unbiased is obvious when one notes that the brain was given to Bonfiglio by Alzheimer. It apparently details the findings described by Alzheimer the previous year in a syphilitic male. Except for his observation that the plaques originated in nerve cells and for some excellent details, it is probably only of historic interest.

By 1910 Perusini had separated senile dementia from other mental illnesses, and Kraepelin had suggested that the disorder be named after his associate, Alzheimer. Subsequently, Simchowicz (1911) described the granulovacuolar degeneration, and in 1914 Divry described the amyloid changes.

It is always interesting to review original articles when one has been using terms such as "Pick's Disease" or "Alzheimer's Disease." Alzheimer clearly made not only major contributions in descriptive pathology but in the conceptual separation of a confusing group of diseases. Neither Pick's nor Bonfiglio's contribution appears to warrant the historical reward it has been given.

On the Relation Between Aphasia and Senile Atrophy of the Brain

A. PICK

WHEREAS IT IS NOW KNOWN that aphasia and other clinical focal signs often found in early stages of general paralysis of the insane are only occasionally complicated by more prominent local anatomic involvement, the same has so far not been considered with respect to the underlying anatomical basis of simple, uncomplicated senile dementia, namely, cerebral atrophy. This is due in large part to the opinion that all aphasias which accompany senile dementia, with the exception of the so-called amnestic form of aphasia, are complicated by definite focal lesions other than senile atrophy. The contrasting viewpoint is most clearly enunciated by Wernicke in a work where the relationship between "aphasia and psychic disorders" is discussed, when he maintains—although mentioned from a different point of view from the present one—that general paralysis is the only mental disease which during its course can lead to cortical and subcortical focal manifestations and, therefore, it holds a unique middle position between psychosis and organic brain disorders. The following article is meant to show that the same holds true for the cerebral atrophy which underlies senile dementia, thus contributing to the effort to bring neuropathology and psychiatry into closer relationship, making the latter understandable in medical terms.

NOTE: Translated by W.C. Schoene from: Pick, A., "Über die Beziehungen der senilen Hirnatrophie zur Aphasie," *Präger Medicinische Wochenschrift* 17, 16 (1892), 165–67. This translation could not have been done without help from Ingo Winzer and Helmut G. Rennke.

On November 11, 1891 the 71-year-old August H. was admitted to the clinic with the history that following two years of progressive mental deterioration he had begun to show rage and had threatened his wife with a knife. Historical review revealed the following: a family history of apoplexy; for the past three years the patient, who had until then been in good physical and mental health, exhibited progressive memory loss; at the beginning of November 1889 he suddenly became "unconscious" after dinner for several minutes and experienced a similar attack the following day; thereafter he is said to have "talked crazy" for a while, having been unable to express himself properly; he subsequently suffered an intestinal illness which left him much weakened. In January of 1890 he suffered a severe case of influenza, the effects of which lingered until April; during the initial fever he was delirious, misidentified persons and manifested speech difficulties which, according to his wife, became pronounced later; during recent days he threatened his wife, crying "I'll kill you." Aside from this he has been quite infantile of late, playing with suspenders and spoons.

On admission to the clinic the patient demonstrated a profound memory loss and throughout his hospitalization lay quietly on his bed without being very much concerned with his surroundings; he is of medium height, shows pronounced senility; except for a barely perceptible facial deficit on the right side, no motor or sensory disturbance; somewhat heightened knee reflexes; ankle clonus; temperature normal, pulse 72; emphysema and bronchial catarrh. Hearing not noticeably impaired. The patient showed a profound speech difficulty of an apathetic character; speech comprehension is significantly, though not totally, destroyed; simple questions about his general circumstances are understood; other questions he does not understand at all.

Speech: The patient possesses a considerable vocabulary and speaks a lot; however, although sentences are sometimes correct when dealing with simple matters, they generally are nonsensical, partly because of the incorrect arrangement of words, partly because the words themselves are unintelligible. This is due at times to transposition of consonants; e.g., he says "colmotive" instead of "locomotive," "reideklasten" instead of "kleiderkasten."

QUESTION: "What is your name?"
ANSWER: "August H." (correct)
QUESTION: "How old are you?"
ANSWER: "Ten or 12, I don't know. I don't understand, the young girl, the stone in the hall."
QUESTION: "What is your job?"
ANSWER: "Karkal... Kakarl... a man who works with gold... my God" (angrily)... (the rest is entirely unintelligible).
To a random question he answers: "I understand, but I must stand up,

it's leaving my head, my head is made of iron, that's how the beginning starts, I don't know that, I can't start, I don't have it here."

He partially recognizes objects shown to him, but often describes them incorrectly:

Hat: "Felt."

Matchbox: "Filter paper."

Pocket knife: "Umbrella."

Given a woolen glove, he rubs the palm of his hand and says: "Wool."

Spoon: "I know that, that's on some coffee." (places the spoon in his mouth)

He repeats phrases correctly if they are spoken to him slowly; however, as soon as the speed quickens he reverts to the above-described form of spontaneous speech. Apparently, in the first example the patient can follow the individual syllables, whereas in the second example he immediately forgets what is said and continues spontaneously.

He reads aloud slowly, with difficulty and usually incorrectly. *Ostende* is read once as: "Oste . . . ost . . . u te te, Ostus, tentinde." Another time: "Otto, Osto, Otto, tes, en, am de, el." *Prager Abendblatt:* "Parger Pagelage Abeangust." *Prager Tageblatt:* "Pag . . . tag . . . tatalak, te tutel . . . ta . . . tel . . . tel." He reads written names correctly, rapidly skimming over them: *Goldarbeiter:* "August" (his Christian name!) "Gust, gold ,goldvater." He identifies individual latters partly correctly; he recognizes numbers, individual ones correctly, polysyllabic ones partly incorrectly, 1891=1848, 25=85.

Script is apparently not at all understood. Spontaneous writing, copying, and dictated writing all appear to be impaired in a similar manner, i.e., the patient often begins correctly, writes two or three correct letters, then attaches regularly a series of illegible signs resembling an "I," at which time the patient excuses himself, saying that his hand trembles too much.

The above-mentioned findings remained fairly constant throughout the patient's hospitalization until the last days of November, when his pulmonary symptoms worsened; the patient died on November 27 of pulmonary disease, having become progressively more apathetic.

The clinical diagnosis in the preceding case was made without difficulty after the speech disorder was recognized. Since our main concern is with the pathological anatomical diagnosis of the secondary symptom, namely, the speech disorder, the primary diagnosis, that of senile dementia, will not be discussed.

In observing the speech disorder we lay greatest emphasis on the fact that we are not dealing with a disorder which can be exclusively, or even primarily, attributed to the simple amnestic effects of the senile process, but, rather, it more closely parallels those which are the result of focal lesions; it resembles those disorders which Wernicke-Lichthein described as transcortical sensory aphasia insofar as we could determine that the patient's primary symptoms were a loss of understanding of speech and writing, paraphasia and partially retained ability to repeat speech.

More difficult than the clinical diagnosis was the pathological anatomical diagnosis, which had to determine both the site and nature of the disease.

If one held to the prevailing readily available opinion expressed at the beginning of this article, it would seem that the vague prehospitalization history could be weighted to indicate that the patient had suffered one or more apoplectic attacks which left circumscribed focal softenings in the left temporal lobe, leading to what was recognized as a primary sensory speech disorder; it need only be briefly mentioned that this localization accounts for the lack of other motor manifestations; it would also not be too bold to associate the recrudescence of the symptoms after the influenza with such localized foci.

Although the idea of focal softening would agree well with currently accepted views, we considered this only as a secondary possibility; rather, our diagnosis before considering the autopsy was *Atrophia cerebri praecipue haemisphaerii sin. in regione gyri primi lobi sphenoidalis*, with the latter region only considered a secondary possibility; this was based on the prior clinical observations which appear in the *Archiv für Psychiatrie und Nervenkrankheiten* (vol.23,no. 3), and also on the fact that the history indicated a gradual development of the patient's speech disorder to its final degree. The preceding statement, viewed in the light of our published observations on transitory postepileptic sensory aphasia, suggests the possibility that a similar mechanism, though much slower, had been in operation here, and that at a certain point in time a more or less circumscribed type of aphasia could result from a simple circumscribed atrophic process.

Autopsy performed on the 28th of November by my colleague, Dr. Chiari, yielded the following with respect to the brain: the scalp soft and pale, the skull 54 cm in horizontal circumference, thickened, compact; the dura tightly stretched, its sinus slightly filled with fluid, slightly coagulated blood; on the inner surface of the pacchymeninges over the surface of the cerebral hemispheres delicate newly formed connective tissue membranes; the inner meninges somewhat thickened, quite edematous, of medium blood content, everywhere easily removable. The walls of the basal vessels unevenly thick. The weight of the brain after removal of almost all meninges (except those covering the cerebellum) was 1150g; the right cerebral hemisphere 500g; the left one 470; the gyri of the cerebral hemispheres clearly narrowed, the atrophy of the gyri of the left side, especially of the *lobus temporalis sin.*, clearly more pronounced than the corresponding ones on the right side; brain substance generally tough, pale, moist. The ventricles enlarged, the ependyma thickened, partially granulated, no focal lesion demonstrated; fresh teased preparations of white matter from the *lobus temp. sin.* do not reveal granulated cells.

If we now advance this new viewpoint of the diagnostic significance of the focal signs in senile atrophy of the brain, it obviously lacks that broad base of case documentation which is the foundation of the prevailing opinion; nevertheless, I find in the literature, which has not yet been thoroughly examined, individual cases which entirely support the previously discussed viewpoint, not only for aphasia but also for other localizing symptoms.

The first case was reported by Bevan Lewis in his *Textbook of Mental Diseases,* 1889, p. 411. A 52-year-old man who eleven months previously had suffered nystagmus and convulsions became ill with what appeared to be senile dementia, having previously shown progressive weakness in the right extremities and speech difficulties; he showed amnestic speech difficulty and ataxic aphasia. Autopsy revealed: brain weight 1270 g; right hemisphere 555, the left 515; the right frontal lobe 327; the left 198. Cloudiness of the meninges, perhaps a slight circumscribed adherence of the meninges to the left frontal and marginal gyri; high-grade atrophy in the frontal and parietal regions, especially on the left side; no focal softening.

The second case taken from the literature comes from the observation by Magnan, which is related to Mlle. Skwortzoff (*"De la cécité et de la surdité des mots dans l'aphasie," 1881, p. 100*) in the chapter on etiology by the few words: "We studied an aphasic patient, where subsequent autopsy revealed atrophy of the entire left hemisphere." The actual clinical observations were as follows: "37-year-old woman who apparently suffered a progressive psychic disorder after a profuse bleeding at age 27; following a psychic shock she became panic-stricken, complained of pain in the right leg, eventually lost the use of nouns, exhibited paraphasia, later only affected speech (she could, however, complete the words of a song sung to her, with which she was familiar) and high-grade dementia, dulling of the senses, muscle weakness without paralysis.

Autopsy reveals a brain weight of 935 g; 770 of which is cerebrum, 415 from the right, 355 from the left hemisphere, 165 from the cerebellum and hydrocephalus externus. The thickened and edematous leptomeninges are easily removed save for some adhesions at the tips of the temporal lobes, especially on the left. The gyri of the left hemisphere are markedly atrophic, except in the motor region; microscopic investigation of cortical grey matter from the third left frontal gyrus and temporal gyrus revealed granular degeneration of the ganglion cells, isolated granule cells and fat granules in the vessel walls.

Although there is no senile but, rather, simple atrophy, paralysis can be eliminated, so that this case, as well, represents support for our thesis that simple progressive brain atrophy can lead to symptoms of local disturbance through local accentuation of the diffuse process. In passing it should be mentioned that this evidence will significantly improve the understanding of other manifestations caused by the diffuse process; just as the understanding of aphasia is also advanced generally by considering the development of the aphasia in the presented case. We do not wish to elaborate further on the pathological-anatomical questions related to the above discussion; these questions should be placed side-by-side with Lissauer's recent attempts to explain similar conditions in general paralysis.

A Unique Illness Involving the Cerebral Cortex

A case report from the Mental Institution in Frankfurt am Main.*

A. ALZHEIMER

THE CLINICAL COURSE and pathology of this distinctive process separate it from the known neurologic disorders.

The patient initially presented at fifty-one years of age with jealousy of her husband. Rapidly progressive memory loss soon followed. No longer finding her apartment suitable, she dragged her furniture back and forth and concealed it. She began to believe that others wanted to kill her, and she would scream out loud.

Following institutionalization she appeared totally bewildered. She was disoriented as to time and place and occasionally stated that she did not understand events around her. She treated her physician as a guest, excused herself and said she was not finished with her work. Following this she would scream aloud that he was trying to stab her with a knife, or indignantly turn him away, fearing that he would violate her. She was intermittently delirious, dragged her bedding about, called for her

*The clinical examination and central nervous system autopsy were performed by Dr. Sioli, director of the institute.

NOTE: Translated by C. N. Hochberg and F. H. Hochberg from: Alzheimer, A., "Über eine eigenartige Erkrankung der Hirnrinde," *Allgemeine Zeitschrift für Psychiatrie und Psychisch-Gerichtliche Medizin* 64 (1907), 146–48.

husband and daughter, and appeared to be having auditory hallucinations. She would scream for hours in a monstrous voice.

She was unable to understand situations and would scream every time someone would attempt to examine her. Only after repeated attempts could an examination be performed.

When shown objects she could name them relatively correctly. However her perceptions were extremely disturbed. Immediately after naming the objects she would forget them. She drifted from one line to the next while reading—either enunciating the individual letters or speaking in a meaningless tone. While writing, she repeated single syllables, omitted others, and quickly became confused. She used perplexing phrases when speaking or made paraphasic errors ("milk pourer" instead of "cup"). She would hesitate during speech. She did not understand some questions put to her. She appeared to have forgotton the use of several objects. Hand functions and walking were undisturbed. Her patellar reflexes and pupillary reactions were preserved. Her radial arteries were rigid. There was no cardiac enlargement or urinary albumin.

Her focal symptoms clearly waxed and waned; but they remained minimal during her illness. However her mental deterioration was progressive. She died after four and a half years of illness. Prior to her death she had become completely apathetic, went to bed in her clothes, neglected her personal hygiene, and developed decubitus ulcers despite nursing care.

The brain sections demonstrated generalized atrophic changes. The major cerebral vessels showed atherosclerotic changes. Neurofibrillary changes were seen in sections stained by the Bielschowsky silver technique. Thick, heavily stained fibrils stood out among the few remaining normal cells. There were many similar fibrillary networks which merged into dense bundles and finally appeared on the cells' surface. In the most advanced stage the cell nucleus and cell body disintegrated leaving only a tangled bundle of fibrils in the site of a former ganglion cell.

These fibrils stained differently from normal fibrils, suggesting that a chemical transformation of the fibrillary substance must have occurred. This transformation may explain the preservation of fibrils despite the cellular destruction. The alteration of the fibrils appears to go hand in hand with the deposit of a previously undescribed material in the ganglion cells. One quarter to one third of the cortical ganglion cells, particularly of the superficial cell layers, had disappeared.

The entire cortex, especially the superficial portions, showed miliary foci resulting from the deposit of a unique substance. This material could be recognized by virtue of its refractivity on unstained sections.

The glia showed numerous filaments and fatty vacuoles. There was no vascular infiltration; but endothelial proliferation and neovascularization were seen.

We feel that this represents a unique entity. In the last few years more cases have been confirmed. These observations suggest that we should not be content to classify a clinical case without exerting maximal effort to investigate it. There are without a doubt many more illnesses than our textbooks describe. In some instances the peculiar features will be confirmed histologically. Over a period of time we will come to the point where we can isolate single clinical cases from the larger classifications and thus more clearly define each clinical entity.

Unusual Findings in a Probable Case of Cerebral Syphilis

F. BONFIGLIO

IN NOVEMBER 1906, Alzheimer[1] presented two remarkable papers at the Tübingen Psychiatric Congress reporting his observations in a case which posed serious problems both clinically and pathologically; the author concluded that his case was unique and could not be ascribed to any of the existing nosological entities.

Having had the opportunity to study a case kindly provided by Dr. Alzheimer—a case which is similar in many respects to the one he reported at Tübingen—I decided to publish a brief account of it.

As regards the clinical history, I must confine myself to transcribing the notes which were furnished to me:

Leonhard of Landshut, a sixty-year-old Bavarian male, was admitted to the Monaco Asylum (Bavaria) on June 20, 1904. Nothing is known about his past medical history. Physical examination on admission revealed that the patient was bedridden on account of his general debility. He was slightly malnourished and suffered from severe diarrhea. His heels slapped against the floor when he walked; bearing down on the soles of his feet resulted in dorsiflexion of the toes. The pupils reacted sluggishly to light. The right knee jerk could only be elicited intermittently and was depressed when present; the left knee jerk was markedly depressed though always elicitable. The patient was euphoric, disoriented, delirious, and dirty (at times). He told fantastic stories about

NOTE: Translated by D. A. Rottenberg from: Bonfiglio, F., "Di Speciali Reperti in un Caso di Probabile Sifilide Cerebrale," *Rivista Sperimentale di Freniatria* 34 (1908), 196–206.

certain monks from his town, stating that one had become a bishop, that another was 106 years old, etc. It was difficult to hold his attention.

During the ensuing days he remained delirious. He saw a monk from his native town on the wall in front of his bed and bade him come down from there at once. He kept up a continuous monologue, conversing with imaginary voices: "You blackguard. Why don't you give me back my son? I'm not a rascal like you," etc. Direct questioning did not provide any further information about his ravings or his psycho-sensory disturbances. He was agitated, shouted, laughed frequently and protractedly, and contended that nobody was stronger or more intelligent than he was.

His condition remained essentially unchanged until August of the same year, when his diarrhea increased; his mental state remained as described above. All day long he insulted various imaginary personages who appeared before him. The name of the chief magistrate of his town recurred often during the course of these conversations. He claimed to have been swindled by the magistrate, that his pension had been withheld, etc. Often he would throw off his clothing and beat on his thighs with his hands. On direct questioning he was unable to point out the imaginary interlocutors with whom he had been discoursing at such length. He was incontinent of urine.

October 6, 1904: Symptomatically unchanged. Serious defects in memory and attention are still apparent, and the patient is disoriented to person, place, and time. He does not remember having been the town clerk in Landshut for thirteen years, when he entered the asylum, or where he lived previously. He is frequently unable to locate the toilet on his ward. At table, after taking his soup course, he forgets that other dishes remain. He is incapable of even the simplest calculations.

October 10, 1904: Both knee jerks are absent. Rombergism is pronounced with his eyes closed, even if his feet are not closely approximated. He is also ataxic in the sitting position; placing one leg over the other causes him to fall supine onto the bed although he attempts to maintain himself in an upright position with his arms. He continues euphoric; only rarely, when contradicted about the existence of his imaginary companions, does he become irritable.

From January 1905 until April of the same year his mental and physical status remained unchanged. In April he suffered from persistent diarrhea, occasionally blood-tinged, and a low-grade fever.

May 10, 1905: He is cured of his diarrhea. His mental state is unchanged except that it is even more difficult to disengage him from his dialogues with the imaginary voices. At night he is frequently incontinent of urine.

September 5, 1905: He is filthy. Slight temperature elevations are recorded in association with a gastrointestinal upset.

December 30, 1905: There is a progressive divergent strabismus the onset of which cannot be dated exactly. Hallucinations persist.

February 3, 1906: The patient's mental status is unchanged. He is continually incontinent of urine and suffers from intractable diarrhea; he is febrile and takes little nourishment. Subjectively he continues to feel extremely well and is euphoric.

March 2, 1906: The diarrhea and fever have abated. The patient is no longer able to walk. Hallucinations continue as before.

April 3, 1906: Vesical lavage for cystitis caused the patient to cry out that the devil take us all, that he has never harmed anyone, and that everybody was abusing him. By nightfall he had forgotten everything and said that nothing had happened to him.

May 25, 1906: Persistent diarrhea has recurred. He takes very little nourishment.

August 25, 1906: The patient is becoming increasingly weak and sleeps a great deal during the day.

October 10, 1906: He is boisterous once again.

December 11, 1906: His general condition has worsened markedly.

January 1, 1907: Death.

Autopsy findings: Bilateral adhesive pleuritis (old), cholelithiasis and purulent cholecystitis, marked (long-standing) atrophy of the right kidney.

The skull is thickened. In places the dura mater is tightly adherent to the bony calvarium and, elsewhere, to the leptomeninges. The brain appears somewhat smaller than usual and weighs 1090 grams. The leptomeninges are focally thickened and at intervals present a gelatinous appearance; at several points they are adherent to the cerebral cortex. The pial veins are dilated and injected. On the whole, the Circle of Willis does not appear sclerotic. The lateral ventricles are dilated and filled with a yellowish serous liquid. The choroid plexuses are injected. The fourth ventricle is not enlarged. Within the fourth ventricle the ependyma is slightly granular; elsewhere it is smooth and shiny.

The vertebrae are soft and friable. At the level of the medulla the left lateral funiculus and both posterior columns are diminished in size. An area of gelatinous appearance and consistency the size of a pinhead is present on the left side in the inferior cervical region of the spinal cord. The anatomical structure of the surrounding parenchyma is preserved. There is a loss of funicular white matter on the left in the lumbar region. In the region of the lumbar enlargement the dura is thickened and adherent to the pia over a distance of five centimeters. Just above that point for a distance of about one centimeter the entire cross-sectional area of the cord appears white, gelatinous, and almost structureless.

Microscopic examination: Numerous blocks taken for histological study from various portions of the cerebral cortex were fixed in alcohol and formalin as described by Alzheimer[2]. Some of the smaller blocks were fixed in Weigert's mordant for neuroglia. Unfortunately, I have not been able to secure blocks of the spinal cord.

The following staining techniques were employed: Nissl, toluidine blue, Pappenheim-Unna, polychrome blue, Ehrlich-Pappenheim (tri-acidic), Herxheimer, Marchi, Weigert (for neuroglia and elastic fibers), Van Gieson, and Bielschowsky (and its modifications). Routine connective tissue stains (Ribbert, etc.) were used. Nerve fibers were demonstrated by the Weigert-Wolters method and neuroglia by an unpublished method of Alzheimer's.

Pathological changes (the essential features of which are summarized below) were neither restricted to specific lobes nor distributed uniformly throughout the crebral cortex; rather, regions in which these changes were marked alternated with regions which appeared relatively better preserved.

The pia is markedly thickened in places. This thickening is produced by connective tissue proliferation without cellular infiltration. Here and there one encounters foci of recent hemorrhage which sometimes involve the most superficial layers of the cortex. Accumulations of pigment and cellular debris are frequently observed.

During the cutting of tissue blocks a homogeneous, roughly spherical mass approximately two millimeters in diameter was observed between the pia and the cortical surface. This mass was lighter in color and appeared more compact than the remainder of the cortical tissue from which it could be easily distinguished. On microscopic examination it does not stain appreciably with basic aniline dyes. With Van Gieson's acid fuscin it appears pale red; homogeneous centrally, a fibrillar structure can be discerned in the periphery. Occasional mast cells, plasma cells, and lymphocytes are encountered within the mass, which is otherwise acellular. It is surrounded by a connective tissue capsule in relation to which one can make out a few plasma cells at a distance from blood vessels. Nearby pial and penetrating vessels present all of the pathological changes (to be described in a moment) observed elsewhere within the cerebral vasculature.

Nerve cells are altered in various ways; however, the basic nature of these alterations is revealed by the presence of large accumulations of pigment and lipid substances. On the other hand, nerve cell destruction is not marked, and the cortical cytoarchitecture is largely preserved. No significant abnormalities are apparent in Weigert-Wolters nerve fiber preparations when these are compared with normal control sections (prepared expressly for this purpose from the cortex of a man of the same age who died of an acute pulmonary ailment without evidence of central nervous system involvement).

Neuroglial changes are largely regressive in nature as indicated by large deposits of pigment and lipid substances. Nevertheless, *gliarasen* are numerous, and here and there one encounters glial nuclei with a proliferate look about them. *Trabantzellen* are frequently observed, five or six of them often surrounding a single nerve cell. Many neuroglial nuclei with abundant protoplasm are associated with blood vessels, around which they often form a continuous ring (Alzheimer's method). In the most superficial cortical layer there is a moderate new growth of neuroglial fibrils.

Rod-shaped cells are found in all of the sections taken from diverse cortical regions. They are not very numerous and are usually of the short variety; basophilic granules are frequently present within their processes.

Marked intimal proliferation is observed within the pial vessels, especially the larger ones; segmental involvement may occur, or, on occasion, the proliferative changes may extend along the entire length of the vessel wall. Where it borders on an area of intimal proliferation the elastic lamina appears to divide, sending numerous fibrillary processes in among the layers of newly formed intima. Pigment deposits occur within the tunica media. In the adventitia one also encounters focal areas of tissue destruction represented by large accumulations of pigment and debris; numerous fascicles of fragmented elastic fibrils course among the areas of tissue destruction.

Endothelial proliferation within the capillaries and precapillaries of the cerebral cortex gives rise, at times, to a subdivision of the vascular lumen and the formation of what Alzheimer has termed "vessel bundles." Hyaline degeneration is sometimes observed in small vessels which course in the superficial cortical layers. Another important finding is the presence of extremely large accumulations of pigment and lipid substances in the vessel walls. Of note is the lack of any cellular infiltration—leukocytic, lymphocytic, or plasmacytic—of the pial or cortical vessels; mast cells are not infrequently observed. There are many leukocytes in the lumina of pial vessels and of the most superficial portions of their penetrating branches.

Having thus outlined the pathological alterations observed in the cerebral cortex, two features remain to be discussed: (1) neurofibrillary degeneration, and (2) the occurrence of unusual miliary foci of necrosis. These features were demonstrated by Bielschowsky's method and are best appreciated in the temporal lobe.

Neurofibrillary degeneration occurs diffusely throughout the cortical gray matter, most often affecting the cells of the external and internal pyramidal layers; in the temporal lobe, where this process is observed with the greatest frequency, approximately one third of the nerve cells are affected.*

This process begins initially at a specific locus within the cell body. In a cell which still retains its normal microscopic appearance several neurofibrils stand out by virtue of their unusual thickness and intense staining (Fig. 1). With further progression of the pathological process all of the neurofibrils—first some, then others—appear to enlarge and join together to form thick bundles which, little by little, work their way to the periphery of the cell, where they become enmeshed and coiled up. The end result is an assortment of skeins or tangles, some pyramidal, some ovoid, some half-moon shaped, etc. (Figs. 2, 3, 4, and 5). At this stage there is no staining of the cellular protoplasm; however, the nerve cell nucleus persists, often appearing degenerated (Fig. 5).

Eventually even the nucleus disappears, and a tangle of thick bundles of neurofibrils is all that remains to attest to the location of the original nerve cell; sometimes a neuroglial nucleus, easily recognizable by its size, shape, etc., becomes associated with the tangle (Fig. 6).

The miliary foci of necrosis have the same distribution as the neurofibrillary tangles. They range in size between 20 and more than 50 micra in diameter, and they do not stain well with any of the usual dyes. The evolution of these plaques may be summarized as follows: Initially a dense meshwork of axis cylinders bearing rounded and fusiform swellings at irregular intervals surrounds a cell which is easily recognizable by its shape as being a neuron, although its internal structure cannot be discerned; some of these swellings, because of their shape and location, bear a strong resemblance to thickened *boutons terminaux* (Fig. 9). Subsequently the peripherally disposed axis cylinders undergo further degeneration; many of the fusiform bodies which contributed to the dense meshwork can no longer be distinguished, and most of those remaining appear to be in the process of disintegration. A nerve cell, still recognizable by its outline, occupies a central position; the entire field is strewn with debris (Fig. 10). In other plaques the nerve cell itself has undergone further degenerative changes and consists solely of lipid globules and detritus. Ultimately only an amorphous or granular plaque can be distinguished centrally; the meshwork of axons has totally disappeared, having been replaced by a zone of detritus within which only an occasional spindle-shaped formation can still be made out (Fig. 11).

In summary we are dealing with the case of a sixty-year-old man who died of inanition two and a half years after his admission to a lunatic asylum. His neurological signs included divergent strabismus,

*Similar changes are not observed in the spinal cord, several sections of which (already stained by Bielschowsky's method) have come into my possession.

ataxia, sluggish pupillary light reactions, and absent knee jerks; euphoria, profound dementia, disorientation, and vivid hallucinations were also prominent.

Noteworthy anatomical-pathological findings included: uniform macroscopic atrophy of the brain; multiple pial-cortical adhesions; circumscribed lesions in the spinal cord and at the pial-cortical junction; nearly complete preservation of the cortical cytoarchitecture, nerve cells, and nerve fibers; regressive changes in the neuroglia; scattered rod-shaped microglia throughout the cerebral cortex (mostly of the short variety); marked proliferative changes involving the cerebral blood vessels; the presence of mast cells; the absence of leukocytic or plasmacytic infiltrates; and enormous deposits of pigment and lipid substances within the walls of blood vessels. Two findings which I have singled out for especial emphasis are: (1) the remarkable alterations in the neurofibrils and (2) the presence of miliary foci of necrosis.

As regards the significance of the fully developed neurofibrillary tangles demonstrated by Bielschowsky's method, the question of differential diagnosis arises only in relation to the pathological alterations in the blood vessels.

One cannot deny that notwithstanding the numerous morphological characteristics of the lesion which can be invoked according to the various shapes of the tangles—among which characteristics the principal ones are: general appearance (vase-shaped tangles as in Fig. 8 or rounded skeins with prolongations resembling nerve-cell processes), number and nature of associated nuclei, etc.—one may remain in doubt at times when confronted with some forms in isolation. For the purpose of differential diagnosis sufficient criteria do exist: on the one hand, a study of transitional forms facilitates the early detection of neurofibrillary degeneration and permits one to follow its gradual evolution; on the other hand, the frequent occurrence of neurofibrillary tangles without associated blood vessels, the simultaneous disappearance of nerve cells and the appearance of mature tangles, and, finally, the location of the tangles at sites previously occupied by neurons are all of diagnostic import.

What significance should be attributed to these two findings? The neurofibrillary changes which I have described are similar in some respects to the changes described by Donaggio[3] following the combined action of cold and fasting; in my case, however, a chemical alteration of the neurofibrils must have occurred since there is no alternative explanation for their staining with basic aniline dyes after fixation in alcohol (Fig. 7), which does not normally occur. And the fact that they continue to stain at a time when the other cellular components can no longer be demonstrated must certainly be attributed to their chemical modification.

As regards the miliary lesions, Redlich[4] was the first to point out their existence, having observed them in two cases of senile dementia. He described them in the cerebral cortex as "miliary sclerosis," homogeneous or finely granular plaques staining intensely with carmine. A peripheral fibrillar layer merged with the surrounding tissue; "nuclear or protoplasmic remnants" were often present at the center. Apropos of the genesis of these lesions, Redlich assumed that plaque formation occurred at sites of nerve destruction; subsequent degeneration of the neuroglia which came to occupy these sites gave rise to the appearances described above.

Alzheimer[5] described similar miliary plaques in unstained preparations; these lesions were well visualized by Bielschowsky's method but did not stain with ordinary dyes. He did not provide a detailed account of these lesions and assumed that they resulted from the deposition of a peculiar substance in the cortex.

In October 1907, Fischer[6] published a detailed study of these focal lesions, which he called "miliary necroses." He found that although they did take up the usual dyes their internal structure was demonstrated to best advantage by Bielschowsky's method. He described a central necrotic plaque surrounded by a zone of radially oriented ovoid, club-shaped, and fusiform structures, which he took to represent the terminations of neighboring axons. Basing his argument principally on the fact that glial stains did not demonstrate the plaques, he rejected Redlich's hypothesis regarding their pathogenesis, and never having observed nerve cells or unequivocal nuclear or protoplasmic remnants at the center of these lesions he considered, as did Alzheimer, that they derived from the deposition of a peculiar foreign substance of unknown composition at the plaque center. He considered the more peripherally disposed fusiform structures as evidence of axonal regeneration. Finally, having encountered these miliary lesions in 12 of 16 cases of senile dementia and in none of numerous controls (45 cases of general paresis, 10 normals, 10 cases of "functional" psychosis) this author came to regard them as characteristic of unusual forms of presbyphrenia.

It would appear that my case and the case previously reported by Alzheimer—neither of which involves senile dementia—demonstrate that Fischer's hypothesis regarding the specificity of these lesions is untenable. Moreover, I have also observed these same focal lesions in other cases (kindly supplied by Dr. Alzheimer), cases which to the best of my knowledge had only a single feature in common, namely, a history of syphilis. It seems to me that the simultaneous occurrence of these focal lesions and the above-mentioned neurofibrillary changes should not be neglected.

As far as the genesis of the pathological process and the nature of the

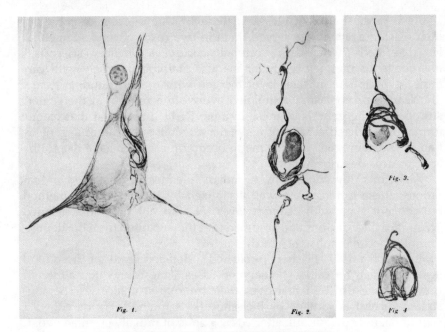

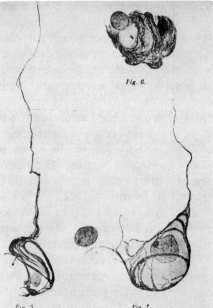

All of the figures were drawn from sections stained by Bielschowsky's method except Figure 7, which was taken from a section stained with toluidine blue.

A Leitz microscope was used throughout: 12× ocular, magnification 1600× (oil immersion).

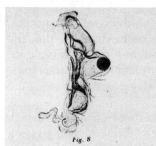

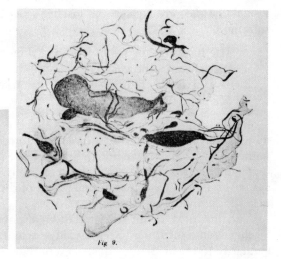

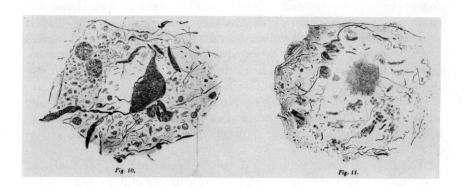

Figure 1.   Large pyramidal cell. Early neurofibrillary degeneration.

Figures 2, 3, and 4.   Cortical neurons at an advanced stage of neurofibrillary degeneration. The nucleus is still visible amidst a tangle of neurofibrils.

Figure 5.   As above. The nucleus has decreased in size.

Figure 6.   As above. A neuroglial nucleus is visible within the skein of neurofibrils.

Figure 7.   Chemical alteration of neurofibrils. A tangle of neurofibrils—almost identical to the tangles depicted in Figures 2, 3, and 4—is stained with toluidine blue (alcohol fixation).

Figure 8.   One of the configurations assumed by the cortical vases.

Figure 9.   A necrotic plaque. Early degenerative changes. A nerve cell is at the center. Surrounding meshwork of axis cylinders; fusiform swellings.

Figure 10.   As above. A more advanced stage of degeneration. A nerve cell is at the center. Large masses of detritus surround the axis cylinders; fusiform swellings.

Figure 11.   A fully developed plaque. An amorphous mass is at the center. Roundabout are numerous masses of detritus.

axonal changes are concerned, Fischer's reasoning is based on two assumptions:

1. The focal lesions result from the deposition of a peculiar foreign substance in the cortex.
2. The axonal changes should be interpreted as regenerative phenomena.

Regarding the first point, a study of the evolution of the process, which I have attempted to summarize, forces us to conclude that the pathological changes are initiated in a nerve cell and in the nerve endings which surround it and that the centrally situated amorphous masses observed only in the terminal phase of the degenerative process are necrotic remnants of the nerve cell itself.

Turning next to an interpretation of the axonal structures which Fischer would attribute to regenerative activity because of their passing similarity to the structures described in regenerating nerves, it seems to me that these structures should be viewed as the result of a destructive, degenerative process. For if it is true that by virtue of their shape and their eventual elaboration of an internal reticulum the spindle-shaped structures associated with miliary lesions may at times resemble similar structures encountered in the proximal stumps of amputated axons, then it is also true that these fusiform structures exist only transiently and degenerate rapidly into amorphous detritus.

Under which of the known nosologic groupings should my case be subsumed? Or should it be set apart in a separate group with the expectation that future research will clarify its relationship to currently recognized disease entities?

The lack of a complete and detailed clinical history precludes an evaluation of the most important symptomatology and the formulation of a secure clinical diagnosis. Furthermore, as regards an anatomical-pathological diagnosis, the fact that the spinal cord, medulla, basal ganglia, and Circle of Willis were not examined histologically obliges me to temper my conclusions with a great deal of reserve.

General paresis can, I think, be excluded with certainty on the basis of the available histological data. The lack of any cellular infiltration of vessel walls and the lack of significant destruction of nervous elements or of the characteristic alterations in cortical cytoarchitecture militate strongly against this diagnosis. One might envision a form of general paresis which is atypical as regards the "quality" as distinct from the "localization" of the pathological process (e.g., Alzheimer's[7] variant as contrasted with Lissauer's). But even this hypothesis can be rejected inasmuch as the pathological changes herein described do not bear any resemblance to those described by Alzheimer in his two cases of stationary paresis; moreover, Alzheimer himself expressed many reservations, raising some doubt as to whether or not such cases should be included within the spectrum of dementia paralytica—or whether, instead, they ought to be considered within another context, namely, within the context of cerebral syphilis.

In point of fact, many of the pathological findings in this case are analogous to those described in some forms of cerebral syphilis: for example, the proliferative changes in cortical blood vessels which resemble the lesions of Heubner's endarteritis; the enormous deposits of pigment within vessel walls, frequently observed in cases of cerebral syphilis; rod-shaped microglia of the same type that predominate in cerebral syphilis (the short variety); and finally, in my view, the circumscribed lesions of the spinal cord and pial-cortical junction.

Alzheimer, summarizing the pathological findings in his case, which, as I noted above, is similar in many respects to the present case, puts forward the hypothesis that he is dealing with "an unusual affection of the cortex."

In recent years, as many investigators have acknowledged the necessity of submitting all cases which come to the postmortem table to a systematic histopathological examination, disease processes not easily ascribed to currently recognized nosological entities have been reported with some frequency.

If I am not mistaken, the present case numbers among those awaiting classification.

In conclusion I wish to express my sincere gratitude to Dr. Alzheimer who, with his accustomed generosity, provided me with this case material, and to Professor Tamburini for his warm hospitality.

NOTES

1. Alzheimer, A. "Über eine eigenartige Erkrankung der Hirnrinde." 37ste Versammlung südwestdeutscher Irrenärzte in Tübingen am 3. und 4. Nov., 1906. *Centralblatt für Nervenheilkunde und Psychiatrie*, vol. 18, March 1907.

2. Perusini, G. "Alcune proposte intese ad un'unificazione tecnica nella raccolta del materiale etc." This journal vol. 33, fasc. 4, 1907.

3. Donaggio. "Effetti dell'azione combinata del digiuno e del freddo nei mammiferi adulte." *Rivista sper. di Freniatria* vol. 33, fasc. 1–2.

4. Redlich. "Über miliare Sklerose der Hirnrinde bei seniler Atrophie." *Jahrbücher für Psychiatrie und Neurologie*, vol. 17, 1898.

5. Alzheimer, "Uber eine eigenartige Erkrankung der Hirnrinde."

6. Fischer, O. "Miliare Nekrosen mit drusigen Wucherungen der Neurofibrillen etc." *Monatschrift für Psychiatrie und Neuropathologie*, October 1906.

7. Alzheimer, A. "Die stationäre Paralyse." Jahresversammlung des Vereins bayerischer Psychiater in München, 21–22 Mai 1907. *Centralblatt für Nervenheilkunde u. Psychiatrie*, vol. 18, 15 Sept. 1907.

ALCOHOLIC DEMENTIA

Introduction

Robert C. Collins, M.D.
Assistant Professor of Neurology
Washington University
Medical School
St. Louis, Mo.

DOES ALCOHOL DAMAGE THE BRAIN? Not directly. The paradox, of course, is that indirectly alcohol leads to neurological disability of endemic proportions. The incidence of head trauma is increased in the inebriated state. Meningitis is not uncommon in chronic alcoholics. The autonomic storm of withdrawal can be fatal. Of major importance, expecially in considering these original papers by Wernicke (1881), Marchiafava and Bignami (1903), and Morel (1939), is that chronic alcoholism leads to or accentuates homeopathic behavior. On the one hand, the alcoholic neglects his diet and becomes depleted of water-soluble vitamins. On the other hand, he engages in recurrent drinking bouts and suffers progressive Laennec's cirrhosis. Such liver disease commonly leads to inadequate fixation of systemic ammonium, and the hepatocerebral syndromes develop.

Wernicke's disease and the Wernicke-Korsakoff Syndrome were long considered hallmarks of alcoholism, even though Wernicke's first case clearly suggested a nutritional etiology. This was a twenty-year-old malnourished seamstress who developed signs of ataxia, ophthalmoplegia, and encephalopathy associated with prolonged vomiting following sulfuric acid ingestion. The experimental work which eventually established thiamine deficiency as the nutritional cause of Wernicke's Disease began with an observation by Eijkman in 1890. He noticed that hens fed on polished rice developed symptoms of nervous system dysfunction.

Working in Batavia (Djakarta), Prof. Dr. C. Eijkman used the pigeon as a laboratory model for investigating the relationship of rice diets to beriberi in man. He made the important observation that the polyneuritis of pigeons was cured by adding back into the diet the discarded rich polishings themselves. In 1911, at the Lister Institute for Preventive Medicine in London, Casimir Funk postulated that the active principle of these rice polishings was present in minute quantities, a vital amine, or "vitamine." The crystallization of thiamine from rice polishings was finally achieved by Jansen and Donath in 1925 in Batavia in the original laboratories where Eijkman had worked. They sent 40 mg of their crystals to his laboratories in Utrecht. He was quickly able to demonstrate its prophylactic and curative potency in pigeon polyneuritis.

While these explorations were being pursued along nutritional and biochemical lines, Rudolph Peters established the clinical details of acute opisthotonus in the pigeon as the biological assay of thiamine deficiency. Working at Oxford from 1929–1939, Peters established the importance of neurochemistry to the study of the pathophysiology of nervous-system disorders. By developing the techniques of decapitation and freezing in liquid air, he discovered that lactate was elevated more in the brainstem than the cerebrum of opisthotonic pigeons. By developing the technique of mincing brain, and with the use of the Warburg respirometer, he discovered a decreased rate of oxidation of pyruvate in the brainstem of these pigeons. He also found that the addition of thiamine increased the respiration of deficient brain tissue and that the essential step was the addition of thiamine pyrophosphate as the necessary cofactor for pyruvate cocarboxylase. In addition to these biochemical observations, he was the first to appreciate the rapid clinical effect of thiamine when given in vivo. In this case, a pigeon who was near death in opisthotonus would be flying about the room just thirty minutes after an injection of thiamine. Sir Rudoph Peters summarized his work in 1936 in a lecture at The National Hospital, Queen Square. Here he first put forth the postulate of the importance of a "biochemical lesion" in neurological disease.

Peters was unable to find histological changes in the brains of pigeons with acute opisthotonus. In an isolated report in 1934, C. O. Prickett from the veterinary laboratories of the Alabama Polytechnic Institute demonstrated the first clear evidence that thiamine deficiency led to neuropathological changes in the brainstem. He maintained rats on a diet deficient in thiamine but supplemented with other vitamins. The animals became ataxic at forty days and died shortly thereafter. Their brains showed bilateral petechial hemorrhages in the floor of the fourth ventricle, predominantly within the nucleus of Deiters, chief vestibular nucleus, nucleus of Bechterew, and nucleus solitarius. He also found similar pathology in deficient pigeons. Prickett was evidently not aware that these findings were similar to those first observed by Wernicke in 1881. Four years later in Boston, Leo Alexander announced the key observation that pulled together these seemingly diverse experimental findings. He demonstrated that experimental beriberi produced in the pigeon resulted in lesions which were identical to those described by Wernicke sixty years earlier in man.

The clinical piece to the puzzle was added independently from the medical wards of the Psychiatric Institute of Bellevue Hospital. Here Jollifee, Wortis, and Fein (1941) reviewed the effects of different forms of nutritional treatment on twenty-seven alcoholic patients with Wernicke's symptoms studied between 1935–1940. They were the first to document the rapid effect of thiamine on ocular palsies, as well as the slower beneficial effects on ataxia and peripheral neuritis. Mental changes, especially Korsakoff's amnesic psychosis, proved to be intractable.

What is the lesson of Carl Wernicke's contribution? One finds here the rewards of a keen eye, a methodical insistence on detail, and a synthetic imagination that saw disease patterns amidst the complex phenomenology of signs and symptoms at the bedside. One recognizes also the first attempts to validate the hypothesis that neurological abnormalities were the result of focal pathology. Upon examining his second case, an alcoholic withdrawing from cognac, Wernicke knew that his patient suffered the same pathophysiological process that studded the brainstem of the malnourished girl he had seen months earlier. Although today we take all this for granted, as we also accept the importance of the prompt use of thiamine when seeing a patient with Wernicke's "acute hemorrhagic polioencephalitis superior," it is instructive to remember the diverse experimental roots that provided this therapy.

A similar history of clinical observation and experimental research is now emerging for the hepatocerebral syndromes and the pathogenetic role of ammonium (Cavanagh, 1974). Several independent workers have found Alzheimer Type II astrocytic changes in laboratory animals with portacaval anastomoses. This work has occurred within ten years after Victor, Adams, and Cole (1965) firmly established liver disease as the basis of the diverse symptomatology of "alcoholic dementia."

One recognizes the characteristic phenomenology of acquired hepatocerebral degeneration in Morel's description of his patients: dementia, fluctuating mental signs, dysarthria, ataxia, choreoathetosis, and tremor. In addition, he describes clear evidence for liver disease in three of his four cases. The only hesitancy in including this rarely cited work as an example of hepatocerebral disease is the topography of lesions. Morel emphasized a laminar sclerosis of layer III of the cortex, an area much less common than the pseudo-laminar necrosis found at the corticomedullary junction. Unfortunately, the peculiarities of Morel's staining technique do not allow a judgment on the fine morphology of the protoplasmic astrocytes. His description of hyperplasia and hypertrophy is probably sufficient, however.

The pathological entity of Marchiafava-Bignami disease—a demyelination in the central portion of the corpus callosum—continues to raise questions that remain unanswered. One can recognize in the clinical descriptions of early cases of "dementia alcoholica progressiva" features similar to hepatocerebral degeneration. The more common occurrence of seizures in Marchiafava and Bignami's cases suggests alcohol withdrawal superimposed. Marchiafava later recognized a more widespread distribution of focal demyelination in his material, especially the centrum semiovale and the cerebral peduncles.

It is possible to formulate a more generous hypothesis for the etiology of this disorder than Italian red wine. If one includes central pontine myelinolysis and alcoholic amblyopia as additional examples of a similar demyelinating process, then the experimental approach would be to find the common denominator in alcohol, malnutrition, and liver disease. Since Alzheimer Type II astrocytes are commonly found in brains with the Marchiafava-Bignami lesion, and since central pontine myelinolysis occurs in liver disease alone, the clinical leads clearly point towards an experimental focus on the liver.

REFERENCES

1. Alexander, L., Pijoan, M., and Myerson, A. (1938): "Beriberi and scurvy." Trans. Amer. Neurol. Assoc. 64; 135.
2. Cavanagh, J.B. (1974): "Liver bypass and the glia." Res. Publ. Assoc. Nerv. Ment. Dis. 53; 1.
3. Eijkman, C. (1890): Geneesk. Tijdschrift Ned. Ind 30; 295.
4. Funk, C. (1911): "On the chemical nature of the substance which cures polyneuritis in birds induced by a diet of polished rice." J. Physiol. 43; 395.
5. Jansen, B. C. P., and Donath, W. F. (1926): "On the isolation of beriberi vitamin." Proc. Klinik. Nederlandse Akad. van Wetenschappen (Amsterdam) 29; 1390.
6. Joliffee, N., Wortis, H., and Fein, H. D. (1941): "The Wernicke syndrome." Arch. Neurol. Psychiat. 46; 569.
7. Peters, R. A. (1936): "The biochemical lesion in thiamin B_1 deficiency." Lancet 1: 1161.
8. Prickett, C. O. (1934): "The effect of a deficiency of vitamin B_1 upon the central and peripheral nervous systems of the rat." Amer. J. Physiol. 107: 459.
9. Victor, M., Adams, R. D., and Cole, M. (1965): "The acquired (non-Wilsonian) type of chronic hepatocerebral degeneration." Medicine 44:345.

Acute Hemorrhagic Polioencephalitis Superior

C. WERNICKE

THE BORDER ZONE between the brain and the spinal cord, the medulla oblongata, has a dual character as regards pathology. On the one hand, we have learned about medullary hemorrhages and softenings, which closely resemble hemorrhages and softenings occurring elsewhere in the brain; and, on the other hand, the medulla differs from the brain in that the grey floor of the fourth ventricle, in particular the motor nerve nuclei, which correspond to the grey matter of the anterior horns of the spinal cord, are the preferential seat of independent diseases of probable inflammatory origin analogous only to poliomyelitis. Insofar as this analogy is real one can speak of a polioencephalitis which runs the variable course characteristic of poliomyelitis. Thus, there is a chronic progressive form, Duchenne's disease; an acute form, so-called bulbar paralysis; and a rarer subacute form, which corresponds to the rare subacute form of poliomyelitis.

However, similar disease processes extend far beyond the limits of the medulla on up into the grey matter of the pons and midbrain, where the involved nuclei are exclusively those of the extraocular muscles. Here, too, the spinal-cord type of disease occurs, and the morphologically indisputable homology of the motor cranial nerves and the ventral roots of the anterior horns is confirmed pathologically. The rostral zone of polioencephalitis extends from the posterior wall of the

NOTE: Translated by W. H. O. Bohne and D. A. Rottenberg from: Wernicke, C., *Lehrbuch der Gehirnkrankheiten*, vol. 2, §47, Theodor Fischer (Kassel and Berlin), 1881, 229–42.

infundibulum in the third ventricle to the level of the abducens nucleus. Here, too, one encounters an acute and chronic form of the disease. It will be useful, therefore, to differentiate between polioencephalitis inferior and polioencephalitis superior depending upon the area of involvement. The border zone between the two is rather ill-defined, however, so that marked involvement of either region is occasionally accompanied by focal symptoms which reflect involvement of the neighboring region.

At this point a short digression into the realm of spinal-cord diseases will not be amiss. It is well known that the diseases grouped together under the name of poliomyelitis are more of a clinical than a pathological entity; the acute form of poliomyelitis was known clinically as infantile spinal paralysis long before the disease of grey matter was discovered. Later, when the study of autopsy material established the anatomical basis of this disease, a more appropriate designation was required. Kussmaul was the first to use the name poliomyelitis, which became universally accepted. In many cases poliomyelitis is—as is any other myelitis—a focal inflammatory softening of the spinal cord, differing from ordinary myelitis only in its characteristic involvement of the grey matter, especially in the cervical or lumbar enlargement. It may, therefore, transiently mimic an ordinary myelitis, the typical picture of poliomyelitis (i.e., myelitis confined to the grey matter) emerging only after the initial phase of the illness. In other cases, where small foci are present from the onset, the characteristic symptoms of a grey-matter disease occur. These symptoms reflect the location of the large ganglion cells, which receive pyramidal-tract fibers and give rise to peripheral-nerve fibers that innervate the musculature of the extremities, in the grey anterior horns. Ganglion cells perish. After a few months the survivors are barely recognizable, severely shrunken calcified structures; only calcified fragments remain of the nerve fibers which are normally so abundant in the grey matter of the anterior horns. These changes were demonstrated by C. Friedländer, who first described similar changes in focal brain softenings. Since spinal ganglion cells are always grouped together to innervate synergistically acting muscles, small destructive lesions lead to the circumscribed loss of specific muscle groups and produce the characteristic symptoms of nuclear disease. If the destruction is more extensive this focality is less apparent, and an entire arm or leg may become involved. Rarely, certain muscle groups gradually regain their function so that the nuclear character of the disease process once again becomes apparent.

There is no need to discuss the other consequences of anterior horn cell destruction. Certainly, the death of a ganglion cell has the same effect on the ventral root fibril which it engenders and on its muscle end-organ as the transection of a peripheral nerve, i.e., immediate paralysis followed, after a time, by atrophy of the denervated muscle fibers. The acute form of poliomyelitis may be contrasted with the sub-acute form in which the same anatomical regions are affected; the sub-acute illness progresses for several weeks or months before reaching the stage at which it becomes arrested, kills, or partially regresses. When such cases come to autopsy one cannot find true myelitic foci, only the residua of probable myelitic changes in the grey matter. In those areas where ganglion cells are usually found one finds no cells at all or only cellular debris; the ganglion cells have been replaced by sclerotic tissue or by an accumulation of spider cells, connective tissue elements that play the role of weeds in the central nervous system and follow hard upon the heels of irreversibly damaged nervous parenchyma. Other very chronic cases, e.g., the so-called progressive muscular atrophy, have been attributed to a simple, primary (sic) atrophy of motor cells. The basic difference in symptomatology, which I wish to emphasize at this point, can be accounted for by the more chronic course of the disease process in that the gradual involvement of single cells necessarily leads to an inability to distinguish between the stage of paralysis and the stage of atrophy: both occur simultaneously. The prevailing tendency to consider all of these forms of motor neuron disease as poliomyelitis cannot be disregarded. I, too, subscribe to this view, because the clinical features of these syndromes are so characteristic. I would also accept the notion that all diseases of the motor nuclei of the spinal cord be ascribed to poliomyelitis and would retain their classification into acute, sub-acute, and chronic progressive forms.

Only the acute form is strictly analogous to disease in the brain, for an acute focal softening in the brain behaves in the same manner as a myelitic focus in the spinal cord. If, therefore, we emphasize the clinical aspects of nuclear disease in the medulla oblongata, as we do in poliomyelitis, then those focal medullary softenings which predominantly or exclusively involve the nuclear regions—regardless of whether they result from vascular occlusion or inflammatory infiltration—correspond to the acute form of poliomyelitis. Thus, Leyden's first case could easily be ascribed to polioencephalitis. Had an autopsy been performed, Hérard's case might well have been ascribed to polioencephalitis, given identical findings. However, inflammatory infiltrates, as in Leyden's case, behave very differently than the softenings commonly encountered in the brain and spinal cord. Both lesions have been reported to occur in the medulla. Only the infiltrating and, consequently, widely disseminated form of red inflammatory softening has been observed in the motor cranial nerves rostral to the medulla.

It soon becomes apparent when one searches for an analogue of the chronic form of poliomyelitis in the brain that softenings in the region of the cranial nerve nuclei assume special significance. One is no longer dealing with a focal softening such as occurs in some cases of acute polioencephalitis—i.e., with a chronic focal softening accompanied by the characteristic findings and course described in section 45 of the text—but rather with the same form of chronic inflammation associated with chronically active foci in the spinal cord, that is, with sclerosing myelitis. As we have seen, sclerosing myelitis (understood in its most general sense) is usually attributed to chronic poliomyelitis. In the region of the cranial nerve nuclei one encounters the same primary neuronal loss that has been described in the spinal cord as well as a marked sclerosis which may be confined to the nuclear zone or may extend to neighboring areas. Thus, the sclerotic process accurately reflects the topography of the chronic forms of polioencephalitis.

These preliminary remarks were necessary in order to put the following three case histories into proper perspective. My notes are most extensive in the last case.

CASE 1

A twenty-year-old seamstress was admitted to the Charité on December 5, 1876 for treatment of sulfuric acid poisoning and was discharged on January 6, 1877. After discharge from hospital she began to vomit; however, she was otherwise well until February 3, 1877, when she became somnolent and took to bed. She yawned a lot and stumbled whenever she tried to get out of bed and walk. She also noted a fall-off in her vision, complicated subsequently by extremely annoying, continuous scintillations, severe photophobia, vertigo, and heaviness in the head. Because her symptoms worsened and her vomiting persisted she sought readmission to the Charité on February 11, 1877. There was no history of infection.

On February 12 physical examination reveals a very pale, somewhat emaciated woman lying in bed with both eyes half-closed. Her palpebral fissures measure only about one centimeter, and even with her eyes shaded she cannot elevate the lids any further. Only when looking up do the eyes open slightly more widely. The right palpebral fissure is narrower than the left, even when looking up. Eye-closure is full but weak and without wrinkle formation; it cannot be improved reflexly by touching the eyes. During forward gaze both globes are motionless and slightly convergent. Upward gaze provokes jerky movements of large amplitude; ultimately, however, the attempted excursion is completed. The same observations apply to downward gaze. Conjugate gaze to the left is significantly impaired. The left eye does not cross the midline despite considerable effort and quivering movements. The right eye can be adducted, but the medial edge of the cornea usually comes to rest at the level of the inferior lacrimal punctum, approaching the caruncula only momentarily. Conjugate gaze to the right is restricted in a similar fashion; that is to say, the right eye cannot be abducted beyond the midline, whereas the left eye approaches the medial palpebral commissure, though falling short of the mark. The same state of affairs obtains during convergence of the visual axes (fixation on the tip of the nose) in that adduction is more complete on the left. Strabismus is not marked in the primary position of gaze, although the visual axes tend to converge. The pupils are midposition, equal, and sluggishly reactive to light. With the face at rest the right corner of the mouth is lower than the left, and the right cheek is somewhat flattened; the nasolabial fold and the fold under the lower eyelid are more prominent on the left. The right corner of the mouth opens less widely than the left. The facial expression is weepy, sullen, and apathetic. The same asymmetries are present during laughter and when the mouth is opened widely. No facial asymmetries are observed during other voluntary movements. No paralysis is demonstrable, but the impression of severe weakness remains. The patient can walk with support. There is no sensory disturbance; the extremities are cold. She complains of extreme fatigue, and her speech is weak and weary. She vomited repeatedly during the course of the day. Temperature (T.) 37.0–37.4.

February 13: Continued somnolence. The patient moans occasionally or calls out the name of her fiancé, is generally disoriented and seems not to know where she is. When stimulated—for example, at mealtimes—she converses coherently with the nursing personnel, suddenly interrupting the conversation to complain of low back pain or of heaviness in the head. She voids small amounts of urine of a peculiar oily consistency containing peptones but not protein or sugar. Cool extremities. T. 36.4–37.2.

February 14: The patient has to be aroused; she answers but remains disoriented. She complains of headache and neck stiffness, manifests extreme anxiety, and expresses fear of falling while she is being carried. Frequent yawning and moaning. She responds only when questioned repeatedly. Her pupils dilate with atropine. Ophthalmoscopic examination reveals bilateral optic neuritis with moderate disc swelling and multiple flame-shaped hemorrhages. Abdomen distended, tense, and painful. T. 37.3–37.5. Pulse (P.) 120 and barely palpable. She was extremely agitated at night and screamed frequently.

February 15: The patient is somnolent and whimpers as if in pain. She does not respond to direct questions. Death in the afternoon.

Autopsy. The gyri are not flattened. The cerebral ventricles contain only a few drops of fluid; the tela choroidea and choroid plexus are bright red in color. A cut through the basal ganglia exposes the entire extent of the third ventricle; its walls are studded with numerous small punctate hemorrhages, and the contiguous brain substance is discolored (pink) to a depth of about 3–5 mm. These changes are bilateral and almost mathematically symmetrical. They are nicely seen in a section through the region of the massa intermedia, which is very well developed and also full of hemorrhages. The colliculi and the cerebellum are not involved. The pia in the region of the medulla oblongata has a smokey grey coloration; the pons and the medulla are not grossly affected, and the spinal cord appears normal macroscopically. Numerous hemorrhages are present in both retinae. The consequences of sulfuric acid poisoning are observed.

Anatomic diagnosis: hemorrhagic encephalitis of the grey matter surrounding the third ventricle, bilateral retinal hemorrhages; pyloric stenosis, chronic distension of the stomach with ulceration consequent upon sulfuric acid poisoning.

Microscopic examination after fixation reveals that the punctate hemorrhages, which vary in size, occasionally attaining the size of a pinhead, usually surround blood vessels. The small vessels and capillaries are filled to capacity and widely distended. The vessel walls appear normal; only rarely does a capillary endothelial cell seem to be swollen or unusually large. Granular cells are observed in the vicinity of the hemorrhages. As regards the distribution of the grey-matter lesions, they do not extend into neighboring structures or fiber tracts. There is an isolated pinhead-sized hemorrhage in the left inferior colliculus. The grey-matter lesions extend inferiorly to the region of the striae acusticae, gradually decreasing in intensity. The basal arteries appear normal.

Case 2

A thirty-six-year-old alcoholic Scots piano teacher, who called himself a professor, had been drinking large amounts of cognac. He was admitted to the Charité in a delirium on June 18, 1877 and spent a sleepless night; he remained delirious but not uproarious. On June 19 his condition was as follows: a well-nourished, somewhat obese man without any diseases of the internal organs; he was covered with perspiration, extremely agitated and tremulous. When forced to get up he was very unsteady and could not walk without support. His gait was broad-based and ataxic, interrupted by jerky and inappropriate movements; his trunk was held stiffly erect. Further examination in bed was impossible because of the patient's agitation, but it was established that he reacted to pinprick over the soles. His hands were not restrained, but their movements were interrupted by tremor. His speech was exceedingly tremulous and, moreover, was difficult to evaluate as he muttered incoherently in Scottish. It was impossible to engage his attention. The pupils were extremely miotic but equal. Extraocular movements seemed to be restricted, but the patient's inability to fixate precluded a more definite statement. The skin temperature was not elevated. The respiratory rate was increased; the pulse, which was difficult to palpate, was rapid and regular.

The patient remained delirious for several days, and his general condition did not give rise to concern. Repeated observations revealed that he hardly moved his eyes at all and fixated objects by moving his head. As the motor agitation subsided he lapsed into a somnolent state associated with such extreme weakness that he could not stand. His pulse, which was always difficult to palpate, became weaker, faster, and irregular. His respirations also became irregular, and he died on June 26 after a prolonged period of stupor. As his restlessness abated it became possible to more closely observe his eye movements, and it was concluded that his eyes were almost completely immobile in the primary position of gaze. Nevertheless, no ptosis could be demonstrated. The pupils, which were usually constricted, could be dilated with atropine. Funduscopic examination revealed that both optic discs were hyperemic but not swollen; a flame-shaped hemorrhage was observed alongside one of the vessels in the right eye.

Autopsy. The findings in the brain are the same as in the previous case. Hemorrhages no larger than petechiae are confined to the central grey surrounding the third and fourth ventricles and the aqueduct. The region of the habenular ganglion is involved bilaterally. Microscopically the changes are exactly the same as in the previous case. The basal arteries are normal.

Case 3

A thirty-three-year-old man was admitted to the Charité on March 10, 1878 following the onset of delirium tremens that morning. A heavy schnapps drinker, especially during the preceding few months. Since the last war he has complained repeatedly of a pulling sensation in both legs. He contracted typhoid fever during an earlier war and was infected once as a young man. During the four weeks prior to admission his gait has been occasionally unsteady. Three weeks prior to admission he experienced difficulty passing his urine. The patient was said to have fallen off a cart, possibly injuring his head, eight weeks prior to admission; however, there have been no sequelae. Occasional headaches and dizzy spells for the past four weeks. He vomits in the morning, especially after having had a lot to drink. Two days prior to admission he became jaundiced and complained of double vision. He has never suffered a stroke or had a convulsion.

Physical examination on March 11 reveals a very strong, well-nourished individual with slightly icteric skin. There is an old bubonic scar in the right inguinal area. A glistening fibrous scar is present on the

neck of the penis. Several sharply demarcated circular patches of de-
pigmentation over both lower legs.

Since admission the patient behaves as if delirious but is oriented to
place and to his surroundings. He has become extremely agitated, continually tugging at his coverlet with his hands. He flings himself about,
turns his head to look at nonexistent persons, calls out for his acquain-
tances, and appears anxious. A coarse tremor appears during animated
gesticulations. His voice is hoarse, his speech hurried and somewhat
tremulous—not, however, slurred or dysarthric. His face is slightly
cyanotic, bloated, and covered with perspiration. Rapid respirations,
perhaps because of the psychological excitement; no coughing. The lips
and teeth are coated with a thick film. The gait is reeling and further
destabilized by sudden ataxic and tremulous movements. He is able to
stand on one foot for short periods.

When asked, the patient complains of weakness in his legs. His head
and trunk are held erect. His tongue, which is somewhat dry and without bite marks, can be protruded in the midline but is markedly tremulous. There is a hint of right-sided facial weakness. He is not stupefied; a
question briefly engages his attention. P. 110–120, regular, fairly full and
very soft; T. 39.3. His urine is free of protein and sugar. The thoracic
organs are normal, and the liver extends two fingerbreadths below the
costal margin.

There is total bilateral abducens paralysis; neither eye can be moved
laterally beyond the midline. All other extraocular movements appear to
be intact. The pupils are midposition and equal, and react bilaterally to
light and convergence. Pinprick is promptly appreciated over the face
and hands; over the feet, however, it is felt only after a delay. A few
moments elapsed before he became aware of a forceful jab with a needle
in his right great toe, and he complained of a severe burning sensation.
On the left most pricks do not elicit a reaction. Percussion of the skull is
not painful, nor is pressure over the spinal column and neck musculature. Ophthalmoscopic examination in the evening revealed extreme
hyperemia of the papillae without swelling; the disc margins were not
entirely sharp, but there were no hemorrhages. Motor agitation and
perspiration is increased. The gait is unsteady, broad-based and stiff-
legged. There is a hint of nuchal rigidity. P. 120, T. 39, Respirations (R.)
28-30.

March 12: At night the patient was quiet but delirious, becoming
somewhat more composed toward morning. He lies quietly with his
eyes closed. Aroused forthwith by the examination he relapses afterwards into a quiet delirium. No further jactitations. R. 24–30; P. 100,
regular and very soft; T. 38.9. He coughs occasionally bringing up
sputum. A vinegar enema yesterday produced large amounts of soft
stool. The neck is still slightly extended, especially when he assumes a

sitting position. Pressure over the spinous processes of the upper thoracic vertebrae and neck musculature evokes considerable grimacing, whereas stroking the skin over the back does not. Hypesthesia in the lower extremities has given way to hyperesthesia, as becomes apparent when the patient's calves are squeezed; this is particularly striking in view of his dazed state. The abducens weakness and facial paresis are unchanged, and the protruded tongue is more tremulous. Atropine dilates the pupils. In the evening T. 38.7, P. 90.

March 13: P. 114, R. 26, T. 37.9. The patient coughs less, mutters under his breath, is disoriented and continues to be delirious. He starts when touched. His muscles are no longer hyperesthetic. He can take a few steps if supported but sways and walks stiffly with a broad base. His eyes and face are unchanged. In the evening P. 100–110, T. 37.8.

March 14: P. 98–100, T. 37.8. The pulse is regular, weak, and very soft. The patient spent the greater part of the night in a delirious state; however, early in the morning he appeared less dazed and better oriented. As he was able to fixate, a more thorough examination of the extraocular movements was undertaken. Lateral movements are restricted as before, and medial movements seem to be impaired as well; upward and downward gaze are intact. When the patient sits up there is obvious nuchal rigidity. In the evening P. 100, T. 38.0. The urine is deeply colored but free of protein and sugar.

March 15: The patient was delirious at times during the night, though quiet most of the time. Now he is stuporous. Intermittent twitching of the arms and legs, sometimes of the whole body. The pulse (approximately 96) is regular, soft, and very weak; it was hardly palpable half an hour ago. Respirations are stertorous and irregular. Progressively deeper inspirations follow long apneic periods, but the regular sequence of Stoke's breathing is lacking. Pressure on the great toe results in brisk withdrawal of the legs and right-sided facial grimacing. The patient starts when touched unexpectedly. The patellar reflex can be tested on the left side and is not elicitable. Once aroused he states that he feels well. His lips are dry, and he complains of thirst. There is no significant speech disturbance. When he sits up there is nuchal rigidity and grimacing. In the evening P. 100, T. 38.2.

March 16: The pulse (96) is intermittently irregular. T. 38.5. The patient's general condition is essentially unchanged. He is weaker and intermittently delirious. Most of the time he lies with his eyes half-closed; only the sclerae are visible. Frequent nonproductive cough. When taken out of bed he exhibits marked weakness, collapsing after a few stiff, unsteady steps. When exhorted he appears alert and oriented and fixates objects held up in front of him. He complains of severe weakness. Extraocular movements are impaired, especially adduction, which is incomplete and jerky. Downgaze is markedly affected, upgaze less so though also somewhat reduced. Funduscopic examination reveals fully developed optic neuritis O.D. The papilla is intensely hyperemic and somewhat swollen with poorly defined margins. The arteries are not visible; all of the veins are distended. One small vessel directed toward the macula is surrounded by a fusiform hemorrhage in the vicinity of the papilla. There are no other hemorrhages. The left disc is hyperemic, its margins somewhat blurred; the arteries and veins and all of their ramifications are filled. The patient expired before noon.

Autopsy. The pia overlying the convexity and the base is uniformly transparent and only slightly edematous. The dura is not tense and appears normal; the pia also appears normal. The hemispheres are not significantly altered, but the cortex is slightly injected. There are no changes at the base. Unroofing the third ventricle, one can appreciate that the massa intermedia is studded with punctate hemorrhages. When the cerebellum is removed, most of the grey areas of the rhomboid fossa are seen to be covered with small red dots, possibly also containing capillary hemorrhages. No other abnormalities are noted. The spinal cord appears normal.

The heart is somewhat enlarged, but its walls are not hypertrophied. On its atrial surface the mitral valve exhibits several old, very hard, knotlike thickenings. Both lungs contain considerable amounts of blood. The pharynx is deeply cyanotic, the laryngeal mucosa thickened, and both vocal cords superficially ulcerated. The spleen is broad, cake-shaped, and increased in thickness. The kidneys are extremely hyperemic.

Anatomic diagnosis: multiple punctate hemorrhages of the massa intermedia, third ventricle and grey matter of the fourth ventricle; pulmonary edema and hyperemia; chronic mitral endocarditis; splenic hyperplasia; fatty infiltration of the liver; and ulceration of the vocal cords. Examination of fixed specimens reveals exactly the same changes as in the previous two cases, although the hemorrhages never attain the size of a pinhead. The inflammatory changes do not extend beyond the floor of the fourth ventricle; in the third ventricle they are not as prominent as in the previous case, but they extend further caudally, to the rostral zone of the calamus scriptorius.

We are dealing with an acute inflammatory affection of the nuclei in the region of the oculomotor nerves which leads to death within 10–14 days. The focal symptoms consist of associated eye muscle paralyses, which develop rapidly and ultimately lead to an almost complete external ophthalmoplegia; the sphincter iridis and levator palpebrarum appear to be spared. The patient begins to stagger; his gait, which combines stiffness with ataxia, usually brings to mind the ataxia of the alcoholic. General symptoms are very prominent and reflect a disturbance of consciousness, which may take the form of somnolence from the outset or, alternately, of somnolence preceded by an extended period of agitation. The optic nerve was involved in all three cases with characteristic inflammatory changes of the papillae. In each case a severe insult antedated the onset of the illness: sulfuric acid poisoning with resultant pyloric stenosis in the first case and the abuse of alcohol to an extraordinary degree in both of the other cases. Whether or not the delirium potatorum in Cases 2 and 3 should be considered as a complication of this illness or as an independent manifestation of it has yet to be resolved. At any rate, ordinary (uncomplicated) delirium tremens did not occur, but rather delirium tremens complicated by polioencephalitis. It should be noted that the characteristic disorientation was also observed in the first case although symptomatic delirium was never present. After having completely misdiagnosed the first patient's illness during life I succeeded in correctly diagnosing the second and third cases despite their atypical presentations. Hence, it follows that we are justified in calling special attention to these cases as a separate disease entity.

Only later did I come upon a single analogous case in the literature. The major symptoms and the pathological findings are undeniably similar, although the latter were not confined to the nuclear region as in my cases. The course (five months) is more consistent with a subacute form of the disease.

GAYET'S CASE

["Affection encéphalique (encéphalite diffuse probable) localisée aux étages supérieurs des pédoncles cérébraux et aux couches optiques, ainsi qu'au plancher du quatrième ventricule et aux parois latérales du troisième," *Arch. de phy.*, 1875.] A twenty-eight-year-old man was admitted on November 23. In mid-September he was working in an engine room when suddenly a boiler exploded not far from him. Although considerable destruction ensued, he himself remained totally unharmed. However, he became extremely distraught, insomniac, and inordinately excited. He continued to work for three days but then noticed that he could no longer read or write properly. Thereafter he lapsed into a state of general weakness, malaise, and apathy; and, subsequently, he developed an incessant craving for sleep.

At the time of admission he responded appropriately if slowly and had to be encouraged. His facial expression was masklike, the orbicularis oris and palpebrarum were flattened against their bony supports, and the eyelids were three-quarters closed; there was bilateral ptosis. In spite of the obvious atonia no facial paralysis could be demonstrated; all facial movements were well performed. Speech occurred as if in isolation, without the participation of the remainder of the physiognomy. There was generalized symmetrical muscle weakness, which was sufficiently pronounced so that the patient was unable to stand or to grasp firmly with his hands. All of the extraocular muscles innervated by both oculomotor nerves were almost completely paralyzed; only the pupils and accomodation were spared. Visual acuity was good. The special senses in general as well as all modalities of skin sensation were normal.

The patient was so lethargic that he fell asleep during the examination, during meals, etc. Only vigorous shaking would keep him awake. His weakness increased until December 18, becoming more pronounced on the right side. His somnolence persisted. Ophthalmoscopic examination on January 5 did not reveal any unequivocal abnormalities; the papillae may have been slightly hyperemic, more so on the left.

A complete right-sided hemiplegia with mild sensory loss supervened on January 8 and persisted until January 18, at which time it seemed to vanish. No longer apathetic, the patient became extremely agitated and complained of pain in his right leg. His facial expression was somewhat livelier. In the evening he ran a temperature, and tracheal rhonchi were heard for the first time. January 19 was a good day. On January 20 he became somnolent once again. His condition did not stabilize until February 7, when it was noted that sensation was impaired over his right side but was normal elsewhere. The special senses functioned normally, and his intellect was normal when he was aroused. The left pupil was enlarged. On February 8 the funduscopic examination was unchanged. Increased weakness and cachexia and urinary incontinence were noted on February 10. An incipient decubitus was discovered on February 15, and the patient expired on February 17. During the month preceding his demise his temperature ranged between 37.4 and 38.5; the elevations were recorded in the morning. Urine taken from the bladder *post mortem* contained neither protein nor sugar. However, a black sediment formed after the addition of an alkaline copper solution; its nature could not be determined.

Autopsy. The central grey surrounding the third and fourth ventricles is studded with capillary hemorrhages. The changes begin rostrally at the anterior commissure and affect the inner walls of both optic colliculi, the thalamic taeniae, the epiphysis, the infundibulum and the tuber cinereum as well as the enormously hypertrophied massa intermedia, the periaqueductal grey and the grey floor of the fourth ventricle as far caudally as the tip of the calamus scriptorius. In addition to the conspicuously injected small vessels and punctate hemorrhages a generalized yellow-grey discoloration is discernible in the illustrations. A transverse section through the peduncular region anterior to the pons suggests that the left crus is involved, whereas according to the text the crura are intact. At any rate, what the author takes to be inflammatory changes are visible throughout the entire cross-sectional extent of the tegmentum including the left superior cerebellar peduncle. Both superior colliculi are involved in a patchy fashion. The changes seem to be more pronounced on the left side, where they extend to the wall of the lateral ventricle. Microscopic sections from the inner surface of the right superior colliculus confirm the presence of an inflammatory process. Careful examination of the vessels fails to reveal any abnormalities.

Laminar Cortical Sclerosis:
A Special Anatomo–Clinical Form of
Chronic Alcoholism

F. MOREL

TECHNICAL DIFFICULTIES in demonstrating normal glia have restricted our knowledge of these cells. The cortical layers of both man and monkey show a particular glial distribution and character, i.e., fibrillary glia (macroglia) in the superior third of the first layer, becoming more protoplasmic as one penetrates deeper. Normally, layers I and V are richest in glial cells followed by layers II and III, where the glia are relatively rare and especially delicate (A. H. Schroeder I).

The normal pattern may be profoundly altered in pathologic states. For a number of years we have systematically studied the glia in 420 brains of patients with oligophrenic dementia praecox, epilepsy, general paresis, various clinical alcoholic states, cerebral arteriosclerosis, and senile degenerations.

We use our own technique in preference to the Cajal gold sublimate. Our method is a modification of Globus's technique. With it we have been able to obtain good representation of glia in most of the above mentioned illnesses.

In systematically applying our method, we were surprised to discover the first instance of a laminar glial band in the third cortical layer. We have discovered only four instances of this special macroglial distri-

NOTE: Translated by F. H. Hochberg from: Morel, F., "Une Forme anatomo-clinique particulière de l'alcoolisme chronique: Sclerose corticale laminaire alcoolique," *Revue neurologique* 71, 3 (1939), 280–88.

bution in the 420 brains studied. These four cases represent an anatomically and clinically distinct entity. In each instance I have confirmed our findings by means of the Holzer technique—which demonstrated this band. However, our method is more sensitive than Holzer's.

CASE 1

Ber... a fifty-eight-year-old man from Geneva with an alcoholic brother. The patient was childish, slightly mentally deficient, and a degenerate chronic alcoholic (a drinker of red wines by his own admission) who produced considerable phlegm. He was first hospitalized at fifty-seven years of age for sweating, anxiety, apprehension, visual hallucinations, and pathologic automatism, e. g., people sending him odors, sensations of electricity. The blood Wasserman was negative. Blood pressure 160/100. The lumbar cerebrospinal fluid was clear with 1.8 cells per cubic millimeter; the albumin was 15 mg/100 ml, the Pandy negative, and the Wasserman ambiguous. Following twenty days of treatment he was much improved. The following year he was rehospitalized with disorientation, marked anxiety, and gross amnesia. He exhibited motor and verbal perseveration (repetitively opening his mouth no matter what he was asked to do and always giving the same answer). He had a severe tremor of his hands and tongue and small fibrillary jerks were observed in one muscle group after another in rapid succession. Urinalysis revealed a small amount of albumin, leucocytes, and casts. The prostate was hypertrophied, and the patient was uremic. He died several days after admission. The brain weighed 1220 grams. The pia mater was transparent and there was a slight degree of fronto-parietal leptomeningitis and subarachnoid edema. The gyri were thin, the sulci deep and large. The carotids contained yellow plaques; the cerebral arteries were normal. The liver had a smooth surface and was slightly firmer than usual. The prostate was hypertrophied and abscessed. Pus was present in the ureters and renal calyces.

CASE 2

Pal... a thirty-seven-year-old man from Geneva with erythematous urticaria of gastrointestinal origin. He vomited frequently and had daily diarrhea. At the age of thirty-five he had developed alcoholic gastritis. He was anxious, his memory poor, and his gait unsteady. Pain sensation was severely impaired over the entire body and he was diffusely weak. The urinalysis was normal. The blood pressure was 100/60. The lumbar cerebrospinal fluid was clear with 0.5 cells per cubic millimeter; the albumin was 30 mg/100 ml. and the Pandy and Wasserman reactions were negative. A guinea pig innoculated with this cerebrospinal fluid remained healthy. The red blood cell count was 4,235,625. The cholesterol concentration in the serum was 180. The Wasserman reaction in the serum was negative. The basal metabolic rate was +5.9 percent. According to his wife, the patient had drunk to excess between twenty and twenty-nine years of age. When hospitalized at age thirty-seven his face was flushed. He was emaciated and had marked acne rosacea. A generalized tremor was present, especially of the jaw and hands. He clung to things and was unable to release them on command. The muscle tone was extremely variable, the normal suppleness being altered by frequent sudden contractions. He carried on an incoherent monologue while remaining in an excited, disoriented, agitated, insomniac, hallucinatory state, and his writing was tremulous—almost illegible. The ankle, cutaneous abdominal, and cremasteric reflexes were absent, the palmo-mental reflex was not elicited, and the plantar reflexes were flexor. Monocular scotomas were present. The pupils were reactive to light bilaterally. Sudden cutaneous paresthesias were noted. A diagnosis of atypical and prolonged delirium tremens was made. He died of pneumonia. At autopsy exam, the pia mater was delicate, and subarachnoid edema was present. The brain was hyperemic but without atrophy, weighing 1480 gm. The basal arteries were not atherosclerotic.

CASE 3

Fia... a fifty-one-year-old Czech man was first hospitalized at age forty-five years for alcoholic gastritis. At that time he was slightly icteric, tremulous, disoriented, hallucinatory, and insomniac; agitated continuously, he fidgeted and performed stereotyped movements (for example, trying to open a window). His writing was almost illegible and markedly tremulous. He had a permanently tonic pilomotor reflex, bilateral monocular scotomata, and transitory amblyopia. The blood pressure was 115/75. There was a trace of sugar in the urine. The lumbar cerebrospinal fluid was clear with a supine pressure of 90 mm of water, 0.3 cells per cubic millimeter, 22mg/100 ml albumin, negative Pandy and Wasserman reactions and a colloidal benzoin flocculation curve of 0000000000000000 [the results with cerebrospinal fluid are similar to those of the colloidal gold flocculation test: Guillain, Laroche, and Lechelle 1920]. His improvement was less complete and less rapid than expected for an attack of typical delirium tremens. On his second admission, at age fifty-one, he suffered from instability of gait which required him to look for points of support. His body was stiff and he exhibited [carphology] continuous hand movements—seemingly picking objects from the air or bed. There was a tendency towards forced movements. His tongue moved continuously in his mouth. The pupils were reactive to light. His writing was illegible. He trembled and was insomniac. The blood pressure was 110/80. On funduscopic exam the discs were a little pale (Prof. Franceschetti). There was urobilinuria. The lumbar cerebrospinal fluid was clear with a supine pressure of 240 mm of water, no cells, 22 mg/100 ml albumin, negative Wasserman and Vernes [a flocculation test for syphilis employing a powder of perethynol treated horse heart and either CSF or sera] reaction, and a colloidal benzoin flocculation curve of 0000022210000000. The diagnosis was atypical delirium tremens. At autopsy, following a terminal pneumonia, the pia mater over the convexity was slightly milky and was raised by underlying edema. The brain weighed 1320 gm. The basal vessels were not atherosclerotic.

CASE 4

Zug . . . a fifty-two-year-old man from Solothurn, for many years a drinker of red wine, eau-de-vie on an empty stomach, and aperitifs. One brother was an alcoholic. The patient had lost his taste for work, became somnolent, and had digital tremors. He developed progressive memory loss and for the last several months of his life experienced daily attacks of leg stiffness, each attack lasting 20–30 minutes, during which he could not take a step. He had formerly complained of calf pains. One month earlier his speech had become confused and vague. He developed insomnia with motor agitation, became emaciated with an ashen color, and had to be hospitalized for eight days. He was an afebrile senile chronic alcoholic who was still oriented as to time and place. His myopic pupils reacted to light and accomodation. His legs were spastic as was his gait, and general muscular strength was diminished. Upper and lower extremity deep tendon reflexes were increased, but there was no clonus, and the cutaneous reflexes were preserved. Lumbar puncture revealed cerebrospinal fluid under a pressure of 56 mm H_2O; the cerebrospinal fluid contained 6.4 cells (all lymphocytes) and 22 mg/100 ml protein. The Wasserman, Pandy, and Takata-Ara reactions were negative. The blood Vernes and Wasserman reactions were also negative. The blood urea nitrogen was 33 mg/100 ml. He was anorexic, and his tongue had a mild quality of stomach foulness [saburra] and exhibited a rhythmic tremor. His abdomen was soft with a liver edge percussed three fingerbreadths below the costal margin. He intermittently responded to questions. His speech was very jumbled. Sometimes ataxic movements of the arm and hand were observed. His somnolence was punctuated by generalized seizures lasting one to two minutes. On funduscopic exam both discs were pale, especially temporally. He was transferred to a convalescent facility (Bel-Air) where he remained for twenty-one days, during which time the episodic contractions of the extremities became so constant as to make gait almost impossible. Astasia, abasia, and motor perseveration were noted, as was motor incoordination. Commands were poorly executed. Transient spells of verbal-motor agitation were reported. He was completely disoriented and falsely recognized items. He confabulated and was amnesic. There was generalized hypesthesia to touch, pinprick, and pinch, and sensory localization was poor. Stereognosis was impossible to test. He was emaciated with seborrheic facies. The above-mentioned involuntary movements disappeared. His demise was preceded by difficulty swallowing and broncho-pneumonia. In summary, the picture was that of an accelerated disorder reminiscent of "generalized alcoholic pseudoparalysis." The autopsy examination revealed thickened meninges over the convexity with subarachnoid edema. The brain weighed 1065 grams and showed frontal atrophy. The cerebral arteries and aorta were smooth with several small atheromatous plaques. The cardia of the stomach contained submucosal hemorrhages.

In summary, we have reported four men: two from Geneva, one from Solothurn, and one Czech dying at thirty-seven, fifty-one, fifty-two, and fifty-eight years of age. The four were chronic alcoholics (red wine, eau-de-vie, and various aperitifs) and presented with severe alcoholic gastritis. Two of the patients had alcoholic brothers. During the last year of life the four had presented signs of alcoholic intoxication including atypical prolonged delirium tremens, from which they never completely recovered, and persistent memory difficulties. Normal muscular flexibility disappeared, the legs became spastic, which interfered with ambulation. The hands trembled grossly [carphology] and moved in a repetitive and involuntary way. There were facial tremors and stammering speech. The progressive decline lasted several months, was accompanied by emaciation, and terminated in death (due to pneumonia in two patients, broncho-pneumonia in one, and complications of prostatic hypertrophy in the fourth).

The negative data are consistent with the positive data I have presented. As to the serologic reactions, the sera and spinal fluid Wasserman reactions were negative in all four, as were the other serologic tests for syphilis. Guinea pig inoculation in one instance was negative, and the spinal fluid pressure, protein, and cells were not increased.

The clinical appearance brings to mind the relatively rare alcoholic dementia referred to as generalized alcoholic pseudoparalysis by the older authors. This was characterized by crises of atypical delirium tremens, associated with a progressive worsening of memory, emotionality, and gait (which was difficult or impossible) along with tremors and dysarthria. Death resulted from pulmonary, cardiac, or renal complications.

From an anatomic point of view the cases had common characteristics: the brain weights were relatively increased: 1220 gm, 1320 gm, 1480 gm, and 1065 gm; all four cases had subarachnoid edema, but there was no leptomeningeal fibrosis as seen typically in general paresis. There was no granular ependymitis or notable cerebral arteriosclerosis. None of the four brains contained senile plaques or Alzheimer cell changes. There were no changes suggestive of general paresis—no perivascular cuffs, rod cells, or neuroglial reaction in the cerebral cortex except in the third cortical layer. I will concentrate on this abnormality that has not been described in general paresis or known forms of chronic alcoholism.

Our four cases presented a clear-cut and systematized neuroglial proliferation. This pseudolaminar proliferation appeared as a continuous sheet of constant density limited to the third cortical layer especially in its external two-thirds (Figs. 1–5), rather than consisting of discontinuous nests or ["fleckweise"] islands of neuroglia.

Symmetrical brain regions always revealed a similar extent and intensity of this proliferation. These alterations were not present in all cerebral regions with the same distinctness. The frontal lobe was always the most affected—particularly the FDm and FDp regions, where the changes were most obvious and characteristic. The laminar proliferation was less distinct in the ascending frontal gyrus. The alterations were more accentuated in the parietal region and tended to disappear near the occipital lobe.

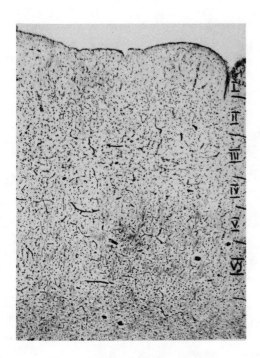

Figure 1. Case Ber. Region FD$_m$ (right), modified Globus method (magnified 23×); glial band in layer III.

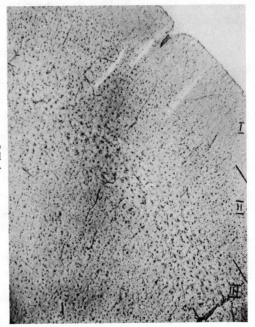

Figure 2. Case Pal. Region FD$_m$ (left), modified Globus method (magnified 23×); glial band in layer III.

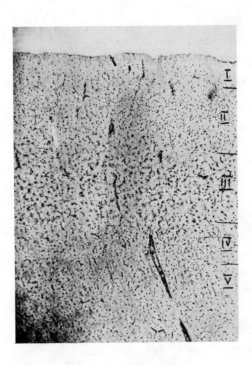

Figure 3. Case Zug. Region FD$_m$ (left), modified Globus method (magnified 23×); glial band in layer III.

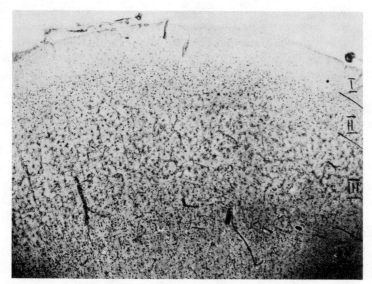

Figure 4.   Case Fia. Region FD$_p$ (left), modified Globus method (magnified 23×); glial band in layer III.

Figure 5.   Case Zug. Region FD$_m$, modified Globus method (magnified 176×); typical astrocytes in the involved third layer.

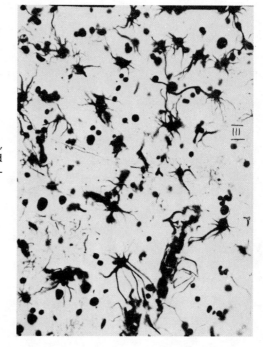

The neuroglia in the third layer were less altered than in general paresis. The astrocytes had numerous visibly thickened vascular foot processes, which were lengthened in the plane of the layer. The changes included hyperplasia, hypertrophy, and alteration of astrocytes of layer III. The microglia of the third layer, normally fine and delicate, became gross, elongated, and rectilinear—oriented parallel to radial fiber— changes also seen in general paresis. The nerve cells of layer III were not characteristically altered but were decreased in the external part of the layer.

The superiorly radiating myelinated fibers, lying external to the third layer, are very difficult to stain and were probably decreased. It is to be noted that none of my four cases had the changes of Wernicke's superior hemorrhagic polioencephalitis in the expected locations. I would like to propose the name *alcoholic laminar cortical sclerosis* for this previously unnamed entity.

A Lesion of the Corpus Callosum in Alcoholic Subjects

E. MARCHIAFAVA AND A. BIGNAMI

WITHIN THE SPACE of a few years we have chanced to observe characteristic lesions in the corpus callosum in the brains of three autopsied alcoholic patients.

The first observation dates from 1897 and was incorporated into Dr. Carducci's doctoral thesis published in 1898. This case was presented and discussed in the School of Pathological Anatomy and was studied histologically in our laboratory under the supervision of Dr. Bignami. The last case was encountered during the current lecture series.

As regards the symptoms which these patients presented during life we have only summary and incomplete notions. Nonetheless, it seems worthwhile to relate what little information we have been able to assemble.

The first patient, S.D., a fifty-year-old peasant, was a heavy drinker who some three years prior to his death exhibited symptoms of mental illness and was diagnosed as suffering from alcoholic mania. In February 1898 he fell into a state of depression, which was succeeded on March 1 by a series of clonic convulsions limited to the right half of the body and associated with loss of consciousness. Other similar attacks lasting four to five minutes occurred subsequently with increasing frequency. In the intervals between attacks the patient could move about and even ambu-

NOTE: Translated by D. A. Rottenberg from: Marchiafava, E., and Bignami, A., "Sopra un'alterazione del Corpo Calloso Osservata in Soggetti Alcoolisti," *Rivista di Patologia Nervosa e Mentale* 8 (1903), 544–49.

late, but he did not speak and was incontinent of urine. Four days before his death he lapsed into coma with his head deviated to the right. His temperature rose to 39°C. Albumin and casts were present in the urine.

At autopsy the only remarkable findings other than those relating to the brain (to be described below) were bronchopneumonia and fibrinous pleuritis.

No clinical information about the second patient is available. All that is known for certain is that he was a heavy drinker.

The third patient, C.T., a sixty-five-year-old man, was admitted to the Santo Spirito Hospital on March 21, 1903, and died there on March 23. According to our best information he was a confirmed alcoholic and had not contracted syphilis or any other venereal disease. Approximately two years prior to his death he suffered from frontal headaches and epileptic attacks. Moreover, the members of his family were aware of a speech disturbance which we cannot further characterize, though the history would seem to suggest dysarthria. Some seven days before his demise he was once again afflicted with severe headaches and convulsive jerks; thereafter he lapsed into coma and expired.

Anatomical-pathological diagnoses included: diffuse arteriosclerosis, bilateral bronchopneumonia, mild cardiac hypertrophy, and finely granular kidneys. The meninges were hyperemic, and the corpus callosum was abnormal as will be described below.

The appearance of the callosal lesions was so constant in the three cases that a single description will suffice. Whereas the cerebral cortex, basal ganglia, cerebellum, pons, and medulla are essentially unremarkable, the entire corpus callosum is pathologically altered. In coronal sections it appears diffusely gray, although the dorsal and ventral surfaces retain the pearly whiteness of normal white matter. The zone of discoloration ends abruptly with well-defined margins a few millimeters beyond the emergence of the fascicles which constitute the corpus callosum from the hemispheric white matter.

The following histological description of the callosal lesions is based on an examination of frontal sections.

Tissue slices were fixed in Müller's solution, passed through alcohol and stained in the usual fashion with carmine, hematoxylin and eosin, and by the method of Weigert-Pal.

The pathological process which we are describing is, as noted above, limited to the corpus callosum, and even this structure is not uniformly affected; two thin zones, one corresponding to the dorsal surface and the other to the ventral surface, are spared.

Thus, in frontal sections through the corpus callosum it is possible to distinguish three parallel zones or laminae, two of which are marginal (one superior or dorsal, the other inferior or ventral) and the third—included between the other two—intermediate. It is in the intermediate zone that the pathological alterations occur.

Low-power examination of a frontal section stained with hematoxylin and eosin or with carmine reveals that the two marginal zones, superior and inferior, are composed of normal nervous tissue; the nerve fibers are clearly seen, and most of them are oriented transversely. In the intermediate zone, which constitutes two-thirds of the thickness of the corpus callosum, the situation is otherwise. Even at low magnification the tissue within this zone may be distinguished by two characteristics: in the first place, it appears somewhat rarefied, less compact, and, in addition, it is manifestly more vascular (containing blood-filled vessels) than the adjacent marginal zones. There is a moderate increase in the number of neuroglial nuclei in the intermediate zone as compared with the two marginal zones.

Examination under higher power confirms the above observations. Moreover, it becomes apparent that vessel walls are not appreciably thickened or infiltrated; that neuroglial nuclei are somewhat swollen, as is the endothelium lining small blood vessels; and that a number of the smaller vessels, especially some of the smaller arterioles, are surrounded by a zone of hyaline substance deriving in all probability from the hyaline degeneration of perivascular neuroglia (perivascular hyalinosis). The great bulk of the tissue is seen to be composed of a meshwork of neuroglia and naked axons (i.e., axons which have lost their myelin sheaths). Evidently, the diminished compactness of the tissue and its gray hue result from the disappearance of myelin.

In some sections one can distinguish a certain amount of cellular infiltration, especially, it seems, in areas where the degenerative changes are less advanced; this increased cellularity is due to the variable presence of granular cells, which also occur as focal accumulations in the vicinity of blood vessels. In those sections or fields in which the degenerative changes are most marked one encounters small, apparently empty lacunar spaces as well as small serous cysts whose borders are circumscribed by neuroglial tissue. Scattered throughout are small hemorrhagic foci, evidently very recent because the extravasated red blood corpuscles are perfectly preserved.

In Weigert-Pal preparations the three previously described zones are readily apparent throughout the corpus callosum; the intermediate zone, which occupies approximately two-thirds of its thickness, appears pale, whereas the two marginal zones or laminae, which are thinner, stain blue-black with hematoxylin. The lesion stains uniformly throughout the extent of the corpus callosum, retaining its characteristic trilaminar appearance. Only in relation to the midsagittal line, that is, along the median raphe of the corpus callosum, does the area of degeneration stain less intensely; this is especially true in the middle and posterior thirds, where many preserved nerve fibers can be distinguished along the median raphe.

At higher magnification it is apparent that the border between the area of degeneration and the marginal zones is quite well defined. In addition, a few varicose fibers are seen to run through the intermediate zone, which contains numerous droplets of deeply stained myelin, the residua of degenerated myelin sheaths.

The thickness of the two laminae of preserved nervous tissue, dorsal and ventral, is fairly uniform in the various portions of the corpus callosum; slight variations in the thickness of the laminae occur only in relation to variations in the thickness of the corpus callosum itself. Thus, the two outer zones are somewhat thinner in frontal sections than in more caudal sections corresponding to the region of the splenium. The zone of degeneration, in contrast, presents approximately the same thickness throughout but is better delimited and somewhat more extensive in the region of the truncus.

Lancisi's striae are preserved.

The zone of degeneration, unaltered histologically, continues for several millimeters into the substance of the centrum semiovale, where it terminates abruptly with well-demarcated borders.

The cores of the gyri on the medial surface of the hemisphere appear normal; similarly, sections of cortex from convolutions on the external surface of the mesencephalon (sic) are unremarkable. The cortical fiber system is normal (Pal's method), as are the nerve fiber bundles which course around the walls of the lateral ventricles.

No pathological alterations are noted within the internal capsule (left or right).

On the basis of these brief anatomical-pathological observations the disease process under consideration can be rather well characterized. Its restriction to the corpus callosum, specifically to the central callosal substance, is especially noteworthy; in all three cases two laminae of nervous tissue, one dorsal and the other ventral, are preserved. Also worthy of consideration are the sharp boundaries of the area of degeneration in relation to unaffected neighboring tissue, a circumstance which recalls the lesions of multiple sclerosis. Finally, we must consider the lack of secondary degeneration.

We are confronted with a disease process characterized principally by the degeneration of myelin sheaths, the formation of granular cells and the proliferation of neuroglia—with relative sparing of axis cylinders.

Such a process is easily distinguished from the common nonsuppurative hemorrhagic encephalidites by a number of features which we shall not undertake to discuss. As noted above, punctate hemorrhages are found within the area of callosal degeneration; however, their appearance suggests that they are of recent origin, whereas the degenerative process itself must be regarded as relatively chronic. Such hemorrhages, moreover, are infrequently encountered and extremely limited in extent and do not in any way resemble the characteristic lesions of the hemorrhagic encephalidites.

Apropos of the pathogenesis of this process, one might discuss the question which has been debated for a long time and which is still being debated with regard to numerous pathological processes within the central nervous system: namely, whether one is dealing with a primarily interstitial process or with a process primarily affecting the nervous elements. In the latter case one might speak of a parenchymal periaxial encephalitis with secondary neuroglial proliferation. The first hypothesis (primary interstitial process) is seemingly confounded by the difficulty in explaining how an irritative and proliferative neuroglial reaction can result in a lesion limited almost exclusively to myelin sheaths, a possibility which various authors refuse to acknowledge. Without entering further into this discussion we shall confine ourselves to expressing an opinion in support of this hypothesis; the difficulty with it, referred to above, does not seem to us to be insuperable, especially when one considers the secondary changes which occur in nerve fibers as a consequence of certain primary glial proliferations (e.g., some of the gliomatoses).

As regards pathogenesis, the influence of alcohol seems indisputable. It is well known that some authors implicate alcohol in the causation of various forms of acute encephalitis (such as the polioencephalitis superior of Wernicke) and of diffuse hemorrhagic encephalitis involving the cerebral parenchyma. The entity which we have described, although totally different from the above-mentioned encephalitides by virtue of its anatomical and pathological characteristics (especially the absence of hemorrhagic manifestations), should, in our view, be added to the better-known encephalidites which develop in the setting of alcoholism.

With respect to the clinical presentation of our patients we shall permit ourselves only a single observation. All of the evidence favors the assumption that the psychic changes, terminal coma, epileptiform convulsions, etc., reflect diffuse alterations in the cerebrum which are not readily detectable by our methods of investigation. The striking callosal lesion evidently represents the only visible pathological alteration in the brains which we examined, and it may be that this lesion is of secondary importance in the pathogenesis of the clinical syndrome observed during life.

From a pathological point of view the corpus callosum is not distinguished by the richness or variety of its lesions. Tumors, as everyone knows, make up the principal part; if one excludes certain exceedingly rare cases of hemorrhage and ischemic softenings (needless to say, the latter process does not apply to our cases), then the remaining alterations observed in the corpus callosum represent only local manifestations of diffuse or disseminated disease processes such as, for example, multiple sclerosis or diffuse nonsuppurative encephalitis. In consequence of the above we have undertaken to provide this account of a unique, sharply circumscribed pathological process within the corpus callosum based on a study of identical lesions discovered post mortem in the brains of three alcoholic subjects.

We have, as a matter of course, focused our attention on the pathological features of the material available to us. Numerous investigations, mostly experimental in nature, have been published by various authors who set out to study the degenerative changes in the corpus callosum which follow removal of all or part of one cerebral hemisphere—or, alternately, the degenerative changes in the cerebral hemispheres which follow longitudinal section of the corpus callosum. Anatomical questions concerning the normal relationship of the corpus callosum to the cerebral cortex and to the various fascicles which are, or are assumed to be, intimately related to it have multiplied considerably as a result of these investigations. Our own observations do not allow us to enter into a discussion of these interesting questions because, as we have repeatedly stated, the pathological changes which we described are limited to the corpus callosum and did not give rise to secondary degenerations.

Epilogue

The first observation of alcoholic degeneration of the corpus callosum by Ettore Marchiafava and Amico Bignami in 1903 stemmed from a surge of interest in the structural changes associated with neurological and mental disease in conjunction with the development of new neurohistological stains. The study of alcoholic degeneration of the corpus callosum was greatly facilitated by the Weigert-Pal staining method for myelin, which had been recently introduced from Germany by Marchiafava.

Following the original description, other features of Marchiafava and Bignami's disease were described in successive publications from the same group. The involvement of the anterior commissure was reported by Bignami in 1907 at a Meeting of the Royal Academy of Medicine in Rome. At the same meeting Bignami classifed the disease as a systemic degeneration of the commissures. The symmetrical demyelination of the middle cerebellar peduncles was reported by Marchiafava and Bignami at a meeting of the Academy of the Lincei in 1910. The following year Bignami and Nazari gave a detailed description of twelve cases in the *Monatschrift für Psychiatrie und Neurologie* (vol. xxix, pp. 181–334, 1911). It was noted that in the less affected cases the lesions had the appearance of symmetrical foci of demyelination on both sides of the midline in the anterior part of the corpus callosum. The symmetrical areas of demyelination in the subcortical white matter of the cerebral hemispheres were first described by Bignami and Nazari in a paper reporting the detailed description of nineteen additional cases (*Rivista Sperimentale di Freniatria*, vol. 41, fasc. 1, pp. 1–70, 1915). Finally, in 1933 a summary of the pathological and clinical features of the disease was provided by Marchiafava in a lecture to the Royal Academy of Medicine in London.

In the present period of increasing specialization and complexity of medical science it is difficult to conceive that many new observations were made at the turn of the century by physicians and surgeons actively engaged, as were Marchiafava and Bignami, in hospital and private practice, who relied mainly on the pathology laboratory for their research. As a first-year medical student in 1949, I used to spend some time every week with a survivor of that period, Dr. Giuseppe Bastianelli, a distinguished physician and outstanding neurologist who collaborated with my grandfather in his studies on malaria. (The experimental demonstration by Bignami in 1898 that human malaria is transmitted by mosquitoes was followed by a description of the life cycle of the parasite in anopheline mosquitoes by Grassi, Bignami, and Bastianelli.)

It thus became apparent to me that the most distinctive feature of the period was the excitement produced in men dedicated to clinical medicine by the opening of new fields of investigation and the expectation that the new tools then becoming available would contribute to the understanding and cure of human disease. This approach obviously resulted in little specialization and may well be impossible at the present time as a result of increasing technical sophistication. However, considering the remarkable results it produced in the past, one may hope that clinical medicine will continue to contribute to medical science, perhaps by exploiting recent discoveries in cellular and molecular biology.

A. Bignami, M.D.
Department of Pathology
Stanford University School of Medicine

MYOCLONIC DEMENTIA

Introduction

E. P. Richardson, Jr.
Professor of Neuropathology
Harvard Medical School

THE DEVASTATING NEUROLOGIC DISORDER now generally known as Creutzfeldt-Jakob disease (with its own acronym—CJD) has, despite its infrequent occurrence, rightly attracted attention because of the recently acquired knowledge that it can be transmitted to animals and that the transmissible agent has remarkable properties shared in common with what are now collectively referred to as slow viruses. Transmissibility has thus become an essential part of the definition of the disease. The transmissible agent, however, still eludes demonstration by immunologic, morphologic, or biochemical methods, so that its recognition still depends on inducing in the experimental animal a disease-state that resembles what the patient had and at the same time has features that are sufficiently typical for it to be consistently identifiable in animal after animal. The delimitation of a recognizable syndrome thus remains of fundamental importance, and for this purpose clinicopathologic criteria must still be used. To decide, therefore, just which clinical phenomena and neuropathologic lesions truly belong to CJD and which do not is still an absolute requirement for studying the disease. In the more than fifty years that have passed since H. G. Creutzfeldt and A. M. Jakob published their case reports, an extensive literature devoted to this very problem of the clinicopathologic definition has come into being. Since all of these writings refer back to the original descriptions by Creutzfeldt and Jakob, it is relevant to the problem to consider just what they had to say.

In the present attempt to make their work accessible to the English-speaking reader, it has been necessary to choose which of their publications to translate. Creutzfeldt's case was the first to be reported. For this reason his name appears first in the current eponymic term, but in earlier writings Jakob's larger contribution—five cases instead of just one—has led to the alternative designation of Jakob-Creutzfeldt disease.

Creutzfeldt published two reports of his case. One of these appeared in an extremely detailed semimonographic form, with many illustrations in color, in the very last issue (1921) of a serial publication originally started by Nissl and Alzheimer and now difficult of access. The other, considered by him as a preliminary communication, appeared a year earlier in one of the standard German neurological journals. This paper, which contains all of the facts in the larger one but more concisely expressed and without the colored pictures, has been used for the translation.

Jakob's cases are divided among three publications. In his first paper, he presented three cases and identified Creutzfeldt's case as being an example of the same disorder. These cases are reviewed in considerable detail in his second paper, which adds a fourth case. It is this paper that has been chosen for the translation, because it presents his observations and ideas fully and yet rather more succinctly than his earlier paper. In a later monograph on disorders of movement [*Die Extrapyramidalen Erkrankungen* (Berlin: J. Springer, 1923)] he added what he considered to be a fifth case. This case, which has features in common with the previous ones, has been reviewed by W. R. Kirschbaum, along with Jakob's other cases and Creutzfeldt's case, in his monograph *Jakob-Creutzfeldt Disease* (New York: Elsevier, 1968).

Jakob has been taken to task for naming the disorder "spastic pseudosclerosis." All he tried to do, though, was to use a noncommittal descriptive term that would be comprehensible to the medical readers of his day and yet, at the same time, point out the combination of mental changes and abnormal movements—reminiscent of pseudosclerosis, as Wilson's disease was then called—with evidence of pyramidal-system dysfunction.

Did Creutzfeldt and Jakob describe CJD? This can be for the reader to decide. In my opinion, Creutzfeldt probably did not—Jakob to the contrary notwithstanding—and Creutzfeldt is said to have disagreed with the identification of his case with Jakob's cases. Jakob's cases, on the other hand, can more readily be fitted into current concepts of the disease without undue strain. Access to the more recent ideas about CJD is provided by a fairly recent contribution by R. Roos, D. C. Gajdusek, and C. J. Gibbs, Jr. (*Brain* 96: 1–20, 1973).

On a Particular Focal Disease of the Central Nervous System (Preliminary Communication)

H. G. CREUTZFELDT

THE PRESENT CASE REPORT lays no claim to giving a fully complete picture of a disease-state. A single case is insufficient for this purpose, as are the kinds of observations and investigations to which this case was subjected. It only became apparent after the patient had been under treatment for some time that we were in the presence of a disease process of a special kind. As the result of this, many questions that otherwise would have been asked were not raised. A similar situation existed with regard to the pathoanatomical examination, which mainly had to be concerned with the identification of tissue changes and their distribution in the central nervous system. The result of this was that questions as to localization, which arose when one tried to determine the meaning of many of the symptoms, could not be answered. The purpose of this publication, therefore, is merely to call attention to a peculiar disease picture that I have not found to be described elsewhere, yet whose clinical resemblance to other spastic disorders allows one to expect that up to now cases of this kind may have likewise been sailing under a false flag. This case, too, was at first thought to be multiple sclerosis, and it was only the later course of the illness that made it necessary for us to change the diagnosis and put it into more general terms—until, at last, the

NOTE: Translated by E.P. Richardson, Jr., from: Creutzfeldt, H.G., Über eine eigenartige herdförmige Erkrankung des Zentralnervensystems," *Zeitschrift für die gesamte Neurologie und Psychiatrie* 57 (1920), 1–18.

autopsy and the histological examination allowed us to recognize that the severe and remarkable tissue changes that we saw were the expression of the morbid process that formed the basis for the clinical symptoms.

The patient, Bertha E., was twenty-three years old at the time of her admission to the Neurological Clinic of the University of Breslau on June 20, 1913 (born December 8, 1890, in Grunau, Silesia).

She was the youngest of five siblings, two of whom were in an institution and are currently under family care and considered as not being normal mentally. At age nine, the patient entered Köppernig Orphanage where she remained until age sixteen, without having shown signs of a nervous illness. After that, she was in the Convent of the Good Shepherd in Breslau. Her mother, who died in 1904 at fifty-five with an unidentified disease, had not had any nervous illnesses. At the Convent the patient stood out because of her childish and stubborn nature; she was lively and much occupied with dolls and childish play. She was industrious at work. Two years before admission to the Clinic she refused nourishment for a period of time under the pretext that she wanted to become slender. Her behavior always had something indecisive about it, and, in general, she was easily influenced. Her gait was remarkably awkward. Almost exactly one year before admission, from the end of June until the beginning of August, 1912, she was under treatment at the Dermatological Clinic of Breslau University for what, in the view of the Clinic, was a hysterical exfoliative dermatitis which symmetrically affected first the face and both hands, then the perineal region and both feet. Allegedly this skin condition had been present for eight weeks before she came to the Clinic. She was found to have signs of spasticity in the legs with patellar and ankle clonus; there was a generalized tremor; the Babinski sign could not be elicited on admission; at discharge it was weakly but definitely present. Following the examination the patient had a major hysterical attack characterized by cautious falling, stiffness of the legs, and pronounced *arc de cercle*. After the attack, she was said to have been entirely without signs of spasticity. Indeed, the stiffness of gait that she had shown and the spastic changes, which were variable in their occurrence, could mostly be made to disappear by energetic exhortation. Ovarian pain [ovarie] was distinctly present.

After her discharge from the Clinic, the stiffness of her gait was especially noticeable at the Convent; gradually this improved. In May 1913 the patient again began to walk unsteadily; in addition to this a mental change appeared. She no longer wanted to eat or to bathe, she neglected her appearance, became dirty, complained of pressure in the region of the heart, assumed peculiar postures, in that she bent over to her left and pressed her hand against her heart. The unsteadiness of gait increased rapidly, and fourteen days before admission the patient fell over while standing, without losing consciousness. The menses were very irregular, with metrorrhagia for several weeks. There was no evidence of fever. Three days before admission she suddenly screamed out that her sister was dead, that she was to blame, that she was possessed of the devil, that she herself was dead, that she wanted to sacrifice herself. During the night before admission she was very excited and over-talkative, and laughed and sang. Only rarely were sensible answers to be obtained from her.

Findings and Course: Patient is of medium height, somewhat emaciated; she is unable to walk or stand without support. A continual fluttering involves the facial muscles. There are ticlike jerks in the arms, and intention tremor. The pupils react promptly to light and on accommodation; there is distinct nystagmus. The periosteal and tendon reflexes are fairly definitely increased. Babinski bilaterally positive; abdominal reflexes easily exhausted. There is generalized hyperesthesia and hyperalgesia. The musculature of the arms and legs is hypertonic. No ataxia. Partial negativisms, which, however, vary greatly in localization. Abundant menstrual flow. Temperature elevated (38.9°). The patient is extraordinarily inattentive; her verbal productions are wholly incoherent. She is disoriented as to time and place, believes she is at the Good Shepherd; her speech has something of a disjointed (staccato) quality. Her mood is very variable, often euphoric. In general, the patient presents a dazed, stupefied impression. Her answers to questions are wholly incoherent. Testing of her intellectual capabilities reveals that they are restricted to matters of the greatest simplicity. Her comprehension is clearly slowed; there are marked perseverations.

During the period of observation her behavior is found to be very variable. At times the patient acts in a silly way, with a tendency to jocularity; she makes word associations in a distractable, entirely superficial manner; for example, from gold in a watch she came to the song "Gold and Silver I Do Love." Often she appears distracted, makes all sorts of grimaces, speaks in an odd, stilted fashion as if she wanted to emphasize even more the scanning quality of her speech. Frequently there are unmotivated outbursts of laughter, which give the impression of being purely a motor activity. Her attention lapses rapidly, even when momentarily she is aroused to greater alertness. Evasiveness in speech and behavior shows itself, and at times there is a suggestion of cataleptic manifestations. The muscular jerking twitchings must often be characterized as more than pseudospontaneous. At times these irritative phenomena are pronounced in the upper extremities and face, and at other times they are more distinct in the legs. The nystagmus and the other somatic symptoms vary continually; on many days no nystagmus can be demonstrated. When left to herself the patient is entirely apathetic, but between times there are states of motor excitement; for instance, the patient screams out the name of her former attendant all day long— both spontaneously and when spoken to. Then again she presents the picture of a stuporous state. Sometimes, after having been more accessible for a while, the patient more or less abruptly starts speaking inappropriately and incoherently. When attempts are made to get her to read, she maintains that she is no longer able to do so. All this gives the impression that a sudden failure of her mental capacities has occurred. In the middle of July her condition becomes increasingly worse. One sees continual cortical twitchings, sometimes more marked on the left, sometimes more on the right. The spastic weakness becomes correspondingly worse, whereas at first the patient had still been able occasionally to walk a few steps with support. Again, the hyperalgesia becomes more severe. The patient misidentifies people around her; echopraxia is seen a few times, also echolalia with word perseveration and stereotyped attitudes. Examination at the Ophthalmological Clinic established the presence of early temporal pallor (?). The manifestations of hypertonicity in the muscles of the face, arms, and hands are relatively pronounced in comparison with those in the legs; in early August a sort of status epilepticus develops. Twitches of cortical type, involving especially the left half of the face and the left arm, occur in lightninglike fashion; sometimes they are followed by a residual tonic state, while at times the attacks are tonic from the start. Her facial appearance is stiff and expressionless. Responses are obtainable only to painful stimuli.

On August 6 a genuine epileptic attack occurs, beginning with clonic jerkings in the right arm, then involving the right half of the face; on the left, relatively less severe contractions in the musculature of the shoulder, chest, and face are the only signs of involvement; towards evening, a second attack, exactly similar to the first. In the ensuing days, the patient lies in a severely obtunded state, with constant cortical twitchings which at times occur only on the right and at times are bilateral; now and again the twitchings seem to be more generalized, quite like those seen in the epileptic attacks. At about the same time, an erythema multiforme bullosum makes its appearance in the vicinity of the left ear, in an area closely corresponding to the territory of the third division of the trigeminal nerve, the first signs of which appear as herpetiform small vesicles. In the last hours, stupor deepens, swallowing is impaired; death ensues on August 11, in status epilepticus.

On lumbar puncture, two lymphocytes per cu. mm. are found on one occasion, seven on another; the protein content is not pathologically increased. The Wassermann test is negative in blood and CSF on two examinations.

Although at first the physical signs of the disease—nystagmus, a suggestion of temporal pallor of the optic discs, spastic paresis, weakness of the abdominal reflexes, intention tremor (though not typical), scanning speech, forced laughter, and relapsing course—led us to think of multiple sclerosis, we soon set this possibility aside. Our main reason for doing so was the emergence of irritative phenomena, the motor aspects of which we saw in the form of lightninglike jerkings and pseudospontaneous movements and the sensory aspects as hyperesthesia and hyperalgesia. To be sure, Gussenbauer has described irritative states of this kind, apparently of cortical origin, in multiple sclerosis; yet this has been so restricted to isolated cases that in my view such symptoms are more against multiple sclerosis than in favor of it. Moreover, the concurrence of physical and mental symptoms indicated to us that in this case the cortex itself must be diseased, and thus we provisionally restricted ourselves to assuming the presence of a disease—perhaps focal—in the central nervous system that was mainly located in the gray matter. The spastic symptoms and the manifestations of cortical irritation made it seem probable that the Rolandic region must be especially severely affected. Because of their amential coloring we grouped together the mental symptoms under the heading of symptomatic psychosis (symptoms of delirium, incoherence, incoordination, inappropriate answers, occasional states of stupor, and impaired consciousness). That there were close relationships between the somatic and mental symptoms was recognizable to us by the parellelism that they showed in their intensity. In this regard, the peculiar transition from mental derangements to purely motor mechanisms allowed us to suppose that there were rather close associations between them. We therefore believed that we were dealing with a probably multifocal disease of the central nervous system that had a relapsing course—a disease which, in one of its acute exacerbations, with the superaddition of amential symptoms, led to death. We had very little knowledge as to the cause; neither hereditary predisposition nor an exogenous injurious factor of infective or toxic origin could be demonstrated with certainty.

Autopsy: Cranial cavity: slight asymmetry of the skull, left greater than right; slight hydrocephalus externus; moderate cloudiness of the pia over the convexity. Brain weight: 1375 gm.

Pial adhesions along the intrahemispheric fissure bilaterally. Falx cerebri atrophic all the way to its anterior and posterior insertions. Basal vessels very thin-walled, especially at the circle of Willis.

Left precentral convolution remarkably thick and resistant, especially inferiorly and in its midportion. Frontal convolutions somewhat narrowed. In one place in the central region, indistinct definition between cortex and white matter; a similar place in the postcentral convolution stands out above the plane of section. Similar small foci in the right Rolandic region. Lateral ventricles definitely enlarged, ependyma somewhat thickened, no granulations; choroid plexus densely adherent locally to the surface of the thalamus. No white-matter lesions; pyramidal tracts homogeneously somewhat discolored.

Thoracic cavity: bronchopneumonia in right lower lobe; diffuse bronchitis.

Abdominal cavity: gallstones; ovarian cyst; hyperemia of kidneys.

Skin: erythema bullosum with crust-formation in and around the left ear.

Microscopic examination: The methods used for the examination were those employed by Nissl and Alzheimer and their school. Fundamental was Nissl's equivalent-picture; the methods for demonstration of breakdown-processes, fibrils, myelin sheaths, glial structures, and blood vessels added the details. Samples were taken from all regions of the central nervous system.

Survey views of Nissl sections taken from the macroscopically altered regions, especially from the Rolandic region, show foci of nerve-cell loss. The structure of the cortex, which contains abundant well-stained ganglion cells, apparently is abruptly interrupted by paler elements which are so arranged that the architecture of the cortex is still recognizable, yet which, from their shape and staining qualities, appear to be nonneuronal in type. (Figs. 1 and 2). Foci of this kind are to be found throughout the entire cerebral cortex and equally distributed on the two sides, yet they are most numerous in the Rolandic regions and their vicinity; they are also frequent in the frontal convolutions, while the posterior parietal region and the temporal and occipital lobes show relatively few of them.

The crowns of the convolutions are less frequently affected than the walls and depths of the sulci. The areas of cell loss vary in size from microscopic foci to lesions which extend over two adjacent sides of a sulcus. The third layer of Brodmann is consistently diseased, and from it the process seems to extend into other layers, yet the second and fourth Brodmann layers—the external and internal granular layers—show greater resistance and often remain, especially the internal granular layer, as preserved dark bands of intensely stained ganglion cells within the pale focus.

In addition to these extensive cortical lesions there also are miliary lesions consisting of glial stars and rosettes (Fig. 3), together with miliary focal areas of devastation in the cortex, the central nuclei, and the gray matter of the spinal cord—which will be discussed below in another connection.

With higher magnification one recognizes that the transition from sound to diseased tissue is not always as abrupt as the survey view leads us to suppose. Instead, one finds here pathologic changes in the tissue elements in this region, which suggest the possibility of determining how the lesions arise (Fig. 4). The pyramidal cells in the third layer are

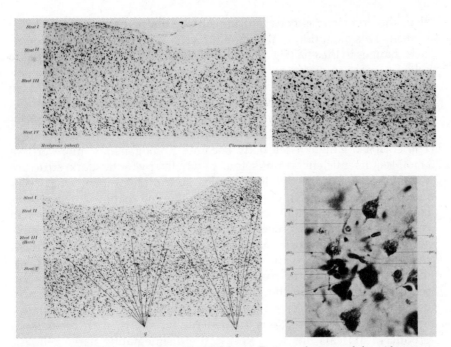

Figure 1. Glial focus in Brodmann's third layer. Bottom of picture, left, with arrows: border of lesion (sharp); bottom of picture, right, with arrow: zone of transition with normal tissue.

Figure 2. Focal lesion with vascular proliferation in Brodmann's third layer (agranular cortex). Lower right, with arrow: border of lesion indefinite.

Figure 3. Miliary focus in the thalamus. Glial rosettes and stars as coffins of nerve cells. r, glial rosettes.

Figure 4. From the border region of a focal lesion in the third layer. gaz$_1$, ganglion cell with beginning tigrolysis; gaz$_2$, enlargement of the nucleus (upper cell), margination of chromophilic cytoplasmic components; gaz$_3$, meshwork formation in the cytoplasm; N, glial rosette with a homogenized, almost colorless ganglion cell and its pyknotic nucleus (gglk) in the middle; g, blood vessel; pglz, glial-cell cytoplasm in rod-cell form, apparently conforming to the configuration of an apical dendrite; glz, glial cells with multiple processes.

diseased. They show central dissolution of the Nissl bodies; the nucleus is indistinctly demarcated, dark, with a poorly defined chromatin network; it has come close to the edge of the cell; the nucleolus is mainly unaltered. The cell processes are visible for a long distance, and they still contain Nissl bodies in their proximal part (Fig. 4, gaz$_2$). The unstained tracts are distinctly seen along the borders of the cell and in the processes. In other cells we see how this tigrolysis has affected the entire cell, which seems to be filled with dark dust (Fig. 4, gaz$_1$). The nucleus is homogeneously opaque, the nucleolus is often displaced from its central position. The dendrites have become pale; fine stainable granules outline their course. The unstained intracellular tracts are no longer visible;

also, the connections between the cell and its processes appear to be broken. This alteration in the ganglion cells is accompanied by progessive changes in the glia (Fig. 4, gaz). The glial cells, especially the satellite cells, increase in numbers, mitotic figures become frequent, the cytoplasm becomes visible, the cell bodies enlarge and send out processes, so that the diseased ganglion cells are surrounded by numerous glial nuclei which lie in a kind of syncytium (Fig. 4, N). This glial syncytium encircles the nerve cell. Within it are basophilic and metachromatic granules. The enclosed ganglion-cell body becomes homogeneous, more or less colorless, its nucleus shrinks into a wholly pyknotic dark structure within which tiny basophilic granules surround the somewhat paler nucleolus (Fig. 4, gaz K). In its final stage this cell change closely resembles the homogenization described in Purkinje cells by Spielmeyer in cases of typhus, spotted fever, and malaria. (Professor Spielmeyer himself noted this similarity in my sections, and he, too, considers that it is a related process.) Later, the ganglion cell disappears, and in its place there remains a star- or rosette-shaped glial syncytium. Yet a mass-reaction of this kind in the glial elements does not always occur; frequently a single glial cell enwraps a pyramidal cell with its cytoplasm, becomes loaded—as sections stained for fat show—with breakdown products, and eats up, so to speak, the disintegrating nerve cell. Although this happens rarely, undoubtedly there are ganglion cells which disintegrate without participation of the glia, as Spielmeyer has also shown in the case of Purkinje cells. What the reasons might be for these differences in the behavior of the glia is not discernible in my sections.

Along with the ganglion cells, the nerve fibers and the myelin sheaths are, likewise, almost wholly absent in the lesions. Only a few tortuous fibers, some pale and stout, some very fine, are to be found in the Bielschowsky preparation. Fusiform enlargements also occur. The Spielmeyer preparation reveals the almost total disappearance of myelin sheaths; only occasionally do tangential fibers traverse the field, and of the radial fiber bundles a few short stumps remain. One may say that in the lesions the neural parenchyma has disappeared in its entirety. The glial elements have come forth to take the place of the neural ones. We first see the above-described rosettes and stars, from the periphery of which, whiplike, drawn-out, finely granular cytoplasmic masses with elongated nuclei, apparently following the processes of the enclosed nerve cell, become differentiated and, in fact, become wholly detached from their site of origin. These, thus, become rod cells (Fig. 5, stz), which are extraordinarily frequent in all of the lesions. Both the origin and the location of these rod cells indicate their close relationship with the degenerated nerve-cell processes, of which they are the architectonic substitute. This is especially beautifully shown in Fig. 5, in which we can see the columnar structure of the cortex, normally effected by the radial

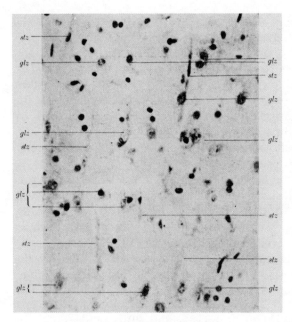

Figure 5. Organized focus. stz, rod cell perpendicular to the cortex; glz, large glial cells with multiple processes in layered arrangement (protoplasm-rich glial rosettes); the smaller nuclei are all glial.

fibers and the apical processes, preserved in shadowlike fashion by means of rod cells that are perpendicularly oriented to the surface of the cortex.

Along with the rod cells, other forms of glia of the most varied sorts are found in the lesions: small elements with scanty cytoplasm; often nuclei alone, which appear to be isolated and which are not infrequently pyknotic and shrunken; small cells with multiple radiating processes and a fine-meshed cell body with a clear zone around the nucleus; epithelioid elements with dark cloudy cytoplasm, and large cells with multiple processes, resembling the large-bodied cells considered by Nissl probably to be fiber-forming (Fig. 5, glz). They are often situated at the site of the disintegrated ganglion cells and frequently have taken on their form, so that the columnar structure, effected by the vertical lamination of the cortex, appears to be preserved only by means of the rod cells. They possess one to three large clear nuclei with a fine chromatin network and, when they are multinucleated, betray their origin from the neurophagic glial syncytia that have been described as glial stars and rosettes, the nuclei of which, in the border regions of the lesions, always show regressive changes. In the well-defined lesions, at any rate, the rosettes are wholly lacking, and the large cells just described are all that remain. In lesions which I should like to designate as old scars one also sees regressive changes—along with nuclear changes of every sort, all the way from active mitoses to phenomena of shrinkage and dissolution, depending on the freshness of the process. In Brodmann's first layer, also, there are occasional rather large glial cells resembling "plump [gemästete] glial cells, "but only once in the first layer have I found a lesion that consisted of several confluent clumps of glial cells, and this was separated from the lesion in the pyramidal layer by the intact external granule-cell layer. Increased fiber formation is not demonstrable by any of the methods. Occasionally a somewhat more dense feltwork of fibers has formed around the vessels. Especially noteworthy is the fact that the large cells do not show any evidence of fiber formation (Weigert, Ranke, Heidenhain-Mann preparations).

The blood vessels in the lesions are often not at all affected by the disease process; in many lesions, however, they participate very actively in the reparative processes and, indeed, show the signs of most vigorous progressive alteration (Fig. 2, g). Many nuclei are in the process of division; sprouting endothelial cells branch off laterally from the capillaries, and in many of the older lesions increased vascularity still is clearly recognizable. The later regressive changes in the fully developed lesions are a phenomenon that probably may be considered as parallel with the regressive glial changes.

I have not been able to establish the presence either of a connection between the other lesions and the vessels or of inflammatory changes in the vessels themselves. Only rarely are there a few lymphocytes in the adventitial spaces, yet these infiltrates are not situated in any direct or approximate relationship to the tissue changes. The adventitial cells frequently are, as fat stains show, densely laden with fat particles, and even in the Nissl preparation they show a markedly vaculolated cytoplasm often containing a yellow-greenish pigment. Many vessels in the white matter, which from their location bear a relationship to the lesions, are especially heavily laden with breakdown products. Often they are surrounded by a broad, regressively altered girdle of connective tissue fibers that had at one time undergone proliferation, in which there still remain numerous macrophages [Körnchenzellen]. Proliferation of argentophilic fibers is not demonstrable.

Along with these focal degenerative lesions of the cortex there is a diffuse abnormality of the neural elements of the gray matter which appears to affect the larger cell forms, or at any rate occurs in those younger cortical and nuclear regions where the larger ganglion cells are located. I have in mind the sixth layer of the cerebral cortex, the basal ganglia (thalamus), the pontine and oblongata nuclei, the dentate nuclei, and the gray matter of the spinal cord, particularly the anterior horns. Yet the cells of the third layer of the cerebral cortex are affected also; the only cells wholly free of these changes are the cells of the substantia nigra and the Purkinje and the olivary cells. This cell change is one which in every respect resembles what has been designated as retrograde degeneration or, as the case may be, primary irritation [primäre Reizung]. We see extreme swelling of the cell, central tigrolysis, clearing and homogenization of the interior of the cell, which finally gives the impression of deposition of an extraneous substance in the outer part of the cell. The nucleus is displaced laterally and flattened into a half-moon shape (Fig. 6,k), and the cell pigment, together with remnants of the Nissl substance, is likewise displaced to the edge of the cell. At their origin the processes are visible for a considerable distance; but they soon disappear, and so the cell takes on the appearance of a rounded disc or an irregularly shaped structure with a rather dark periphery containing more or less coarse remnants of chromatic substance and a central clear zone of homogenization. In the Bielschowsky preparation one sees the internal fibrils, for the most part, to be undergoing dissolution; the midportion of the cell is filled with an argentophilic mass of dust, yet this, too, loses its stainability, and, finally, all that is seen is a homogeneously pale disc, which at times may be surrounded by a few external fibrils. Again and again one sees that the glia behaves in an almost refractory way toward this particular disease of the ganglion cells; at most, the satellite cells are filled with breakdown products which appear as metachromatic granules or fat droplets. Often, however, the glia participates actively in the changes in the neural elements, resulting in neuronophagic pictures and the formation of what, for the most part, are very impressive glial stars and rosettes (Fig. 3), which then correspond exactly to those we have seen at the margin of the lesions. Moreover, the engulfed ganglion cells show the same picture of homogenization that Spielmeyer has described in Purkinje cells

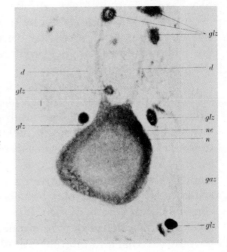

Figure 6. Betz cell with central homogenization and peripheral accumulation of diffuse chromatic masses. glz, glial cells; gaz, ganglion cells; ne, nucleolus of the ganglion cell; n, nucleus (pyknotic and flattened) of the ganglion cell; d, dendrites.

as "homogenizing cell-disease." Tiny miliary foci of this kind are found in almost all of the localities where the diffuse ganglion-cell change dominates the picture.

The axis cylinders in these regions likewise show expansions with central homogenization and lateral displacement of the outer fibrils and, thus, are reminiscent of the picture presented by the ganglion cells. This may, perhaps, indicate the presence of a particular form of reaction affecting similarly the cells and axons in response to a damaging factor as yet unknown to us. Spatz, at any rate, in his transection experiments on the spinal cord, likewise has seen the picture of retrograde degeneration in the anterior horn cells in association with similarly swollen, centrally homogenized axons, and he believes that this too represents a form of reaction that is shared in common by the cell and the axon. The myelin-sheath sections show dilatations and, at times, a beaded configuration conforming to the axons situated within them.

The glial changes in the vicinity of the rosettes are the same as at the borders of the lesions. Yet in those regions where cell loss is clearly recognizable, e.g., in the anterior horns of the spinal cord, there are large-bodied cells with abundant processes and one to three nuclei, which probably occupy the site of disintegrated nerve cells. The vessels, except for fat deposits in the adventitial cells, show no reaction. In the convolutional white matter and especially in the territory of the pyramidal tracts the picture of secondary degeneration is seen, from the earliest stages to the final stage of sclerosis. The myelin-stained sections show distinct thinning out of the pyramidal tracts throughout their entire course.

The pia is proliferated and greatly thickened. This change is not clearly dependent upon the presence of lesions. Moreover, inflammatory changes are not demonstrable in the pia.

As additional findings I should particularly like to mention a cicatricial shrinkage of one cerebellar convolution, with loss of Purkinje cells but without reparative glial proliferation, and a fine fibrillary gliosis of the alveus in Ammon's horn.

From the histologic findings it is apparent that one is dealing with a *noninflammatory process. Exudative phenomena affecting the vessels are wholly lacking.* The extremely sparse infiltrates, found in two sections without any relationship to the lesions, have no relevance to the essential nature of the disease. Instead, this is a *disease of the neural parenchyma involving the gray matter of the central nervous system* which is characterized histologically by two features. First, we are dealing with *focal destruction of the neural tissue* which, insofar as it is at all extensive, is situated in the cerebral cortex where, in turn, it preferentially affects the pyramidal-cell layer and only then extends to other layers, leaving intact for the most part the external and internal granular layers. The removal of the disintegrated neural elements is often effected by neuronophagia, which is performed by the glial cells and glial syncytia. At the edges of the lesions, and even in the lesions themselves, we have seen how extraordinarily abundantly the glial cytoplasm is filled with metachromatic and lipid breakdown products, and how rich in macrophages the vessel walls are in the lesions—and even at some distance from them. The replacement of the neural parenchyma is likewise brought about by the neuroglia, mainly by rod cells and large cells with multiple processes, which to a certain extent grow into the framework previously formed by the neural elements, inasmuch as they conform morphologically to the shapes of the structures that have been destroyed. Thus, in place of the cortical columns (normally made up by radial fibers and apical processes) we see rod cells, and in place of the layers of ganglion cells we see glial cells with abundant cytoplasm. A large number of the lesions, thus, are characterized by outfall of the neural parenchyma and its replacement by glial elements. I shall designate these as *glia-lesions* (Fig. 1). In other lesions one sees very active vascular proliferation which, even in the late stages of the process, results in the presence of multiply convoluted, twisted-up blood vessels that traverse the lesion, as can be seen in Fig. 2; these I shall call *vascularized lesions*. Along with these differences in the relative degrees of participation of the tissue elements in the formation of the lesion there is also a difference in the age of the lesions. At their borders many of them show very active degenerative processes with glial proliferation, and, to the extent that they are abundant in vessels, progressive changes in the vessels; within the lesion itself the processes of shrinkage are not recognizable, but, instead, the multinucleated glial cells predominate, nuclear division and nuclear disintegration are found, and breakdown products are abundant in glial and mesodermal cells. This is the picture of *newer, fresher lesions*, which, for the most part, are fully developed only in the third layer. In others, which I consider to be old lesions (scars), there is a *distinct shrinkage of the entire tissue* which manifests itself as puckering of the cortical surface, peripheral convergence of the adjoining healthy cell columns and deflection of the preserved layers in the direction of the lesion.

Together with these more extensive lesions one finds that *miliary foci have developed* (Fig. 3); these are associated with the second form of destruction or disease state in the neural parenchyma. These miliary lesions are present nearly *everywhere where gray matter is affected by what has been called the diffuse alteration of the gray substance*—in the cortex, in the nuclear structures, in the gray matter of the spinal cord. They consist of individual or confluent glial rosettes that have formed around a disintegrating nerve cell and are thought to be *recent foci*. In favor of this view is their resemblance to the changes that are found only at the borders of larger recent cortical lesions. The question as to whether larger lesions may develop from these miliary foci can only be answered by pointing out that, on the one hand, the frequent development of glial stars in the third layer may perhaps indicate that there is a lesion here in the process of evolution, but, on the other hand, that in the rest of the gray matter the small foci only occur sporadically and in miliary form and remain so. One does find at any rate that a constant result is *loss of individual cells, in association with which large pale glial elements occupy the location of ganglion cells that have disappeared.* These could be *old miliary lesions.* Moreover, foci of devastation of this kind are demonstrable everywhere in the cortex, so that it is impossible to state with certainty what the outcome of such a recent miliary focus might be.

We are no more justified either in concluding from the findings in our case that all possibilities regarding the disease process have been exhausted. On the contrary, the diffuse changes indicate that one is not dealing here with a process that has come to its end. With regard to these changes, we should distinguish between the involvement of the large elements and that of the smaller ones. Whereas the large ones undergo a morbid change that is the equivalent of the pictures which, being a form of reaction of the cell to interruption of the cellulifugal conduction pathways, we designate with the name "primary irritation," what we see in the smaller ones are simple processes of liquefaction in which central homogenization occurs extremely infrequently. While in relationship to the largest cells (Betz cells, anterior horn cells, cells of motor nuclei) the glia shows relatively little in the way of scavenging or of progressive alterations, around the somewhat smaller cells of the thalamus, the trigeminal nucleus, the pons, and the dentate nuclei we see abundant evidence both of tissue breakdown and of proliferation of the glia. So we must ask ourselves whether some aspect of these diffuse changes is not capable of recovery. In view of the presence of many individual instances of nerve-cell outfall and of the earlier attacks of the illness as shown by the previous history, it seems to me justified to infer the presence of a diffuse cell disease of this kind at an earlier period, in response to which individual cells succumbed but others recovered. Perhaps, also, this generalized disease state was less extensive then. On the other hand, this is not a necessary interpretation. A considerable number of extensively homogenized cells still have a nucleus that is so well preserved that one cannot rightly believe that these are condemned to destruction; the refractory behavior of the glia, furthermore, may be in favor of this possibility. The fact that cells with what is known as primary irritation and with the similar change described here recover from these states may likewise support the view that in our case also recovery of at least some of the nerve cells is possible.

Although a morphologic distinction can be made between the focal and the diffuse changes, in all probability they are closely related pathophysiologically. Which of these two processes is to be considered as cause and which as effect cannot be stated with certainty. I have elsewhere attempted to take a position with regard to this question.

The question as to the etiology of this disease can be answered only to the extent that *an infectious or toxic cause that might give rise to the illness can neither be established clinically nor proven anatomically*. Moreover, this undoubtedly is not a hereditary affection in the narrower sense. As to the presence of a familial disease, the fact that two siblings were mentally abnormal is not conclusive. This fact may well indicate, though, that there is some degree of hereditary predisposition. For the reasons already given it is only possible to correlate the clinical picture with the anatomical changes to a limited extent. This, at least, is definite: that the *cortical sites of origin of the pyramidal tracts are the locations of the most severe changes,* and this is in keeping with the predominance of cortical motor symptoms. Also, the hyperalgesia with marked radiation of stimuli has its anatomical substrate in the changes in the central sensory region and thalamus. Further, I would like to point out the alterations in the trigeminal nucleus and the herpes zosterlike erythema in the territory of the second division of the trigeminal nerve. To what extent the mental symptoms can be correlated with the changes in the frontal region, with the disorder of the association pathways, and with the diffuse disease in the cerebral cortex, cannot be decided even though it is probable that some of the symptoms, particularly the psychomotor ones, were the result of the histologically demonstrated cerebral cortical lesions. The available facts as to the childhood of the patient do not provide us with any data from which we can determine the onset of the disease. There must already have been some disturbance of gait before she was sixteen. The first attack of the disease as reported to us seems to have occurred at age twenty, but only the mental aspects were noted at the time. The next episode followed when she was twenty-one, in which, along with the spastic symptoms, the hysteriform behavior of the patient and the trophoneurotic disorder of the skin, considered to be hysterical, stood in the foreground. The next attack was the one that led to admission to the Neurological Clinic, and this ended with her death. Between the individual attacks there were periods of considerable recovery. This relapsing course fits in with the anatomical findings, which indicate to us the presence of old and fresh lesions and point out that even earlier more or less diffuse cell changes together with foci of outfall in the neural parenchyma probably occurred in the attacks. The long-lasting fever can be interpreted as a kind of resorption fever brought about by the flooding of the organism with disintegration products from the central nervous system.

The fatal outcome is to be attributed to the severe convulsions, which are to be understood as the result of the disease in the motor region.

In clinical differential diagnosis probably only multiple sclerosis comes into question, but this must be excluded on the basis of the predominance of cortical irritative manifestations in our case. Anatomically, separation from multiple sclerosis is easy because of the presence of the lesions in the gray matter, the lack of inflammatory phenomena, and the absence of loss of myelin sheaths with preserved axis cylinders. Moreover, our case differs from those of focal disease resulting from arteriosclerosis in that, first of all, atheromatous changes are lacking in the vessels in our case, and, in addition, the focal lesions as well as the diffuse changes are independent of the vessels.

Thus, we are dealing with a disease process which occurred in a female patient at a youthful age, and which is characterized by the following features:

1. Unknown cause (perhaps familial predisposition).
2. Relapsing course with remissions.
3. Cortical symptoms referable to the motor and sensory centers (spasms and hyperalgesias).
4. Mental symptoms of the type of intellectual deficit with predominance of psychomotor manifestations.
5. Progressive course.
6. A noninflammatory focal disintegration at the neural tissue of the cerebral cortex with neuronophagia and reparative glial proliferation (partly with vascular proliferation).
7. A noninflammatory diffuse cell disease with cell outfall throughout almost the entire gray substance.

These are the main characteristics of this peculiar disease picture. I have restricted myself to a simple statement of the findings because I believe that in a single case all of the possible manifestations of the disease group to which it belongs cannot have developed, and, primarily, I do not want, by ill-based attempts at interpretation, to lead studies of similar cases into all too narrow a track. And yet I believe that I have found here some important distinguishing features which in connection with new observations may justify the establishment of a hitherto undescribed disease picture.

REFERENCES

1. Alzheimer. *Histologische Studien zur Differentialdiagnose der progressiven Paralyse.* Histologische und histopathologische Untersuchungen über die Grosshirnrinde.
2. Kraepelin, *Psychiatrie,* 1909, 8th edition.
3. Müller. *Die multiple Sklerose des Gehirns und Rückenmarks.* Jena, 1904.
4. Spielmeyer, "Über einige anatomische Ähnlichkeiten zwischen progressiver Paralyse und multipler Sklerose." *Zeitschrift für die gesamte Neurologie und Psychiatrie* 1 (1910), 660.

Concerning a Disorder of the Central Nervous System Clinically Resembling Multiple Sclerosis with Remarkable Anatomic Findings (Spastic Pseudosclerosis)

Report of a Fourth Case

A. JAKOB

IN RECENT YEARS, collaboration between the clinic and the pathologic-anatomical laboratory has led to significant progress in the area of pathology of the movement disorders. If we set aside the motor symptoms resulting from cerebellar or frontal lesions, which clinically and pathogenetically have been fairly well analyzed, there is then a particularly interesting group of disorders of movement which differ in striking fashion from ordinary hemiplegia and are not attributable to a lesion of the movement-controlling pyramidal system. Whereas the classic pyramidal symptoms are manifested by lively exaggeration of the tendon reflexes, reflex spastic states with positive Babinski reflex, and ab-

NOTE: Translated by E.P. Richardson, Jr., from: Jakob, A., "Über eine der multiplen Sklerose klinisch nahestehende Erkrankung des Zentralnervensystems (spastische Pseudosklerose) mit bemerkenswertem anatomischem Befunde. Mitteilung eines vierten Falles," *Med. Klin.* 17 (1921), 372–76.

sent abdominal reflexes, together with states of paresis, in certain other disease processes we find that there are abnormalities of movement that mainly take the form of rigidity, a tendency to contractures and postural abnormalities, a certain decrease in muscular power, slowing of movement, peculiar trembling, and athetoid movements, with absence of alterations of the reflexes, and there frequently are involuntary contractions together with a marked immobility of facial expression.

These disorders of motility have been studied clinically in some detail mainly in the work of von Strümpell, Bonhöffer, Kleist, Anton, Wilson, and others, and von Strümpell has introduced for them the term amyostatic symptom complex. The amyostatic symptom complex, which appears in especially pure form in Westphal-Strümpell's pseudosclerosis, in Wilson's disease, and in the various forms of chorea, is pathogenetically attributable to a lesion of the basal ganglia, principally of the striatal system (caudate nucleus and putamen) and the corresponding nuclei of the thalamus, on the basis of the investigations of numerous authors (Anton, Kleist, Alzheimer, C. and O. Vogt, Wilson, von Economo, von Stauffenberg, Spielmeyer, and others). To C. and O. Vogt and Bielschowsky we are especially indebted for valuable studies of the pathophysiology of these parts of the brain, which, in view of their principal function, can concisely be brought together as the extrapyramidal motor system.

Recently I have been able, on the basis of my studies, to report three cases which, in view of their unique clinical aspects and their pathologic-anatomical findings, cannot be brought into any of the hitherto recognized groupings of diseases. They display a lurid mixture of symptoms, in particular true pyramidal symptoms combined with those referable to the extrapyramidal system, so that, on the one hand, they are reminiscent of multiple sclerosis and spastic disorders, and, on the other, show certain relationships with the striatal disease processes such as pseudosclerosis or the varieties of chorea. Associated with these symptoms are striking mental changes which complicate the disease picture even more. In these cases I was able to discern histologic changes that were well characterized both as to localization and nature, and which served to emphasize more clearly the unique position of these cases. I am now in the position of being able to report a fourth case which undoubtedly belongs also with this disease group.

Since we are dealing with forms of nervous and mental illness which up to now have not been correctly diagnosed, I should like in the following to give a brief summary of the main clinical and anatomical features of the previously studied cases, and to present the clinical classification and anatomical characterization in the way that I attempted to do in greater detail in my previous study on this same theme,[1] which is still in the press. After this, I shall sketch in the additional recent case, which essentially is a confirmation of my previous findings and views.

A short summary of the histories of the first three cases gives the following:

This fifty-one-year-old woman, whose previous history showed nothing remarkable and who, moreover, knew nothing of a syphilitic infection (blood Wassermann test negative in the husband) became ill in the spring of 1918 with weakness and pains in the legs. In recent years she had complained frequently of cramplike pulling in her legs, particularly in the feet. Soon there appeared—along with general depression—dizziness, fatigue, and numbness in the legs, which often became stiff as she walked. Neurological examination showed nothing remarkable at first, but the abdominal reflexes were unobtainable; the Wassermann reaction was positive in blood and also in the cerebrospinal fluid, with negative phase I and normal cell count. After transitory improvement (remission), pains and weakness in the legs recurred. The reflexes were decreased in the lower limbs. The abdominal reflexes were absent, and the blood Wassermann test was again positive. From the beginning of 1919 on, her condition became worse, with the addition of states of depression, feelings of pressure in her chest, and marked derangement of gait with hypotonia and ataxia of the lower extremities. The tendon reflexes were normal. Mentally, apathy and total lack of will were outstanding. In walking, she allowed herself to fall, and her legs gave way under her. Finally clear-cut bulbar symptoms appeared, aphonia and dysphagia, slight hemiparetic disorders with positive Babinski and pseudospasms without true paralyses, and pseudospontaneous movements reminiscent of athetosis in the presence of total inability to walk or stand. With certain noises she startled, whereupon her entire body went into a kind of rigidity. On a background of increase in psychomotor restlessness and worsening of the anxious-depressive confusional state, death, with fever and signs of a hypostatic pneumonia, finally occurred after a duration of illness of one year. A repeated blood test was negative.

The second case is that of a thirty-four-year-old woman who already for a considerable period had suffered from digestive disturbances and from weakness of bowel and bladder and disordered gait (and ? dizziness) and had become markedly emaciated. In April 1920, while under treatment for a contact eczema from lubricating grease, she began to show pronounced psychomotor abnormalities (flexibilitas cerea, negativism, echolalia, auditory hallucinations, psychomotor restlessness), reminiscent of dementia praecox. Soon thereafter there appeared bowel and bladder incontinence, marked Romberg phenomenon, a broad-based spastic gait, rigidity of the limbs without definitely spastic reflexes but with left-sided Babinski. The abdominal reflexes were absent. The eyegrounds were normal. Speech was slow and monotonous. The facial expression was masklike. Her dull affectless state was soon superseded by anxious confusion with transitory and surprising lucid intervals, and, after the development of pronounced cerebral irritative phenomena (twitchings in the left half of the face, grinding of the teeth, an epileptic attack with some hemiparetic features), the patient died after an evolution of the severe nervous and mental symptoms of about six weeks. The Wassermann reaction was negative in blood and CSF. The CSF showed only a slightly positive phase I.

The third case, a forty-two-year-old man, whose past history showed nothing remarkable, became ill while a soldier in Rumania, with rheumatic symptoms, dizziness, attacks of weakness, and digestive disturbances; following transitory improvement (remission!), disturbances of ocular movements, of speech and of handwriting appeared, together with distinct ataxia of the limbs. Six months after the onset of the illness he gave an impression of total confusion with marked impairment of attention (Korsakow symptom complex). Neurologically he showed ocular paralyses, positive Romberg, static and locomotor ataxia, dysarthria with very lively tendon reflexes in the limbs, and a suggestion of the Babinski sign bilaterally. The patient was admitted here as a taboparetic. In the next three months he showed increasing mental deterioration, mainly in the form of anxious confusion with visual hallucinations, associated with areflexia, hypotonia of the lower extremities, absence of the abdominal reflexes, a speech disorder of bulbar character, occasional suggestive Babinski sign, and gradually developing muscular atrophy in the lower limbs. Wassermann test negative in blood and CSF; in the CSF there was only a slightly positive phase I. Death, with myocardial failure, occurred after a duration of illness of about nine months.

When the whole development of the illness is taken into account, none of these three cases can be classified readily with any of the diseases recognized up to now. In individual cases one thinks of taboparesis, dementia praecox, amyotrophic lateral sclerosis, choreatic disorders, and yet other conditions; but in their symptomatology they are most reminiscent of multiple sclerosis, from which, however, they differ because of the lack of the cardinal symptoms (eyeground changes, nystagmus, pronounced intention ataxia, scanning speech, etc.). Yet the most likely possibility was thought to be an atypical form of multiple sclerosis.

In these cases I was able to demonstrate remarkable findings that were, with respect to localization and nature of the changes, the same in all. The abnormality consists of a pure parenchymatous degeneration without any inflammatory phenomena. When these are present, as in the third case, they have no relationship to the parenchymatous lesions. In the face of essentially normal macroscopic findings in the central nervous system, in which only a slight atrophy of the brain is manifest, on microscopic examination we find severe, extensive histologic changes throughout the entire central nervous system which, in general, develop in two directions. Thus, one can distinguish a diffuse parenchymatous process from one that is more focal and localized.

The diffuse parenchymatous lesions, which are similarly widespread in the brain, brainstem, and spinal cord, manifest themselves as a degeneration of ganglion cells, partly chronic with marked fatty change, partly subacute with a tendency to swelling, together with a generalized proliferation of protoplasmic glia (Fig. 1). The changes in the ganglion cells, in the form of marked swelling and chromatolysis to the point of total disintegration of these elements, are especially frequently seen in the large pyramidal cells of the entire gray matter, but are at times present in the smaller elements also. Not infrequently we encounter marked enlargement of individual ganglion-cell processes (Fig. 2), with more or less inconspicuous changes in the ganglion-cell bodies. Because of the fact that in many regions of the cortex and in the nuclear groups of the brainstem, the basal ganglia, and the spinal cord, individual nerve cells in many places have been lost, there is everywhere a certain spotty appearance to the cellular pattern of the structure, without there usually being, however, a derangement of the architecture.

Tissue breakdown products are increased. Diffuse outfall of myelinated fibers is discernible mainly with the Marchi method.

The focal lesions, which from their localization give insight as to the sites of predilection of the entire process, manifest themselves as an abundance of gliogenic neuronophagias, as characteristic syncytial glial rosettes with numerous nuclei, profusely found in gray and white mat-

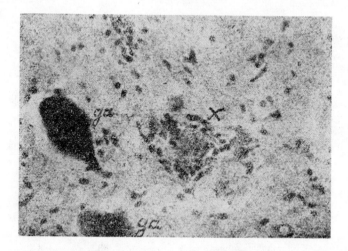

Figure 1.   Ganglion-cell swelling (ga) and glial-rosette formation (x) at the site of a disintegrating ganglion cell. Generalized protoplasmic glial proliferation. Anterior horn, spinal cord. Nissl stain. Microphotograph.

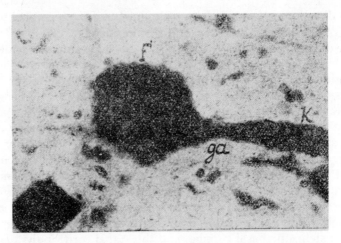

Figure 2. Marked enlargement of a ganglion-cell process (F); ga, ganglion cell; K, nucleus of the ganglion cell. Anterior horn, spinal cord. Nissl stain. Microphotograph.

ter, and as small foci of devastation in the gray matter marked by small collections of proliferated protoplasmic glia.

In the chronically developing lesions, along with the thinning out of ganglion cells one is struck with areas of proliferation of protoplasmic glia, in which several glial elements, at times in a grapelike arrangement,

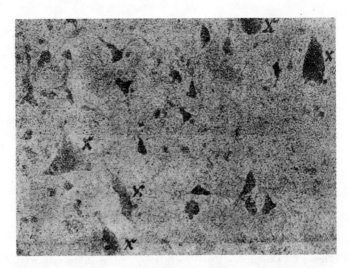

Figure 3. Characteristic degenerative manifestations in the Betz cells (s) in the precentral convolution. Nissl stain. Microphotograph.

and within which large profusely stippled nuclei stand out, show fusion of the cytoplasm into a single structure. Here, also, there is widespread fatty degeneration of ganglion cells. We regularly encounter the neuronophagias as well as the rosettes and the small scarred foci of cell loss in particular parts of the central nervous system, each lesion taking the form corresponding to its age. They are especially frequent in the precentral gyrus, in the anteriormost parts of the caudate nucleus, in the medial nucleus of the thalamus, and in the motor nuclei of the brainstem and spinal cord. The posterior parts of the frontal and temporal regions are likewise severely affected. The foci of devastation in the cortex, which are especially characteristic of the precentral gyrus, are mainly located in Brodmann's third layer, but they occur in the lowermost two layers as well. Only rarely do they acquire a more widespread distribution, as in the temporal lobe of the third case, in which the columns of Clarque (sic) in the spinal cord, the spinocerebellar tracts, and the Purkinje cells of the cerebellum showed more or less severe degenerative changes. The precentral gyrus with its diffuse alterations—the isolated foci of ganglion-cell loss, the small areas of devastation, and the severe manifestations of degeneration in the pyramidal cells of Betz, characterized by swellings and chromatolysis to the point of cell-shadow formation—presents in all instances a characteristic, very striking picture (Fig. 3). The diffuse loss of myelinated fibers becomes more visibly apparent in the pyramidal tracts. Foci of hermorrhage, softening, or macrophage accumulation are nowhere encountered.

Thus, in all three cases we are dealing with an organic disease of the central nervous system, the anatomic substrate of which is clearly distinct from that of all hitherto-known disease processes.

There apparently does exist some rather remote relationship with a few isolated cases reported in the literature as instances of "strange disease." The only one that I should like to consider as identical with my cases is Creutzfeldt's case, published after the completion of my studies, of a "particular focal disease of the central nervous system,"[2] which conforms in all essential points to my cases; for I do not believe that the more widespread distribution of the cortical destruction in Creutzfeldt's case, in the presence of an otherwise identical development of the tissue process both as to its nature and localization, constitutes a fundamental difference, especially since the clinical picture in this case shows distinct similarity with my cases.

Thus, in my three cases and with the addition of Creutzfeldt's case, we are dealing with illnesses of a particular sort, for which, in view of the clinical evolution of the disorder and the anatomic substrate displayed, a separate status cannot be denied. Along with this, the anatomic process in the central nervous system shows itself mainly to be a severe, purely parenchymatous degeneration of which the particularly characteristic features are the occurrence of numerous neuronophagic foci, the development of glial rosettes, frequently extensive, in gray and white matter, and the presence of circumscribed foci of devastation with a preferential localization in particular regions (precentral gyrus, anterior part of the striatal system, medial nucleus of the thalamus, the motor nuclei of the medulla oblongata and spinal cord, the posterior frontal region, and the temporal region). Accompanying these changes are degenerative changes in ganglion cells—chronic and diffuse, with a tendency to fatty degeneration, and subacute, with various forms of swelling—and a diffuse loss of myelinated fibers together with generalized proliferation of protoplasmic glia.

On the basis of this accumulated experience I thought it possible to characterize the clinical picture of the disease as follows: this is a disease of middle and late life which begins with progressive—slowly at first—disturbances of the motor apparatus and of sensation. The patients complain of weakness and pains in their legs, which become stiff. In walking, their legs often give out under them and they fall down; meanwhile, objective findings on examination at first are lacking. A suggestion of spasticity may already be detectable at this stage, however, and the abdominal reflexes seem early to show a tendency to become decreased or absent. At the very beginning of the illness the variability of the symptoms, with remissions, is most clearly apparent. Gradually more definite disorders of movement appear which apparently represent a peculiar mixture, difficult to analyze at first, of spastic and striatal symptoms. Without showing demonstrable paralyses, the patients' gait is strikingly uncoordinated; the patients collapse and fall down, and, finally, standing and walking become impossible. Muscle spasms can occur, but hypotonic states predominate. Clear-cut striatal symptoms, in the sense of pronounced impoverishment of movement and characteristic tremors, need not always be striking. Speech is slow and monotonous and is generally impaired in a dysarthric fashion. The tendon reflexes are usually exaggerated, but they may be normal and can even be absent. The Babinski sign is, at least in certain phases of the evolution of the disease, suggestively present or positive. The abdominal reflexes are decreased or absent. The eyegrounds are always normal. Examinations of blood and cerebrospinal fluid are generally negative. During the period when the neurologic manifestations are becoming more distinct, striking mental changes appear, in the form of apathy, negativism, and delirious and hallucinatory confusional states; depending on the duration of the illness, these changes can progress to marked mental deterioration. Finally, cerebral irritative states with disorders of function of the bulbar nuclei come to occupy the foreground, and these, progressing rapidly, with signs of severe obtundation often subsequent to epileptiform attacks, and febrile temperatures, bring the illness to a close. The course of the disease is subacutely progressive, with a range of duration, from the onset of the more severe symptoms, of several weeks to a year.

In accordance with its histologic uniqueness, the disease process may be characterized as an encephalomyelopathy with disseminated foci of degeneration. On the basis of the findings up to the present, the outstanding features are a regularly occurring affection of the entire pyramidal system and of the striatal system together with the anteromedial nucleus of the thalamus. Diffuse though the changes may be, there still is a certain tendency to a systematized distribution which chiefly manifests itself as a partial disorder of the pyramidal and extrapyramidal motor systems.

Thus, from a pathophysiological and clinical point of view, this disease occupies a place between the spastic system diseases, particularly amyotrophic lateral sclerosis, and the disease processes primarily localized to the striatum, particularly Westphal and Strümpell's pseudosclerosis, Wilson's disease, and chorea. From the standpoint of symptoms it comes closest perhaps to multiple sclerosis, from which it differs sharply on the basis of the histologic substrate. Thus, the disease can be classified as a special subgroup of pseudosclerosis and may most reasonably be set apart from the other pseudoscleroses with predominantly striatal localization, as spastic pseudosclerosis, whereby recognition is given to the striking changes in the pyramidal system.

These findings and ideas of mine have now received full confirmation by an additional case from my present material. The microscopic sections from this case, which had been in my collection for many years, had always seemed remarkable to me; until now, however, I had not been in a position to evaluate them adequately. As a result of the above-cited observations my attention was again drawn to them, and a renewed detailed study of the entire brain with special consideration of the basal ganglia showed that there was an extreme degree of similarity with the disease process described above. Moreover, the clinical picture also shows interesting points of agreement.

The case is as follows: The patient, Jac., born in 1869, a mason, was admitted on January 13, 1912 to the Friedrichsberg Insane Asylum. From his past history, obtained from his wife, the following information was received. The patient's father was a heavy drinker. The patient had previously been a very strong man, always healthy, and at the time of his marriage in 1891 he drank but little. His wife was healthy; she had had seventeen children, of whom four were living; the others had died at an early age of general debility and pulmonary tuberculosis. No miscarriages. The living children were all physically and mentally healthy except for the youngest, who was somewhat retarded and had to attend a special school. Syphilitic infection was denied.

A few years after marriage he began to drink heavily. He drank spirits (schnaps) in large amounts and could tolerate it well, but he often was drunk nevertheless. He became more irritable and—especially after taking alcohol—was very irascible and violent; but at the same time he showed no true psychotic manifestations in the sense of delusions, hallucinations, delirious states, or the like. When he was sober he was easy to get along with. He was an industrious, competent mason. In 1906, while in a drunken state, he fractured his right hip so that he had to be under treatment at the Eppendorf Hospital for several months. Following his discharge from the hospital he did not return to work; at first he needed two crutches for walking, but after two years he was able to get along quite well with one crutch. He had never worked since this injury. Following the injury he did not drink as much as before and was only rarely drunk. In the latter half of 1911 he drank practically no more spirits, as he complained of gastric symptoms and had no more desire for alcohol. During this period of time a physical and mental change was observed in the patient. He complained frequently of his stomach, he had no appetite, he lost weight and felt fatigued. At the same time he was normal mentally, although very irritable and at times excited. In mid-October he complained of increasing weakness in his legs, saying that they felt heavy and that he was unable to move them in walking and that he no longer had normal feelings in his legs. In bed, he could move his legs quite well, being able to flex and to extend them, but he could no longer get out of bed unassisted and, on attempting to walk, could no longer move his legs, so that he let himself be dragged along with his legs dangling beneath him. Meanwhile he complained that his legs were getting shorter and that the tendons were tightening, particularly in the popliteal fossa. He said, moreover, that his legs became stiff when he wanted to use them in walking. He had no particular pains in his legs. After transitory improvement, which lasted through approximately the first half of November, his condition became worse again. He began having headaches and fever in addition to the difficulty in walking and the digestive complaints, so that at the end of November he came under medical treatment in his home, and a diet and compresses for his head were prescribed. Soon thereafter nocturnal delirium set in, with intense anxiety and excitement. He continually demanded that he have a knife in bed with him, thinking that someone was going to do him harm. Almost every night he soaked through the bedclothes with sweat. At the same time he recognized his surroundings and was entirely calm in the daytime. His facial expression became more rigid. As his nocturnal excited state became worse and he no longer was able to get about, he was admitted on December 30, 1911, to the Neurological Division of the Eppendorf Hospital. From the history that was taken at the time, the following points are excerpted: Initially, no definite abnormalities were found on physical examination; the abdomen, however, was moderately tender to pressure. The stomach contents were normal to aspiration. The neurological examination likewise showed nothing remarkable at first; the only possibly abnormal finding was that the patellar reflexes were very lively, but without clonus. Although the patient passed urine spontaneously at the time of admission, he was unable to urinate over the four ensuing days and was catheterized. The urine itself was normal. Soon he began having states of psychomotor excitement in the hospital, alternating with periods of wholly calm behavior. At times he gave "a very strange impression. He looks fixedly at the physician, gives meaningless answers to questions, speaks abusively to the doctor, and suddenly begins shouting harshly and loudly without purpose or reason. He hears voices and answers them." In his quiet periods he had no recollection of these periods of excitement. Because of the fact that these sudden attacks of excitement, in which he tore his bedclothes to small pieces, became more frequent, the patient was transferred on January 13, 1912, to Friedrichsberg with a diagnosis of ? catatonia. Here the noteworthy findings were as follows: The examination of the visceral organs was still negative. His state of nutrition was poor. His facial expression was rigid. At the same time there was a general restlessness of the facial musculature. The pupils were not quite round but were bilaterally equal and reacted promptly. There were no pareses referable to the cranial nerves. There was a slight tremor of the hands. The legs could be moved actively but there was a not inconsiderable weakness of the extensors of the lower legs and probably of the peronei also, with tenderness to pressure of the large nerve trunks in both legs. "The patient can neither stand nor walk without support; if supported for walking, he does not move his legs from the floor." He reacted to painful stimuli, but sensation, in view of his confusional state, could not be accurately tested.

The patellar reflexes were very active ($+++$), the Achilles reflexes likewise; no definite clonus; a suggestion of Babinski bilaterally, sometimes $+$. The abdominal reflexes were unobtainable. During the physical examination the patient was very fearful; he was brought screaming loudly into the examining room and resisted being examined. The stiff, empty facial expression at times was enlivened by distinct grimacing. Periods in which the patient lay quietly and rigidly in bed alternated with episodes of severe psychomotor restlessness. The patient repeatedly acted as if deaf and dumb; when dealt with energetically and firmly he immediately showed appropriate behavior and answered questions. In his answers he showed himself to be temporally and spatially disoriented, confused, euphoric, and apprehensive. He frequently confabulated and was subject to auditory misinterpretations. For short periods at times he gave correct answers as to time, place, and person, but he fatigued easily and showed pronounced impairment of attention.

Over the ensuing days the patient remained in the same state of anxious confusion, and he died on January 24, 1912, with fever and signs of bronchopneumonia.

Thus, in this patient's case we are dealing with a forty-three-year-old man who, as a son of a heavy drinker, was in earlier years subject to alcoholic abuse. In later years he drank less and was reported not to have drunk any alcohol at all in the last six months before his illness. The disease began with digestive disturbances, increasing weakness of the legs, stiffness of the legs and an odd disturbance of gait. The patient became unable to mobilize his legs for walking, although there was no actual paralysis. After a transitory improvement (remission) in the neurologic symptoms, he began having nocturnal states of anxious delirium, and in the hospital the outstanding features essentially were the rigid facial expression, a periodic restlessness of the facial musculature with definite grimacing, and the inability to stand or walk in the absence of definite evidence of paralysis. At the same time there were pronounced pyramidial-tract symptoms with absent abdominal reflexes. Periods during which the patient lay quietly and rigidly in bed and seemed to behave more or less appropriately alternated with others that were characterized by anxious hallucinatory states of confusion. The variability of the mental symptoms was striking. Amid increasing restlessness and evidence of fever and bronchopneumonia, death occurred after a three-month period of evolution of the more severe nervous and mental symptoms.

This case also cannot immediately be brought into any of the recognized categories of disease. The initial diagnosis of catatonia is wholly unsatisfactory, and the possibility of a disorder due to alcohol must, in view of the history and the particular clinical features of the illness, also be rejected, because the mental and nervous derangements that develop on a background of alcoholism ordinarily arise in immediate association with alcoholic intoxication, and in their disease picture and course they show features other than those seen in our patient. The diagnosis of multiple sclerosis likewise cannot be supported. Thus, this case also remains unexplained from a clinical standpoint.

At autopsy, except for foci of bronchopneumonia and a slight degree of brain atrophy (brain weight 1335 grams), nothing remarkable was found. The microscopical study of the central nervous system showed findings that were surprisingly similar to those in the previously described cases. In this case, also, we are dealing with a purely parenchymatous disorder which, in its particular features and its localization, wholly conforms to the picture of our disease process, the only differences being that on the whole the glial rosette formation is somewhat less, and fatty degeneration of ganglion cells dominates the histologic picture to an even greater extent. The precentral convolution especially is the region that reproduces in all details the same structural changes as in the other cases (cf. Fig. 3). In the posterior frontal region and in the temporal regions the cerebral cortex in this case also shows small foci of devastation with proliferation of protoplasmic glia. Extensive lesions of the cortex are nowhere to be found.

I have carried out a thorough study of the basal ganglia, which were kept in formalin, using fat stains and Bielschowsky, Van Gieson, and myelin-sheath preparations, and here, also, was able to confirm the findings of the earlier cases. In these nuclear groups, isolated foci of ganglion-cell loss with proliferation of protoplasmic glia and an extraordinarily severe degree of fatty degeneration of ganglion cells are the outstanding changes. Here, too, the sections stained for fat are what give the best appreciation of the extent of the process. In this new case the previous experience that the alterations undoubtedly reached their most extensive development in the anterior parts of the striatal system, together with the medial nuclei of the thalamus, is confirmed; but the remaining parts of the basal ganglia also are similarly altered, although to a far lesser extent. In the medulla oblongata, again it is the motor-cell columns that show severe ganglion-cell changes. A partial degeneration of the pyramidal tracts is distinctly recognizable.

So, on the basis of the histologic examination there can be no doubt but that this case also belongs with our disease process. The clinical picture, too, in its essential features, conforms to the particular characteristics of the earlier cases.

Of particular interest still is the etiology of the disease, which at first seems to display no features of uniformity. In the first two cases some indications of a possible syphilitic infection are given. In the third case one may perhaps have to consider a chronic latent malarial infection. In Creutzfeldt's case an endogenous predisposition stands out. In my newest case chronic misuse of alcohol must be taken into etiologic consideration. It is striking that almost all of the patients had digestive disturbances at the onset of the illness. The possibility may perhaps not be excluded that with regard to this disease process we are dealing with complicated toxic manifestations of varied causation and of intrinsic metabolic origin which finally give rise to the severe disease of the parenchyma of the central nervous system and, together with this, the remarkable mental and meurologic disease picture.

NOTES

1. A. Jakob, Concerning Peculiar Disorders of the Central Nervous System with Remarkable Anatomical Findings (Spastic Pseudosclerosis–Encephalopathy with Disseminated Foci of Degeneration). Z. Neurol. Psychiatr., 1921.
2. Z. Neurol. Psychiatr. 57 (1920), 1–18.

DYSPHASIA, DYSPRAXIA, AND DISORDERS OF THE BODY IMAGE

Introduction

Norman Geschwind, M.D.
James Jackson Putnam Professor
of Neurology
Harvard Medical School
and
Director, Neurological Unit
Beth Israel Hospital

THE THREE PAPERS in this section all share certain characteristics. Each of them aroused great interest at the time of publication, an interest which has continued until the present day. On the other hand each aroused controversies concerning the interpretation of the author's findings that still rage unabated. Their interest is therefore more than antiquarian since each one is at the core of a major area of concern to those interested in the more complex functions of the human brain. The historian of ideas can dispassionately rate each one as of major historical importance, but no dispassionate judgment is possible as to their ultimate significance.

Of the three, Broca's paper was certainly the most influential. Although there are earlier descriptions of aphasia even dating to antiquity, this publication led almost immediately to a tremendous output of work concerned with the loss of language functions after brain lesions, an output that continued steadily through the next half century. Broca's teaching that lesions of part of one hemisphere could lead to aphasia is almost universally accepted. But certain parts of his argument still remain in dispute. Broca thought that the third frontal convolution has a special importance for language production. Some, such as Pierre Marie later denied this, arguing that only lesions of the temporal speech areas lead to aphasia. Many others accept Broca's view, but even among these there is no agreement as to whether only the foot (or pars opercularis) of this gyrus constitutes the language area, or whether the more anteriorly lying pars triangularis should also be included. Thus, over one hundred years later, the limits and significance of Broca's area remain active questions.

Babinski's paper became a landmark contribution to the borderland field between neurology and psychiatry by calling attention to the remarkable phenomenon of patients who showed gross unconcern with or indeed even overt denial of striking neurological deficits. The clinical phenomena he described are well known to every neurologist, but their interpretation remains unsettled. At one extreme are the purely "psychiatric" theories which deny any importance to the brain lesion itself and regard denial as an emotional response to an unbearable deficit. The great majority of neurologists regard denial of hemiplegia as the direct result of brain lesions. There remain, however, deep disagreements even among the neurological theorists. Most authors (but not all) accept the finding that denial of left hemiplegia is much more common than denial of right hemiplegia. Some argue, however, that denial of right hemiplegia is simply masked by the aphasia which is usually present. The most commonly advanced theory of denial of hemiplegia might be termed the "perceptual" theory, i.e., that a lesion in the parietal lobe in one hemisphere leads to inattention to the opposite side of external space and of the body itself. Other investigators, however, support a radically different view. They argue that the right hemisphere is dominant for the more refined aspects of emotional response and that the change in emotional state resulting from right sided lesions, either frontal or parietal, leads to a widespread change in behavior, of which unconcern with illness is only one manifestation.

Of the three papers in this section, Gerstmann's has certainly been the most controversial. Most authors, however widely they may differ in their opinions concerning the anatomical localization and mechanisms of the phenomena, at least agree that the clincial pictures described by Broca and Babinski exist. Gerstmann's observations have, by contrast, been subject to the harshest criticisms at every level. His syndrome has even been labelled as a fiction—as a group of phenomena singled out arbitrarily, with no localizing significance. The depth of the controversy is, however, most vividly apparent when one realizes that others have just as strongly argued that the simultaneous presence of all four components is an excellent predictor of a focal lesion in the left temporo-parieto-occipital junction.

The past quarter-century has witnessed a great revival of interest in the intellectual and emotional effects of brain lesions. This revival has been associated with a resurgence of the controversies raised by these papers. Whatever the ultimate resolution of these issues, the three papers reprinted here will have to be credited as major stimuli to the deeper analysis of the neurological foundations of mind.

Contribution to the Study of Mental Disturbances in Organic Cerebral Hemiplegia (Anosognosia)

J. BABINSKI

I WISH TO DRAW ATTENTION to an observation I have had the opportunity to make of a mental disturbance associated with cerebral hemiplegia, in which the patients ignore, or seem to ignore, the existence of the paralysis that afflicts them.

I have excluded cases with diminished intelligence where the patient had only a vague notion of events occurring around him. I have also discarded those instances in which a notable, but not profound, alteration of intellectual functions occurred.

I would like to remind you of the observation published by Dr. Barat: "Replacement of Sensations by Impressions. Report of a Case with Multiple Hallucinations and Illusions" (*Journal de Psychologie normale et pathologique*, March–April 1912). His patient had a left hemiplegia and blindness. Although the patient's judgment and reasoning were only minimally affected, she was unaware of her paralysis. Evidence of confusion was noted: "She is completely disoriented in time and space" and "has obvious visual hallucinations in which she sees lamps close to her which she asks to be taken away because they are damaging her eyes; she also has auditory illusions and possibly auditory hallucinations."

My observations, while similar to those I have mentioned, have dis-

NOTE: Translated by F. H. Hochberg from: Babinski, J., "Contribution à l'étude des troubles mentaux dans l'hémiplégie organique cérébrale (Anosognosie)," *Revue neurologique* 22 (1914), 845–48.

tinct differences. I was unable to study the patients' mental status in detail, but my evaluations and those of others suggested that there was no mental confusion, confabulation, or hallucinations despite the fact that their mentation was not completely in order.

One of the patients in question, examined by Dr. Langlois of the faculty, had a left hemiplegia and over several months preserved essentially intact intellectual and emotional faculties. She recalled past events, spontaneously expressed sensible ideas in a correct fashion, interested herself in news of her friends, and remained involved with her family as before her illness. There was no confusion, confabulation, ravings, or hallucinations. In striking contrast to her apparent intellectual preservation was her ignorance of her almost complete hemiplegia; for many years prior to her hemiplegia she had expressed fear about someday being so afflicted which she neither complained about nor alluded to. She moved her right arm immediately after being asked to. When asked to move her left arm she did nothing, remaining silent, as if the request had been made to another person.

Sensation on the paralyzed side was altered but not abolished; she had some position sensation and sometimes complained of pain in her left shoulder.

Significant mental disturbances subsequently appeared, and the patient died after having been demented for some time.

One other patient first seen by Dr. Larcher and me following a left hemiplegia of sudden onset presented a similar clinical picture over several months. As in the preceding case, no hallucinations, confusion, or confabulations were noted during this period. However, she was a little overexcited, her thinking was changed, and according to her chambermaid of many years she occasionally had strange thoughts. Her memory was excellent, her conversation lively and interesting, and she joked, reminding her doctor that he had always cured her previous illnesses but this time "his science was powerless."

When she was asked precisely what bothered her, she stated that she had a backache or that she suffered from an old phlebitis (she had previously had a phlebitis) but never mentioned her arm which was completely paralyzed. She performed all right-sided movements that were asked of her. When asked to move her left arm, she either did not respond or simply said "there, it's done." Several days after the question of electrotherapy had been discussed in front of her, she told her physician: "Why do you want to use electrotherapy? I am not paralyzed."

The patient showed profound left-arm anesthesia, not perceiving even passive arm movement. I learned later that her intelligence progressively worsened, she became demented, and died.

I will permit myself the use of a neologism in calling this state anosognosia.

I have also observed several hemiplegics who, although not ignoring the existence of their paralysis, seemed to attach no importance to it as if it were an insignificant bother—a state that might be called anosodiaphoric (indifference, insouciance).

How can we interpret these facts?

It might be supposed that the patient's ignorance, the anosognosia, is feigned, it is well known that patients by affectation of self-esteem seek to conceal their problems; but in this situation concealment is in vain as the paralysis is visible to everyone. Even if there was an attempted concealment, the persistence with which the patients carried it out was amazing, as for several months they did not falter in the role they played.

Must we admit the anosognosia was real? I cannot be sure, and it was impossible for me to question the patients in a way that would allow me to resolve this point. In fact, in my two cases, the families considered the observation to be providential and asked us to avoid all questions that would enlighten the patients and thereby disturb their peace. If it (anosognosia) is real, then sensory troubles play an important role in its genesis.

I would like to note that my cases had a left hemiplegia. Perhaps anosognosia is a feature of right hemispheric lesions. Whatever hypothesis one accepts, the phenomenon is remarkable, and I will study it more deeply if the occasion presents itself.

Dr. Souques: I recently observed a case similar to that of Dr. Babinski's. One morning, one of our colleagues suffered an attack of vertigo followed by a left hemiplegia without loss of consciousness. I examined him the next day and three times a week for the next two months. He had a hemiplegia accompanied by a complete superficial and deep hemianesthesia. The patient, a very cultivated and shrewd man, did not *seem* to have appreciable intellectual difficulties. I did not examine him sufficiently to say his memory was intact, but he was perfectly lucid. Three days after the attack he showed interest in the newspapers and brochures that he read or that were read to him. Nothing in his conversation betrayed a notable intellectual decline. However, from its onset and during the next month he had no notion of his hemiplegia. His family and I were amazed by his silence and inattention to his complete paralysis. One day, when I used the term hemiparesis he paid no attention to it. He was neither playful nor resigned; rather he seemed to have forgotten his left side. I wonder if the anesthesia did not play some role in his mental state. Whatever it is, this case is reminiscent of the findings that Dr. Babinski has designated as *anosognosia*.

Dr. Dejerine: The patients of Dr. Babinski and Dr. Souques present altered sensation in their paralyzed limbs—an alteration that perhaps plays a role in their indifference to their disability.

Dr. Pierre-Marie: I wonder if it is not the place to consider that we see the same sort of psychological trouble in visceral problems, as well as in those of the nervous system: for example, patients with severe urinary tract problems, who ignore them.

Dr. Gilbert Ballet: Dr. Babinski's data are very interesting. One sees a similar indifference in patients with cerebral tumors who stop complaining of a previously bothersome headache, which we might think is now gone, and state they have no visual problems when they are in reality totally blind. In these cases, one should formally study retentive memory.

Dr. M. Henry Meige: It is both remarkable and true that certain hemiplegics show a kind of indifference to their infirmity. It seems that they disinterest themselves in their body parts which they either no longer control or control with pain. Surely there exists a disproportion between their physical disability and the mental reactions that result. It is common to see an aphasic patient upset and complaining during an unproductive effort to speak; however, the hemiplegic complains rarely of the immobility of his arm or leg. Does this resignation reflect a desire to hide his disability from himself or others? It occurs in certain cases, but in others one is dealing with a true psychopathic disorder.

I have often been struck by the rapidity with which hemiplegics seem to have lost the function of their paralyzed extremity.

Even intelligent and young patients who are perfectly able to understand the therapeutic goals sometimes fail to show motor rehabilitation. This failure does not result from weakness, negligence, or lack of confidence in the results. With the transitory cessation of motion all memory of function seems ended—as if the paralyzed extremities never existed. The hemiplegic ignores the extremities, and nothing seems to incite him to perform spontaneous motion. Even when motor activity is regained in certain muscular groups, the patient neglects to make otherwise possible movements. Ten years ago I suggested that a *functional motor amnesia* exists among hemiplegic patients. Dr. Babinski's presentation relates to a similar psychopathic process: anosognosia caused by a functional motor amnesia.

Dr. Henri Claude: Regarding the sensory difficulties to which the ignored hemiplegia has been attributed, I observed sensory changes in a patient with a left hemiplegia and right apraxia that I reported to the Société Medicale des Hôpitaux [no reference given]. This man, whose intelligence was sufficiently preserved, was incapable of localizing cutaneous stimuli. He could feel a pinprick but would localize it to a region far distant from the stimulus. I thought there was a problem in the topographic representation of body parts and have designated this trouble by the term topo-anesthesia. It is possible that in the situations noted by Dr. Babinski it was equally a question of the loss of representation of the paralyzed limb which can no longer be brought to the patient's attention by motor or psychomotor stimuli.

Remarks on the Seat of the Faculty of Articulate Speech, Followed by the Report of a Case of Aphemia (Loss of Speech)

P. BROCA

I.

THERE IS A GENERAL FACULTY of language that governs all these modes of expressing a thought; it may be defined as the ability to establish a constant relationship between an idea and a symbol—whether the symbol is a sound, a gesture, a figure, or some kind of tracing. Furthermore, every sort of language depends upon the functioning of certain organs of *emission* and *reception*. The organ of reception may be the ear, the eye, or sometimes even the skin (touch). As regards the organs of emission, they are activated by voluntary muscles such as those of the larynx, tongue, palate, face, upper extremities, etc. All normal language, therefore, presupposes the integrity of: (1) a certain number of muscles, their motor nerves, and that part of the central nervous system (CNS) where these nerves originate; (2) a certain external sensory apparatus, its afferent nerves, and that part of the CNS where these nerves terminate; and (3) that part of the brain which subserves the general faculty of language as I have just defined it.

NOTE: Translated by C. Wasterlain and D. A. Rottenberg from: Broca, P., "Remarques sur le siège de la faculté du langage articulé, suivies d'une observation d'aphémie (perte de la parole), *Bull. Soc. Anat. Paris*, 2ᵉ série, 6 (1861), 332–33 et 343–57. Section I of the original article is irrelevant to Broca's argument, and only a single excerpt has been translated—Eds.

The absence or abolition of this last-mentioned faculty renders any sort of language impossible. Congenital or traumatic lesions of the organs of reception or emission may deprive us of the particular kind of language which presses these organs into service; but if the general faculty of language and a sufficient amount of intelligence remain, we can compensate with another sort of language for the sort which has been lost.

The pathological conditions which deprive us of the means of communication usually deprive us of either emission or reception; the organs of emission and reception are rarely affected simultaneously. For example, the adult who becomes deaf continues to express himself verbally, but we employ a different language—gestures or writing—in order to communicate an idea to him. The reverse holds true when the muscles subserving speech are paralyzed; the patient whom we address in spoken language replies in another language. Thus, the various systems of communication may substitute for one another.

This is nothing more than elementary physiology; but pathology has enabled us to carry the analysis a step further as regards articulate speech, which is the most important and probably the most complex language of all.

There are cases in which all of the muscles—including those which subserve phonation and articulation—are under voluntary control, the auditory apparatus is intact, and the general faculty of language remains unaffected, but in which, nevertheless, a cerebral lesion abolishes articulate speech. It seems to me that this loss of speech in patients who are neither paralyzed nor demented is singular enough to warrant a special designation; therefore, I shall name this symptom *aphemia*(α, privative prefix; φημί, I speak, I utter) because these patients lack only the ability to articulate words. They listen to and understand everything that is said to them, and they retain all of their intellectual faculties. They utter sounds with ease. With their tongue and lips they execute far more extensive and energetic movements than are required to produce speech, yet, nonetheless, the perfectly sensible response which they wish to make is reduced to a few articulated sounds—always the same ones, and always in the same order. Their vocabulary, if one can call it that, is composed of a short series of syllables, sometimes of a monosyllable, which expresses everything, or rather nothing, because this unique word is usually foreign to all vocabularies. Certain patients do not even retain this vestige of articulate speech; they try in vain to utter a single syllable. Others possess, as it were, two degrees of articulation. Under ordinary circumstances they invariably utter their favorite word. When roused to anger, however, they become capable of articulating a second word, most often a crude oath which, in all probability, they habitually used prior to their illness; after this final effort they fall silent. . . .

II.

Aphemia of twenty-one years' duration produced by a chronic, progressive soft-ening of the second and third convolutions of the superior part of the left frontal lobe

On April 11, 1861, a fifty-one-year-old man named Leborgne suffer-ing from a diffuse gangrenous inflammation of the entire right lower limb, from the ankle to the buttock, was admitted as a surgical patient to the general infirmary of the Bicêtre. When I questioned him the next day about the onset of his illness his only response was the monosyllable "tan," repeated twice in succession and accompanied by a movement of the left hand. I inquired into the past history of this man, who had been at the Bicêtre for twenty-one years. His attendants, fellow patients, and those relatives who came to visit him were interviewed in turn, and the following story finally emerged.

Leborgne had been subject to epileptic fits since his youth, but he worked as a lastmaker until the age of thirty, when he lost the power of speech and was admitted to the hospice of the Bicêtre as an invalid. It is not known whether he lost his speech suddenly or gradually, or whether any other symptoms were present at the onset of his illness.

When he arrived at the Bicêtre he had been unable to speak for two or three months. He was intelligent and in excellent general health, suffering only from the loss of articulate speech. He came and went in the hospice, where he was known by the name of Tan. He understood everything that was said to him; in fact, his hearing was excellent. But regardless of the question put to him, he always answered "tan, tan," qualified by various gestures through which he managed to express most of his ideas. When his gesticulations were not understood he would lose his temper and supplement his vocabulary with a single expletive, the same one I mentioned earlier in connection with Mr. Au-burtin's patient. Tan was considered self-centered, malicious, and vindictive; his companions disliked him and accused him of stealing. These faults may have been due in large part to his cerebral lesion. They were not sufficiently marked, however, to appear pathological, and, although the patient was at the Bicêtre, there was never any question of transferring him to the psychiatric ward. On the contrary, he was con-sidered as being entirely responsible for his actions.

Ten years after he lost the ability to speak, a new symptom appeared: the muscles of his right arm gradually weakened and eventually became completely paralyzed. Tan continued to ambulate without difficulty, but the paralysis slowly spread to involve the right lower extremity; after dragging his leg about for some time, he finally took to bed. Some four years elapsed between the onset of the paralysis of his arm and the time when he became completely unable to stand because of leg weakness. Tan had been confined to bed for almost seven years when he was transferred to the Bicêtre infirmary. We know very little about that period of his life. As he had become unable to work any mischief, his companions ignored him, except, on occasion, when they amused themselves at his expense (which made him very angry). He even lost whatever fame the unusual nature of his illness had earned him. It was observed that his eyesight had become noticeably worse during the last two years of his life, this being the only change in his condition after he took to bed. He never became senile. As his sheets were changed but once a week, the diffuse inflammation which prompted his admission to the infirmary on April 11, 1861, was first noticed by the nurses only after it had invaded the entire right lower extremity from foot to buttock.

It was exceedingly difficult to study this unfortunate man who could neither speak nor write (his right hand was paralyzed). Moreover, his general condition was such that it would have been cruel to torment him with lengthy examinations.

I established, nevertheless, that somatic sensation was preserved throughout, though patchily. The right half of his body was less sensitive than the left, which undoubtedly contributed to lessen the pain of his phlegmonous cellulitis. He did not suffer a great deal as long as the inflamed limb was not disturbed, but palpation was painful; the few incisions I had to make increased his agitation and caused him to cry out.

Tan's right arm and leg were completely paralyzed. He retained voluntary control of his left arm and leg, which, although weak, were able to execute any movement without hesitation. Urination and defecation were normal. Swallowing was somewhat difficult, but mastication was well performed. His face was symmetrical at rest; however, when he inflated his cheeks the left cheek ballooned out slightly more than the right, indicating a slight weakness of the facial muscles on the left side. There was no suggestion of strabismus. The tongue moved freely and did not deviate; the patient was able to protrude it and to move it in all directions. The two halves of the tongue were of equal thickness. The above-mentioned difficulty in swallowing was due to incipient pharyngeal paralysis and not to paralysis of the tongue, as only the third stage of deglutition was laborious. The laryngeal musculature seemed normal: the patient's voice had a natural ring to it, and his monosyllables were clearly articulated.

Tan's hearing remained acute; he heard the ticking of a wristwatch perfectly well. But his eyesight was poor. When he wanted to see what time it was he would take his watch with his left hand and place it in a peculiar position approximately twenty centimeters away from his right eye, which appeared to be stronger than his left.

It was not possible to reach any firm conclusions about Tan's intellect. Certainly, he understood almost everything that was said to him. But as he was reduced to expressing his ideas and desires by motioning with his left hand, my moribund patient could not make himself understood as well as he understood others. He fared best with numerical answers, which he communicated with his fingers. I asked him several times how many days he had been ill; sometimes he replied five days, sometimes six. How many years had he been at the Bicêtre? He opened and closed his hand four times in succession and held up a single digit; this meant 21 years, which, as noted above, was perfectly correct. The next day I asked the same question again and obtained the same answer. But when I repeated the question a third time, Tan understood that I was testing him; he became angry and uttered the aforementioned expletive, which I heard from his mouth only this once. I showed him my watch on two successive days. The second hand was not working, and, consequently, he could only distinguish the three hands by their shape and length. Nevertheless, after examining the watch for a few moments he was able to indicate the correct time on each occasion. There can be no doubt, therefore, that this man was intelligent, that he was able to think, and that he had retained in some measure his memory for past events. He was even able to comprehend rather complex ideas. For example, I asked him in what order his limbs became paralyzed. First, he made a short horizontal movement with his left hand, which meant "understood!" Then he showed me in succession his tongue, his right arm, and his right leg. This was perfectly correct, though he attributed his loss of speech to paralysis of the tongue, which was only natural.

However, Tan was unable to answer various questions which a man of average intelligence would have managed to answer with a gesture, even with only one hand. At times his answers were incomprehensible, a circumstance which seemed to annoy him considerably. Occasionally the answer was clear but erroneous. For example, although he had no children he insisted that he did have some. Thus, it appeared that Tan's intelligence had been profoundly affected by his cerebral lesion or by the fever that consumed him, but he undoubtedly retained more than enough intelligence to be able to speak.

It was obvious from the history and from the results of my examination that this was a progressive cerebral lesion, which at the outset and during the first ten years of Tan's illness had remained limited to a rather circumscribed region, sparing the motor and sensory organs [sic] and that after ten years the lesion spread to involve one or more motor organs; subsequently, somatic sensation was affected together with vision, especially in the left eye. Since Tan's right side was completely paralyzed and since sensation in his right limbs was slightly impaired, the principal cerebral lesion must have been in the left hemisphere. The partial paralysis of the left facial muscles and of the ipsilateral retina confirms this formulation, for it is well known that paralyses of cerebral origin are crossed with respect to the trunk and limbs and ipsilateral with respect to the face.

It remains, however, to determine more precisely, if possible, the seat of the original lesion. Although the validity of Mr. Bouillaud's doctrine* was impugned at the last meeting of the Anthropological Society, I decided to predicate my arguments on the correctness of his teachings; anticipating an autopsy, this seemed the best way to put his theory to the test. Since Mr. Auburtin had declared a few days earlier that he would repudiate Bouillaud's doctrine if shown a single well-documented case of aphemia without a lesion in the frontal lobes, I invited him to observe my patient in order to learn what his diagnosis would be and whether or not he would accept the outcome of this case as conclusive. In spite of the complications which had ensued during the previous eleven years my colleague found the patient's past history and present condition sufficiently unambiguous to affirm without hesitation that the lesion had to originate in one of the frontal lobes.

Given the above, in order to localize the lesion I recalled that the corpus striatum was the motor organ closest to the frontal lobes. The hemiplegia, then, resulted from an extension of the original lesion into the corpus striatum. Thus, the probable diagnosis was: primary lesion of the left frontal lobe with subsequent extension into the ipsilateral corpus striatum. Regarding the nature of this lesion, all of the facts pointed to a slowly progressive, chronic softening; the absence of any signs of compression ruled out an intracranial tumor.

The patient died at 11 A.M. on April 17. The autopsy was performed as soon as possible, that is, twenty-four hours later. It was cool, and the body showed no signs of putrefaction. The brain was shown to the Anthropological Society a few hours after it was taken, whereupon it was placed in alcohol. This organ was so altered that exceptional precautions were required to insure its preservation. After two months and several changes of alcohol the specimen began to harden. Today it is in perfect condition in the Dupuytren Museum (*Nervous System*, No. 55a).

I shall not attempt a detailed description of the phlegmon. The muscles of the right arm and leg were replaced by fat and reduced to a small volume. All of the internal organs were normal except for the brain.

The skull was opened carefully with a saw. All of the sutures are fused. The skull bones are slightly thickened, the diploë replaced by compact tissue. The internal surface of the cranial vault presents a fine, worm-eaten appearance, an infallible sign of chronic osteitis (No. 55b).

The external surface of the dura is red, or extremely vascular; the

---

*that the faculty of articulate language resides in the frontal lobes—EDS.

membrane itself is quite thick, vascular, and fleshy and is lined internally by a serous pseudomembrane having a lardaceous appearance.
The dura mater and the false membrane together have an average thickness of 5 mm (minimum 3 mm, maximum 8 mm)—from which it follows
that the brain must have lost a considerable amount of its original bulk.

With the dura mater removed the pia mater appears generally thickened and very vascular in places; some areas are opaque owing to the
deposition of a yellowish plastic material that resembles pus but is solid
and (under the miscroscope) does not contain any purulent globules.

Over the lateral aspect of the left hemisphere near the Sylvian fissure
the pia is elevated by a transparent serous collection which occupies a
large depression in the cerebral substance. When the cyst was
punctured and its contents drawn off the pia collapsed revealing an
oblong cavity the size of a hen's egg, which coincides with the Sylvian
fissure, separating the frontal and temporal lobes. It extends back as far
as the Rolandic sulcus, which, as we know, separates the anterior or
frontal convolutions from the parietal convolutions. Thus, the lesion is
situated anterior to the central sulcus, and the parietal lobe is intact (at
least relatively so, since no part of either hemisphere is perfectly normal).

After incising and reflecting the pia overlying the above-mentioned
cavity it became immediately apparent that the latter represents a loss of
cerebral substance rather than a superficial depression. The fluid contents had been secreted *in situ* to fill the enlarging void, as occurs in
chronic softenings of the superficial layers of the cerebrum and cerebellum. A study of the convolutions delimiting the cavity reveals that they
are the seat of one of those chronic softenings that progresses sufficiently slowly to allow the cerebral molecules (dissociating, as it were,
one by one) to be reabsorbed and replaced by a serous secretion.[1] A
considerable portion of the left hemisphere has been gradually destroyed by this process; but the softening extends far beyond the limits
of the cavity, which is not circumscribed and cannot be compared to a
cyst. Its walls are, for the most part, irregular and fissured and are
formed by the cerebral substance itself, which is extremely soft; the
innermost layer, in direct contact with the serous secretion, was in the
process of slowly dissolving when the patient expired. Only the lower
wall is smooth and relatively firm.

It is apparent, therefore, that the cavity marks the site of the original
softening and that the disease process spread by degrees through the
neighboring tissues; the earliest lesion must be sought where the loss of
substance is more or less complete and not where the tissue is soft or in
the process of softening. Consequently, after examining the structures
that delimit the cavity I shall draw up a list of those that are missing.

The cavity that I am going to describe is located, as previously mentioned, in the region of the Sylvian fissure; it is situated, therefore, between the frontal and temporal-sphenoidal lobes. If the structures that surround this cavity were merely displaced without being destroyed, it should be limited inferiorly (temporally) and superiorly (frontally) by the *inferior marginal convolution* and the *third frontal convolution* respectively;[2] its floor should abut on the insular lobe. But such is not the case. The inferior wall of the cavity is bounded by the second temporosphenoidal convolution, which is preserved in its entirely and is rather firm; thus, the inferior marginal convolution has been completely destroyed down to the level of the *parallel fissure*. Moreover, there is no trace of the insula in the depths of the cavity; it has been entirely destroyed, together with the inner half of the extraventricular nucleus [sic] of the corpus striatum. The loss of substance extends inward to involve the anterior portion of the ventricular nucleus (of the corpus striatum) in such a manner that the cavity communicates with the left lateral ventricle by means of an irregular opening half a centimeter long. Finally, the superior border—or, rather, the superior wall—of the cavity encroaches upon the frontal lobe, which is deeply indented. The posterior half of the third frontal convolution has been completely eroded. The second frontal convolution is slightly less affected; its outer two-thirds (at least) have disappeared, and the inner third, though still present, is extremely soft. More posteriorly, the inferior third of the transverse frontal convolution has been completely destroyed back to the Rolandic sulcus.

In summary, then, the following structures have been destroyed: the small inferior marginal convolution (temporosphenoidal lobe); the small convolutions of the insula and the subjacent portion of the corpus striatum; and, finally, in the frontal lobe, the inferior portion of the transverse convolution and the posterior half of the two large convolutions known as the second and third frontal convolutions. Of the four convolutions which form the superior aspect of the frontal lobe, only one—the first and most medial—is anatomically continuous, though softened and atrophic. If one mentally replaces all of the convolutions that have disappeared, one finds that at least three-quarters of the cavity has been carved out of the frontal lobe.

It remains now to determine where the lesion originated. An examination of the cavity produced by the loss of cerebral substance clearly reveals that the center of the focus was in the frontal lobe. Assuming that the softening advanced at an equal rate in all directions, the disease process should have begun in the frontal lobe. But we must be guided by the condition of the surrounding cortex, which is variably softened, as well as by the boundaries of the area of cavitation. Thus, the second temporal convolution, which limits the lesion inferiorly, presents a smooth and rather firm surface; it is softened superficially but not too much. On the opposite side of the lesion, in the frontal lobe, the cortex is diffusely softened. The cerebral substance becomes gradually firmer as one moves away from the area of cavitation, but the softening extends for a considerable distance and involves virtually the entire frontal lobe. The frontal lobe, therefore, bears the brunt of the pathologic process; other areas were almost certainly affected later.

For the sake of greater precision it should be noted that the third frontal convolution has suffered the greatest loss of substance, having been transected near the anterior limit of the Sylvian fissure; its entire posterior extent has been destroyed, accounting for nearly half of the total loss of brain substance. Moreover, the second or middle (frontal) convolution, although profoundly altered, preserves its continuity internally. It seems likely, therefore, that the softening began in the third frontal convolution.

The remaining parts of the cerebral hemispheres appear relatively healthy; they are, indeed, a little less firm than usual—and it is fair to say that the entire cortical surface of both hemispheres is markedly atrophic—but their appearance, configuration, and anatomical continuity are preserved. As regards the deeper structures, I elected not to study them in order not to mutilate the specimen, which I wished to deposit in the museum. However, as the opening of the cortical cavity into the anterior horn of the left lateral ventricle became enlarged during the dissection of the pia mater (despite my precautions), I was able to partially examine the internal surface of the ventricle, and I observed that the entire corpus striatum was more or less softened but that the optic thalamus was of normal color, size, and consistency.

The whole brain together with the pia mater weighed only 987 grams after the fluid was drained from the cavity, nearly 400 grams less than the average brain weight of a fifty-year-old man. This considerable loss of substance derived from the cerebral hemispheres almost exclusively. It is well known that under normal circumstances the remainder of the brain never weighs more than 200 grams, and usually weighs less than 180 grams. In the present case the cerebellum, pons, and medulla, though small, are certainly not much reduced in size; and to suppose that they have lost a quarter of their normal weight (which is unlikely) would explain only a small fraction of the total weight loss.

The destruction of the gyri surrounding the Sylvian fissure of the left hemisphere undoubtedly accounts for much of this weight loss; however, I removed a similar amount of tissue from a normal brain, and the excised mass weighed barely 50 grams. It is very likely, therefore, that both cerebral hemispheres are considerably atrophic. This likelihood becomes a certainty if one considers that the meninges and false arachnoid membrane attain a thickness of 5–6 mm in certain areas.

Having described the lesions and having attempted to determine their nature, location, and evolution, it is important to compare the pathological findings with the clinical observations in order to establish, if possible, a relationship between the patient's symptoms and their anatomical substrate.

The anatomical examination indicates that the lesion was still enlarging when the patient succumbed. Thus, the lesion was progressive, but it advanced very slowly, requiring twenty-one years to destroy a rather restricted region of the brain. One may conclude, therefore, that the lesion was confined to the organ [sic] where it originated for a long period of time after the onset of the illness. As we have seen, the disease process began in the frontal lobe, most probably in the third frontal convolution. From a pathological-anatomical point of view the illness evolved in a biphasic manner: during the first phase a single frontal convolution (probably the third) was affected; later the disease process spread by degrees to involve other convolutions, the insular lobe, and the extraventricular nucleus of the corpus striatum.

Turning now to the succession of symptoms, we can also discern two phases of the illness: an initial phase lasting ten years during which the faculty of speech was lost, all of the other cortical functions remaining intact; and a second phase lasting eleven years during which the right upper and lower extremities were paralyzed in turn, partially at first but later completely.

Given the above, it is impossible to ignore the parallel between the two anatomical phases and the two symptomatologic phases. It is well known that the cerebral convolutions are not motor organs. The corpus striatum of the left hemisphere is, therefore, of all the organs affected the only one wherein a lesion could account for the paralysis of the right arm and leg. The second clinical period, during which motility was affected, thus corresponds to the second anatomical period, when the softening, spreading beyond the limits of the frontal lobe, reached the insula and the corpus striatum.

Hence the first ten-year period, characterized clinically by aphemia as the sole symptom, must correspond to the period during which the lesion was still confined to the frontal lobe.

Until now, in drawing a parallel between symptoms and lesions I have not spoken of disorders of the intellect or of their anatomic substrate. As noted above, Tan's intellect, which remained intact for a long time, began to deteriorate at some point that cannot be precisely determined and was markedly impaired when I first examined him. Lesions which adequately explained this deterioration were discovered at autopsy. Three of the four frontal convolutions were profoundly damaged over a considerable area; the entire frontal lobe was more or less softened. The cortical mantle over both hemispheres was atrophic, collapsed, and considerably softer than normal. It is difficult to imagine that the patient retained any intelligence at all, and it seems unlikely that one could survive very long with such a brain. I personally believe that the generalized softening of the left frontal lobe, the generalized atrophy of both cerebral hemispheres, and the chronic generalized meningitis are relatively recent; I am inclined to believe that these lesions occurred long after the softening of the corpus striatum, so that one can subdivide the second phase into two periods and summarize the patient's illness as

	Lesions	Symptoms
Phase I (10 years)	Softening of one frontal convolution (probably the third)	Simple aphemia
Phase II (11 years)	a. Spread to the left corpus striatum	Crossed motor paralysis
	b. Softening of the entire left frontal lobe; generalized hemispheral atrophy	Weakening of the intellect

Facts such as these, which bear on important theoretical questions, cannot be set forth in too much detail or discussed too minutely. I avail myself of this logic in order to excuse my lengthy arguments and lackluster prose. A few words will suffice to summarize my conclusions from this case:

1. Aphemia, i.e., loss of speech without intellectual impairment or motor paralysis, resulted from a lesion in one of the frontal lobes.

2. This case, therefore, confirms the opinion of Mr. Bouillaud, who localizes the faculty of articulate speech in these lobes.

3. Previous case reports, at least those accompanied by clear and precise anatomical descriptions, are not sufficiently numerous to definitively establish the localization of a particular faculty in a specific lobe, but such localization is extremely probable.

4. Whether the faculty of articulate speech resides within the frontal lobe taken as a whole or within one of the frontal convolutions—whether, in other words, cerebral faculties are localized by faculty and by convolution or merely by groups of faculties and by groups of convolutions—is a much more difficult question to answer. Additional cases must be collected in order to resolve this issue. The exact name and location of the affected convolutions must be specified, and if the lesion is very extensive the point, or, rather, the convolution where the disease

process began must be determined, as far as possible, by anatomical examination.

5. The lesion in the present case originated in the second or third frontal convolution, probably in the latter. Thus, the faculty of articulate speech may be located within one or the other of these convolutions. But the question is still unresolved, inasmuch as previous authors do not comment on the state of particular convolutions; and one cannot even make an educated guess, since the principle of localization by convolution has not yet been firmly established.

6. At all events, one need only compare the present case with those previously reported in order to dismiss the notion that the faculty of articulate speech resides at a fixed point or is located under some bump on the skull. Lesions associated with aphemia have been found most often in the most anterior reaches of the frontal lobe, not far from the brow and above the roof of the orbit, whereas the lesions in my case are much more posterior, closer to the coronal suture than to the superciliary arch. This discrepancy cannot be reconciled by any system of bumps; it can, on the other hand, be explained within the context of localization by convolution, since each of the three major convolutions of the superior aspect of the frontal lobe courses in its anterior-posterior extent through all of the regions where, to date, the lesions producing aphemia have been found.

NOTES

1. Such is not the case when a softening begins in the convolutional white matter; only when a lesion begins beneath the pia mater, that is to say, within the cortical layer, is the softened and slowly resorbed brain substance replaced by serum. I have observed the various stages of this process in the cerebellum as well as in the cerebrum. The first specimen that I collected (presented to the Anatomical Society in January 1861) perplexed me initially, but several others have since satisfied my doubts.

2. To ensure comprehension of what follows I shall briefly review here the arrangement and relations of the cerebral organs which figure in the discussion.

   The frontal lobe includes that portion of the hemisphere which lies above the Sylvian fissure and in front of the Rolandic sulcus; the Sylvian fissure separates the frontal lobe from the temporal-sphenoidal lobe, and the Rolandic sulcus separates it from the parietal lobe. The position of the Rolandic sulcus is specified in an earlier note. Its orientation is nearly transverse; from the midline it courses in a straight line with a minimum of meanders and ends below just short of the Sylvian fissure, which it approaches at nearly a right angle behind the posterior border of the *insula*.

   The frontal lobe is made up of two *tiers*: an inferior orbital tier formed by several *orbital* convolutions, which rest on the orbital roof (and about which I shall have nothing further to say), and a superior tier located beneath the squama of the frontal bone and the most anterior part of the parietal bone.

The upper tier consists of four primary convolutions, the *frontal convolutions* proper: one posterior and the other three anterior. The posterior frontal convolution, which is not very flexuous, forms the anterior border of the Rolandic sulcus and is, therefore, nearly transverse. It ascends from without inward, from the Sylvian fissure to the great longitudinal fissure, which contains the falx cerebri; hence, it may be designated alternately as the *posterior, transverse,* or *ascending frontal convolution.* The other three convolutions of the superior tier are extremely tortuous and very complex, and a certain amount of practice is required in order to distinguish them throughout their length, to avoid confusing the primary sulci that separate convolutions with the secondary sulci that separate second-order gyri; the latter are subject to individual variation according to the degree of complexity, i.e., according to the degree of primary convolutional development. These three frontal convolutions are oriented antero-posteriorly and, coursing side by side, run the entire length of the frontal lobe from front to back. They begin at the level of the superciliary arch, where they make a bend in order to join up with the convolutions of the inferior tier, and end posteriorly at the transverse frontal convolution, into which all three merge. They are known as the *first, second,* and *third frontal convolutions;* though one may still refer to them as *internal, middle,* and *external,* the ordinal names have gained acceptance.

The *first frontal convolution* skirts the great longitudinal fissure. In man a constant more or less continuous antero-posterior sulcus divides the convolution into two second-order gyri. The convolution is thus subdivided into two convolutions, but comparative anatomy teaches us that the two gyri form only a single basic convolution.

The *second frontal convolution* does not present any special features. Such is not the case with the *third,* which is the most external. It presents a superior (internal) border, which is adjacent to the undulating border of the middle convolution, and an inferior (external) border, the relations of which differ according as one examines them anteriorly or posteriorly. In front, the inferior border is in contact with the external border of the most external of the orbital convolutions; behind, it lies free, separated from the temporal-sphenoidal lobe by the Sylvian fissure (of which it forms the superior rim). Because of this latter relationship, the third frontal convolution is sometimes called the *superior marginal convolution.*

I might add that the inferior rim of the Sylvian fissure is formed by the superior convolution of the temporal-sphenoidal lobe, which, in consequence, is called the *inferior marginal convolution.* This thin, nearly rectilinear gyrus, which courses antero-posteriorly, is separated from the second temporal-sphenoidal convolution by a fissure that runs parallel to the Sylvian fissure, designated the *parallel fissure* (the implication being that it is parallel *to the Sylvian fissure*).

To conclude, if one separates the two marginal convolutions (superior and inferior) of the Sylvian fissure, one exposes a broad sloping eminence, the summit of which gives rise to five short, simple convolutions—or rather, to five rectilinear gyri arranged in the shape of a fan. This is the *insular lobe,* which overlies the extraventricular nucleus of the corpus striatum; arising in the depths of the Sylvian fissure, its cortex is continuous with that of the deepest parts of the two marginal convolutions, its medullary substance with that of the extraventricular nucleus of the corpus striatum. As a result of these relationships, a lesion which spreads from the frontal lobe to the temporal-sphenoidal lobe—or in the reverse direction—almost invariably traverses the *insula* and is likely to spread from there to the extraventricular nucleus of the corpus striatum, inasmuch as the insular gyri (which separate this nucleus from the surface of the brain) are quite thin.

The Symptoms Produced by Lesions Of the Transitional Area Between the Inferior Parietal and Middle Occipital Gyri[1]

The Syndrome: Finger Agnosia, Right-Left Confusion, Agraphia, Acalculia

J. GERSTMANN

DURING THE PAST YEARS Pötzl published a number of articles describing approaches to the localization of circumscribed lesions of the parietal-occipital convexity. He emphasized (as was theoretically expected) that localization of lesions in the parieto-occipital cortex depends on the major symptoms that appear. The nature of these symptoms differs from one case to another, reflecting variations in the areas involved. I trust that the reader is aware of Pötzl's work on the anatomy and connections in this region.

I will discuss "finger agnosia"—a subject I described several years ago (1924).[2] This symptom complex includes the inability to recognize, name, and select individual fingers of both hands. This difficulty may apply to both the patient's and the examiner's fingers. As a result of this

NOTE: Translated by C.N. Hochberg from: Gerstmann, J., "Zur Symptomatologie der Hirnläsionen im Übergangsgebiet der unteren Parietal- und mittleren Occipitalwindung (Das Syndrom: Fingeragnosie, Rechts-Links-Störung, Agraphie, Akalkulie," *Nervenartzt* (1930), 691–95.

abnormality there is an apraxia (lack of facility of individual movements and difficulty with coordinated movements) which is associated with right-left disorientation (for right and left sides of the patient and examiner), agraphia, and acalculia of varying severity.[3] These features are the basis of a well circumscribed neuropathologic syndrome. This syndrome stems from a focal lesion in the area of the parieto-occipital convexity. Pötzl and Herrmann localized this to the transitional area between the inferior parietal (angular) and middle occipital gyri.

Since my first observation and description of this syndrome (finger agnosia, right-left disorientation, agraphia, and acalculia) I have seen many cases with the same findings—either alone or, more seldom, as part of the residua of a more complex neurologic state.[4] My review of the literature indicates that this syndrome is not at all rare.

In my experience the syndrome appears in a characteristic manner. The patients were all physically and intellectually sound, or at best only slightly impaired; aphasia, apraxia, agnosia, or other similar (general) disturbances, which could have been attributed to the symptom complex, were not recognized or were absent during the period of observation. The other symptoms seen in conjunction with the syndrome (such as hemianopia or hemiamblyopia, absence of opticokinetic nystagmus, amnesic dysphasia, impaired ability to read, disturbed color recognition, dyspraxia, disturbed balance) can be classified as distinct from the syndrome, as they occurred only occasionally and were of minor significance. The finger agnosia, always present as a limited disturbance of the recognition and orientation of the fingers of both hands (patient's and examiner's) along with right-left disorientation, is often associated with loss of facility of practic functions (innovatory-practical functions).[5] The patient remains able to recognize and orient other parts of his body. The association of finger agnosia with agraphia and acalculia is comprehensible if one remembers the important role that the individual fingers and right-left discrimination play in the development of the skills of writing and calculation.

My observations indicate that finger agnosia should only appear with agraphia and acalculia and the associated right-left disorientation. This is to say that I have never found finger agnosia to be associated with other disturbances of writing or calculation (as are associated with the complex aphasia or apractic syndromes). This does not mean that every case shows agraphia and acalculia associated with finger agnosia and right-left disorientation. (Although the appearance of these together is most often the case.) It should be emphasized that one should always test for the appearance of finger agnosia and right-left disorientation in cases of isolated writing and calculation disturbance.[6] The proof that my observations of finger agnosia, right-left disorientation, agraphia, and acalculia form a syndrome comes from the work of Pötzl and

Herrmann,[7] Schilder,[8] Kroll,[9] and Johannes Lange.[10] Pötzl and Herrmann performed an autopsy on a patient with a well-localized tumor and showed that the syndrome of finger agnosia and agraphia correlated with a lesion in the transitional area between the inferior parietal (angular) and middle occipital gyri.

After my initial case with finger agnosia I felt that the lesion was most localized in the left inferior temporal lobe, namely in the angular gyrus. I was unable to prove this on account of the insufficient anatomic evidence. Since the symptoms of my cases were extremely similar to those of Pötzl's and Herrmann's autopsied tumor cases, I assume that they had similarly localized lesions. The findings of Pötzl and Herrmann have been confirmed by two additional autopsies of patients I had seen along with a case seen by Lange (which had the complete syndrome: finger agnosia, right-left disorientation, agraphia, and acalculia). This latter case provided concrete proof. One of my cases had a glioma diffusely involving the parieto-occipital convexity and extending into all of the transitional area between the angular and the middle occipital gyri. My second case was a several-month-old cortical lesion which involved the same transitional region.[11] The onset of this lesion coincided with the onset of the symptom complex discussed in this paper.

The same area of involvement (although more extensive) was found in Lange's autopsied case (lesion in the transitional zone of the angular and middle occipital gyri). The frequent simultaneous expression of the characteristic parts of this syndrome suggests that they are related not only in terms of localization but, also, in terms of pathophysiology and psychopathology. It is possible that this syndrome, in addition to involving a distinct area, produces symptoms which share a common functional disturbance. Recently, Lange tried to determine which of the disturbances was the fundamental one. He concluded that the basic defect might be in the "conceptual and creative organization of space," involving direction in space and spatial interrelationships (as a function of direction). He postulated that the entire syndrome did not represent a completely physical disturbance (i.e., hemiparesis) but, rather, a functional disturbance (i.e., psychologic). After having reviewed Lange's research, I have to agree with many of his impressive explanations. It is impossible to say that his explanation of the basis for the syndrome is the only possible one. Many other options still exist. It is certain that Lange's work will stimulate interest in the psychopathology and pathophysiology as well as the anatomic localization of the syndrome.

I have already mentioned that the syndrome finger agnosia, right-left disorientation, agraphia, and acalculia appears more frequently as the primary disturbance but can also occur as the residua of a more complex brain lesion. (This observation is of importance in view of the subject of this meeting.) One of my patients, following a stroke, developed an extensive sensory or pseudosensory aphasia along with parietal or parieto-occipital symptoms, which dominated the clinical picture. Following the gradual disappearance of the sensory aphasia, and despite the rather extensive recovery of reading ability, the syndrome of agraphia-acalculia became evident and remained as a residual defect. The syndrome persisted along with a right-sided hemianopia, which had been present since the initial stroke. In addition, I have seen the syndrome in question develop after being disguised as tactile agnosia, apraxia, alexia, and color agnosia. Obviously, the direct or indirect appearance of the syndrome depends on the degree of involvement of the transitional zone in comparison to other areas. Involvement of the transitional zone between the angular and the middle occipital gyri is mandatory for the development of the syndrome. The more localized the lesion is to this transitional area, the more likely the syndrome will appear as a more localized finding. The more extensive the lesion, the more likely the more subtle findings of finger agnosia and right-left disorientation will be hidden, only to become evident upon the disappearance of the more serious defects.

It should be emphasized that with the exception of the tumor case of Pötzl and Herrmann, which revealed a lesion in the right parieto-occipital transitional zone, all of my cases (as well as those of others) which demonstrated finger agnosia, right-left disorientation, agraphia, and acalculia showed lesions localized to the left side. Of some interest is the fact that the patient of Pötzl and Herrmann not only had a tumor which might have affected the contralateral side, but was, in addition, ambidextrous. These facts explain the exceptional findings in that case. It appears that the findings of finger agnosia and right-left disorientation are related to left hemispheric lesions in right-handed persons.

In conclusion, I would like to direct attention to the value of knowing this syndrome (finger agnosia, right-left disorientation as the dominant symptoms) as a means of localizing lesions in the parieto-occipital area. Pötzl and Herrmann used the occurrence of the syndrome in their tumor case to localize the lesion (to the transitional zone of the angular gyrus and middle occipital gyrus) for surgical intervention. This localization has since been proved by both autopsy and surgery. I will conclude by stating that the depicted observations are worthy of further analysis and our pathologic observations suitable for further study.

NOTES

1. Speech given at the 20th annual conference of the German Neurologic Association on September 18–20, 1930. Dresden.
2. Fingeragnosia. *Wien. Klin. Wschr.*, 1924, No. 40.

3. Fingeragnosia and Isolated Agraphia. *Z. Neur.* 108 (1927).

4. Patients with this symptom are incapable of selecting individual fingers of both hands, although they are aware of this defect and able to see.

5. In the past I have stated that the finger agnosia accompanied by right-left disorientation is directly related to changing the relationship between spatial sense and body sense. I have chosen this way of explanation to support the understanding of this disturbance. I have explained this approach in *Z. Neur.* 108.

6. For the authors who do not believe there is a difference between this isolated agraphia and acalculia associated with finger agnosia and *any* general disturbance of writing and calculation in other conditions, I would like to emphasize that I use the former terms in a special sense. These special forms of agraphia and acalculia only accompany finger agnosia.

7. *Über die Agraphie und ihre lokaldiagnostischen Beziehungen,* Berlin: S. Karger, 1926. *Mschr. Psychiatr.* 70, 1928.

8. *Z. Neur.* 113 1928 (gemeinsam mit Isakower).

9. *Die neuropathologischen Syndrome,* Berlin: Julius Springer, 1929.

10. Fingeragnosie und Agraphie. *Mschr. Psychiatr.* 76 1930.

11. Near this old walnut-size lesion in the left parieto-occipital region were two fresh right hemispheric areas of softening; a smaller one was near the base of the occipital lobe extending 4 cm forwards. The second lesion was a 4-cm long (anterior-posterior extent) hemorrhage in the inferolateral frontal lobe. These two foci do not provide data as to the localization of the syndrome of finger agnosia, agraphia, etc., as they occurred on top of the well-developed syndrome (of finger agnosia, agraphia, etc.) and resulted in the occurrence of *new* common and local clinical signs which partially disguised the syndrome.

The Syndrome of Apraxia (Motor Asymboly) Based on a Case of Unilateral Apraxia

H. LIEPMANN

THE CASE upon which the following discourse is based is so extraordinary that I believe a detailed case report does not require any further justification.

So far as I know, it has not yet been observed—or at least not yet reported—that a human being might act with his right extremities as if he were a total imbecile, as if he understood neither questions nor commands, as if he could neither understand the value of objects nor the sense of printed or written words, yet prove by an intelligent use of his left extremities that all of those seemingly absent abilities were in reality present.

I would not consider it permissible to draw the conclusion that such a case has never before occurred.

It would be an error to assume that the condition which was eventually recognized was conspicuous at the outset. On the contrary, for reasons to be given below, the essence of the disease was hidden in such a way that it was recognized only after two and a half months. The patient gave the impression of being a severely demented sensory aphasic, and his appearance furthered this impression. No other diagnosis was considered by the various physicians who had observed him previously. In one hospital in Berlin, where he was treated for seven weeks, the

NOTE: Translated by W. H. O. Bohne, K. Liepmann, and D. A. Rottenberg from: *Monatschrift für Psychiatrie und Neurologie* 8, 15–44, 1900.

diagnosis was "mixed aphasia and dementia following apoplexy." The commission paper with which he was admitted into the Dalldorf Institute read "aphasia and mental derangement."

A long time elapsed before the difference between his right and left hands was discovered because the patient preferentially used his apractic right hand.

Beginning with a certain set of questions which derived from my experience with the asymbolic syndrome, I forced the patient to use his left arm by holding on to his right arm. Thus, the essence of the disturbance became apparent. By taking advantage of a peculiarity of the patient's illness it was possible to establish a system of communication, and the patient's mental state was thereby unveiled in a stepwise fashion.

Before I pass on to the various examinations performed, I should like to provide the previous medical history.

PAST MEDICAL HISTORY

Mr. T., a forty-eight-year-old senior civil servant in one of the Reich's government agencies, suffered from vertigo and fainting spells since the summer of 1899. He complained frequently of occipital headaches, could no longer follow discussions, and could not master his work. While conversing he would often stop talking, mispronounce words and lose his train of thought. One day he wrote *Brunne Rstr.* instead of *Brunnenstr.* and did this several times in a row, although he noticed the mistake and laughed at it. His memory fell off, and he began to lose his way. The morning of December 2, 1899, the patient walked towards the bathroom, turned around and sat down on his wife's bed. As he looked distraught, she asked him if anything were the matter. He replied, "Nothing, nothing" and answered all further questions with "yes, yes." Shortly thereafter he fell down. He was fully conscious when he was picked up but could stand only with support. This inability to stand or walk without support was supposed to have persisted for several days. He was put to bed. He sat in front of his food without knowing what to do and, consequently, had to be fed. According to his wife, he was "anxious, moved his head, opened his eyes widely, and made snapping movements with his mouth," but he could move his arms and legs normally. His wife stated further that he repeatedly used his right hand to bring down his left hand, which he would raise to scratch the back of his neck. (See below for an explanation of this statement.)

We have these further statements about the patient's prior medical history: His family is healthy, as was he except for an inguinal hernia, which he acquired in 1874, and syphilis, which he contracted in the early

'80s. He drank as much "as is customary in society." He married in 1886. In that year his wife was treated with mercury for syphilis. A macerated child was stillborn in 1887. His wife subsequently had a miscarriage in the third month of pregnancy. A girl, the product of a full-term pregnancy, died at fifteen weeks of age after an episode of projectile vomiting. A boy, born in 1895 following a breech delivery, suffers from congenital weakness of the left arm but is otherwise healthy.

When the patient was at university he fenced with his right hand. He also wrote and ate with his right hand. However, he is reported to have used his left hand when playing cards.

Two years ago he had a bladder ailment and was unable to hold his water.

Since all communication with the patient was impossible—he continued unable to speak and remained helpless and, at times, violent—he was taken to the medical division of a general hospital on December 7, 1899. The preliminary report reads "paralysis of the arms" (which was vehemently denied by the patient's wife when she spoke with me).

I excerpted the following from the record of that hospital: "State of almost complete imbecility." Faculties of speech and writing lost, except for a few indistinct words. Does not understand the sense of most questions. "Has completely forgotten how to write." Lies quietly and listlessly in bed without participating; protracted sobbing after his wife's visits. Is incontinent of urine and feces. Left-sided facial paresis, otherwise no signs of paralysis.

The urine contains 1 1/2 percent sugar, no protein.

Four weeks later, on January 8, 1900, considerable improvement is noted. At times the patient cries and sobs a great deal; at other times he appears restless and paces back and forth. For several days he bowed deeply each time anyone approached his bed. He says only "Yes" and "Alas." Once, when excited, he said "Blast." Sometimes he seems to understand and chooses correctly among objects put before him; at other times he makes the wrong choice.

A further entry: His gait is no longer disturbed (there was no previous mention of a gait disturbance). "Can also move both arms quite well." Knee-jerks very weak. Sugar 2 percent.

January 13, 1900. He can now write his name, though he drops some of the letters. He cannot, however, copy either writing or designs. Instead he draws a few M-strokes or curlicues. His comprehension fluctuates. He has learned to write the word "Messer" (knife).

Since then this word flows from his pen whenever he writes. When asked to sign a salary receipt the distraught patient produced the word "knife" though attempting to write his name. "He seems to comprehend nothing of what he reads." Several times he is said to have pronounced single words correctly. "The patient appears to be hallucinating at times; he cries a great deal and looks anxiously in a certain direction."

On January 30, 1900, he moved about the corridor anxiously, weeping, and attempted to escape in the evening. At about eight o'clock in the evening he was found wandering aimlessly in the streets. He was discharged the following day at his wife's request.

The diagnosis was: apoplexy, mixed aphasia, dementia.

Ten days later he was admitted to the Mental Hospital at Dalldorf with a certificate. According to the latter, the initial "mild paralysis of both sides of his body has resolved." "Only the right (undoubtedly a mistake for the "left") side of the face remains slightly paretic; the (?) left arm is also weak." "He seems to understand questions most of the time but does not react to them." Completely unable to answer them.

He is intermittently excited, can not find his way around his own apartment, searches everywhere, and hides objects.

"Mentally disabled as a result of apoplexy, aphasia," etc.

GENERAL FINDINGS IN DALLDORF

February 10, 1900, in Dalldorf. At first he was very restless, especially at night; he got out of bed frequently, ran through all the rooms and wept, but could be led back to bed. He quieted down after two days.

On February 11 it was noted: he wipes his face with the (toilet) paper handed to him after he moves his bowels. He urinates in the corner of the room when he cannot find the chamber pot right away.

On February 12 a salve was prescribed (3 grams per day), also 3 grams of potassium iodide. The latter was discontinued on the 14th, as the patient suffered "an anxiety attack with considerable dyspnea, acceleration and irregularity of the pulse, iodine acne and conjunctivitis."

It should be noted that a similar attack occurred eight days after potassium iodide was reinstituted. Some time after the final discontinuation of the medication on March 6 yet another attack occurred, during which the patient lay rigid in bed and failed to react when spoken to. The fingers of the left hand and the toes of the left foot were observed to twitch. The pupillary light reaction was intact. Both globes were turned to the left.

On March 17 he had an attack without twitching: duration about 15 minutes; severe dyspnea, flushed facies, signs of obstruction.

The sugar varied between 2 and 3 percent.

I would like to record some of the physical findings noted at that time: drooping of the left corner of the mouth, flattening of the left nasolabial fold, stronger innervation of the right orbicularis orus, left pupil slightly larger than the right (both react promptly and fully to light and convergence), full extraocular movements. Gait unremarkable, slight swaying with the eyes closed, grossly normal strength in the lower extremities as far as one can determine.

Patellar reflexes brisk bilaterally.
Hand grip and arm movements seem to be stronger on the left side.
Radial artery not rigid; pulse irregular, rapid (92).
Cardiac dullness normal, heart sounds clear.
Irreducible right inguinal hernia.

I saw the patient for the first time on February 17. He was asked to point at certain objects placed before him and to carry out certain hand movements. He failed in almost everything, handling objects quite absurdly. At first sight it appeared as if the patient did not understand—that he was cerebrally deaf, possibly also cerebrally blind. However, I noticed certain bizarre and distorted movements which he made during the course of the examination; they were confined to the right upper extremity, which the patient used exclusively during the period of observation. This peculiar motor behavior made me wonder if his incorrect responses reflected a basic lack of comprehension (of auditory-verbal or visual-object impressions), or whether these responses related, rather, to faulty motor execution. Arguing against the total absence of speech comprehension was the fact that the patient promptly obeyed commands which he could carry out using the entire body, such as getting up, walking to the window, and walking to the door. To resolve the question I held on to the patient's right hand and forced him to use his left hand. Now, all of a sudden, the picture changed. With his left hand he immediately selected the card that was asked for from among five cards set out before him. His performance with the right hand led in general to faulty responses. I immediately established that the situation was the same as regards the lower extremities. The patient could imitate movements of my foot with his left foot but failed altogether with his right foot. It was established, therefore, that the patient was neither cerebrally deaf nor cerebrally blind.

An examination of his reading and writing ability pointed in the same direction. Thus, a firm basis was provided for the contention that the patient's faulty behavior did not result from faulty comprehension but, rather, from a disturbance in his control of motor communication; more specifically, it was the consequence of a localized disturbance restricted to the right side of the body. The revelation that the patient's left side was intact yielded the key to his inner life. A means of communication was thereby established, and the seeming imbecile was enabled to display a relatively rich intelligence.

One could certainly deduce solely from the above that the patient suffered from a right-sided apraxia in the usual, general sense of the word. Apraxia is used in the sense of inability to use objects correctly. In this general sense the term does not specify why the use of objects is faulty. To the best of my knowledge, the cases of severe apraxia which have been reported to date always exhibited faulty object recognition, i.e., the collective effects of mind blindness (visual agnosia), tactile paralysis, etc. In these cases the apraxia was produced secondarily by another disturbance. If the above supposition is correct—namely, that my patient is not apractic because of a disturbance of receptive functions but, rather, because the motor components of his acts are themselves disturbed—then he is apractic in a narrower and stricter sense of the word. One would then have a disease for which the term apraxia ought to be exclusively reserved, or for which, at least, the term should be further qualified by the addition of the word "motor" (apraxia).

The following discourse sets out to prove that such a syndrome exists as a pure entity, that my patient is apractic in the strict sense of the word, and, more specifically, that he is unilaterally apractic. This very unilaterality makes it possible in our case to ascertain the nature of the disease. A bilaterally apractic patient would naturally be deprived of the proper use of the musculature subserving speech and would have no means of communicating that he understands or comprehends correctly; he could hardly be distinguished from the patient with sensory apraxia.

It will appear that the syndrome under discussion here lends reality to Meynert's notion of a disease first described by Wernicke. On page 270 of his lectures on psychiatry, Meynert refers to "motor asymboly, which will betray itself by the patient's being unable to make use of objects." The case which Meynert adduces in support of this theoretical construct is, however, unsatisfactory, as I shall discuss further. I shall deal with the terms apraxia, asymboly, etc. in greater detail below.

This stricter definition of apraxia closely approximates the literal meaning of the word. Apraxia is, in short, the inability to act, i.e., to move the moveable parts of the body in a purposeful manner, though motility is preserved. There is no reason to draw a sharp distinction between apraxia and parapraxia. For the "a-" does not negate the movement but, rather, the purpose, which two concepts are contained in the verb "to act." Thus, the notion of falsity, counterproductivity, is conveyed by the word apraxia itself. But one might give the name parapraxia to those forms of apraxia in which the characteristics of purposeful movement have not been completely lost, in which elements of a purposeful movement or actions resembling purposeful movements remain (though they do not correspond to the intended purpose).

A patient who is unable to move is, therefore, not apractic. If a specific statement is required, apraxia presupposes that the ability to move is preserved. Several authors have used the expression "soul paralysis" to describe patients who in the absence of paralysis in the strict sense (a mono- or hemiplegia) have lost, or nearly lost, the ability to move an extremity or, alternately, who cannot move an extremity under certain circumstances (e.g., when the eyes are closed). Hence, soul paralysis and apraxia are two different things. The relationship between these two conditions will be discussed below.

A scrutiny of the collective results of various examinations and the exclusion of certain other possible explanations are necessary in order to ascertain that the present case is really an example of "motor" apraxia, that is, of apraxia in the strict sense. Moreover, such a scrutiny will allow us to penetrate more deeply into the character of the disease and to open it up to our understanding.

DETAILED DESCRIPTION OF THE SYNDROME

Since the symptoms and signs of his disease have remained qualitatively the same and have only changed quantitatively, insofar as the disturbance has, on the whole, tended to remit, I shall integrate the findings of various examinations into a single description which corresponds, in the main, to the most florid state of the disease, rather than presenting a chronological account of the patient's illness. Changes which occurred subsequently will be summarized later in a short description of his current status.

The patient gives the impression of a man in his fifties. His hair is grey, his face flushed, and his eyes moist. He strides briskly into the room. He replies to your greeting with a bow. To the question "How are you?" he either smiles affably and says "Yes, yes" or appears moved. His weeping, which occurs frequently when he is asked about his health, is peculiar. The tears stream from his eyes; he sobs without his facial musculature becoming fully involved in the act of crying. His facial expression does not, however, remain unchanged but facial movement lags behind the sobs and tears.

"How old are you?" Stands up, bows, does not answer. "What is your name?" Shows signs of anxiety, says "Yes, oh my God." "Are you married?" "Yes." "Are you a bachelor?" "Yes." (Then with signs of anger) "Oh, well."

Speech function: Further questioning reveals that the patient suffers from motor aphasia. He has never answered a question or spoken spontaneously since coming to Dalldorf. The only exception, during the period of remission, will be discussed below. The only articulated sounds which he produced were: "Yes"; "Yes, indeed"; "Alas"; "Oh, my God"; "Oh, God, yes"; "Ow"; and "Nay." He cannot imitate any sounds except, occasionally, "a." When asked to repeat words spoken by the examiner he behaves rather oddly. He bows and bows again, turns his wide-open eyes upwards, nods, and now and again makes snapping movements. Once, instead of repeating words, he repeatedly gave the examiner a box of matches that was lying in front of him.

The fact that speech comprehension was preserved was so certain and apparent from subsequent examinations that special tests do not have to be reported here.

The patient had been labeled "letter blind" [sic]. This appeared to be the case simply because he could neither read aloud, owing to his motor aphasia, nor carry out written commands with his right side. But with his left hand he even carried out commands written in a foreign language. March 1, 1900: The written command "Donnez le chapeau" is carried out promptly after a short delay (with left hand). It is true that he does not follow longer written commands but, instead, manipulates the piece of paper. When he is told, "Point at the thing written down here," and the name of an object lying on the table is written down, he solves the problem without exception as soon as he is forced to use his left hand.

His reading comprehension is, thus, limited to simple phrases and is not adequate for sentences of any length. In this respect it must be termed restricted. See below as regards his writing ability.

Movements to spoken command: The patient is asked to stick out his tongue. He throws back his head, opens his eyes widely, opens his mouth, and makes snapping movements with his jaw.

He is requested more insistently to put out his tongue. Instead of obeying the command he moves the remainder of his body more vigorously. He draws himself up in military fashion, nods his head repeatedly, bows, and says, "Yes." I should like to note here that the unilaterality of the patient's apraxia, i.e., his inability to employ voluntary muscles purposefully, does not apply to the head; movements of the entire head, movements of the tongue, and movements of the facial musculature are, if apractic at all, bilaterally apractic.

Ocular motility was always completely preserved. It is true that during the first two days of the examination he had much more difficulty moving his eyes to the right on command than to the left. Since, however, this asymmetry was no longer present later in his course, I consider it sufficient merely to mention the earlier observation. Subsequently he was able to carry out all eye movements on command. But eye movements often occurred when something else was requested. It was repeatedly observed that he looked upward when faced with other tasks.

He is asked to sit down. This command must usually be repeated before he obeys.

"Point to your nose, sir."

Once again the military posture, the head nodding, and the repeated bows. The fingers of the right hand perform vigorous ab- and adduction movements; however, the hand is not raised.

"Point to your nose!"

The patient says "Yes" and waves his hand through the air while continually spreading his fingers.

Now the right hand is restrained and the request repeated. He immediately raises his left index finger to his nose while the restrained right hand is engaged in lively but unrelated movements.

"Can't you do the same thing now with your right hand?"

The same game begins again. Bewildered, the patient innervates one muscle after another. During the entire period of observation he never correctly performed this task. The same holds true for the other parts of his face. He cannot carry out these reflexive movements, that is, movements directed towards parts of his own body, not even when they have been performed passively two or three times with his own arm (in contrast to the patient described by Bruns as a case of "soul paralysis," to be discussed below). Even standing in front of a mirror does not alter this behavior.

He cannot usually reach other parts of his body either, when asked to do so; for instance (March 1, 1900): "Point to your left hand with your right hand" (after he had previously done the reverse). He nods his head, says "Yes" and picks up the inkwell in front of him.

"Touch your left sleeve."

Says "Yes," bows, and pushes the inkwell back a little.

"Your left sleeve."

Bows, looks toward the ceiling, and makes a gesture of embarrassment. With his eyes open he occasionally succeeds in pointing to his right knee with his right hand; with his eyes closed, never.

"Put your left hand on top of your right hand."

He does it.

"Now, you should be able to put your right hand on top of your left hand."

Nodding his head, he correctly moves the right hand towards the left hand; instead of putting the one on top of the other, however, he folds his right into his left, the latter remaining passive. He even fails when the body part to be indicated is touched, for instance, the nose, and he is told "here."

In the course of the examination he twice succeeded in pointing to my hand. With his right hand he also succeeded twice in removing my pince-nez on command, once even putting it on his own nose. When asked to repeat this performance immediately afterwards, he turned around instead and looked toward the wall.

"Clench your right hand into a fist." Does not succeed, makes incorrect movements of trunk and arm. "With the left one." Immediately executed.

In the same way he is unable to make threatening gestures or thumb his nose. He does both promptly with his left hand.

"Put on your hat." He does this correctly with the right hand. "Take it off with your right hand." Complete confusion. "With your left hand." This is accomplished.

"Point to my necktie." Despite encouragement six times in a row, this proves impossible. "With the left." Immediately carried out.

Imitation of movements: Instead of verbal requests, he is now asked to imitate movements made by the examiner. He cannot imitate any movement with either side of his face, nor can he protrude his tongue in imitation of the examiner. The examiner stands in front of him and executes some simple movements with both arms. The patient's left arm imitates everything correctly, the right arm performs completely different movements or none at all, again with frequent spreading of the fingers when movements of the entire arm are requested. Clenching a fist, threatening gestures, and reflexive movements are just as poorly imitated with the right hand.

This deficit, also, remained constant. To exclude the influence of a possible hemianopia or unilateral cerebral blindness, all movements are carried out first in the right, then in the left visual field. The result remains the same.

The legs function in exactly the same manner. The left leg correctly imitates flexion and extension of the knee, lateral movements, and toe tapping; the right leg performs incorrectly or not at all. In the latter case, the frequently observed military posture of his.

Sound-directed movements: A bell is rung near his head, and he is asked to point to it. He is completely unable to localize the sound with his right hand.

Touch-directed movements and the coordination of movements with tactile stimuli: I tickle the patient's right external auditory canal with cotton. He reacts by shaking his head slightly and smiling but does not use his right hand to ward off the stimulus or scratch himself. The same stimulus applied to the left external auditory canal immediately brings the left hand up to the ear. I repeated this maneuver on both sides ten times with the same result; never once did the patient bring his right hand up to his ear. He elevated the right hand only once, without, however, bringing it up to the area stimulated. With his right hand he is unable to reach and remove a pin stuck in his right thigh though requested to do so (see below regarding the question of sensitivity and localization).

Spontaneous movements are discussed repeatedly below without regard to the stimulus initiating or directing movement, so that I need not consider them here. For the present I shall disregard the initial stimulus as a classifying principle and, instead, characterize the patient's performance in relation to a number of complicated tasks, without considering the nature of the external or the internal stimuli.

Response to choice: One frequently performed test was primarily designed to determine if the patient was able to recognize objects.

February 20. Five objects are placed on the table in front of the patient: a pencil, the King of Diamonds, a cigar, a watch, and a ring with keys.

Testing the right hand: "Point to the keys." The patient picks up the cigar even before the word "keys" is spoken. He is told to take his time and not to rush. He says, "Oh, God, yes" and nods. "Point to the keys." Again he picks up the cigar. "The keys." Puts down the cigar, picks up the keys, puts them to the right of the cigar. He bows after nearly every request.

"Point to the King of Diamonds." "Yes." Picks it up and puts it to the side.

"The cigar." He picks up the watch and puts it next to the cigar. "The cigar." He picks up the playing card, which is now next to the keys, and puts it on the other side of the cigar. Then he picks up the cigar.

"Give me the King of Diamonds." He hands over the keys. "The King of Diamonds." Gives the cigar. "The King of Diamonds." Now he gives the playing card.

"The cigar." He hands over the cigar. "The keys." Again he picks up the cigar.

The following remarkable response recurred rather frequently during numerous tests of this kind. Instead of the cigar, he first hands over the keys, then the watch, and, while still holding the watch in his right hand, he hands over the cigar with his left hand. Thus, he frequently picks up the correct object with his left hand while still fumbling around perplexedly among the wrong objects with his right hand.

Later, when his condition had improved, he only made mistakes when a large number of objects was offered to choose from. In the beginning he usually repeated the above-mentioned behavior, namely, picking up any one of the objects lying in front of him even before the request had been completed, apparently without any deliberation, taking his chances. Once, after practicing for half an hour, he succeeded in picking up the correct object with his right hand ten times in a row.

On February 23 he was asked to choose from among ten objects. With his right hand he picked up the correct object one-third of the time; two-thirds of the time he did not succeed at all or he succeeded only after having pointed to as many as three incorrect objects. After an incorrect response he usually had to be encouraged to try again. Only later did he begin to be dissatisfied with incorrect responses and continue his search spontaneously.

When he was allowed to choose with his left hand, he almost always picked up the correct object forthwith. Only on certain days, when he was distracted or tired, did he make occasional mistakes.

On February 23 he picked up the watch instead of the keys with his right hand. He then immediately handed me the keys with his left hand. "Surely you can now hand me the same object with your right hand." Even then he frequently failed. If, however, his left index finger was still touching the object being requested, he was usually able to pick it up with his right hand. Similarly, it happened repeatedly that while the right hand was searching in vain for an object the left hand grasped for it; if the right hand picked it up before the left hand reached it, both hands together pushed it toward the examiner.

These tests reveal several extraordinary features of the patient's responses: (1) his precipitous reaction to the command before the essential part of it was verbalized; (2) the fact that he was usually satisfied with his incorrect responses. Only in a minority of cases, especially when his mistake was pointed out to him, did he display embarrassment through a gesture of dissatisfaction or indicate with a sigh that he perceived his error.

The possibility that he had not understood the request seemed excluded by the fact that he responded correctly with his left hand. Did he, perhaps, understand the request only when his right hemisphere began to function, i.e., when he began using his left hand? Arguing against this is the fact that it was not necessary to repeat the command in order for him to respond correctly with his left hand after he had failed with his right hand. It was sufficient to say "Do it with the left." Accordingly, it was indisputably proven that he had understood the command when it was first given.

Was he, perhaps, cerebrally blind? Did he fail to recognize the objects placed before him? Yet he did recognize them when he used his left hand.

That he did recognize objects was also demonstrated in another manner.

February 27. Objects were placed in his right hand and he was asked "Is this such and such?" If one were to accept a nod as "yes" or a shake of the head as "no," one would have to assume that he did not recognize them. However, the reliability of his gestures had already become suspect. He was advised, therefore, to signify "yes" by making a plus sign with his left hand, "no" by a minus sign. It soon became apparent that he recognized all objects, and, at the same time, he was shown to be amimic or paramimic; his nodding did not signify assent, nor did shaking his head signify negation.

In this way he also made it clear that he recognized the incorrect responses made by his right hand. However, he never volunteered this information but admitted his errors only after being urged to do so, when asked, "Is this really the object in question?"

In an attempt to find another means of communication the patient was asked to signify "yes" by raising his left arm and "no" by stamping his left foot. This method was not as dependable as the above. He was usually correct, but not always.

Hemianopia and unilateral cerebral blindness could be unequivocally excluded, as will be reported more fully below. Tactile paralysis, that is, the inability to recognize objects by touch, could not be excluded by his correct left-sided responses since, after all, such a paralysis might exist only on the right side. On the other hand, one could argue that he should have rejected the wrong objects he had handled if he were able to recognize objects by touch.

A special series of investigations was undertaken in order to discover the nature and cause of his faulty responses.

On March 9, 1900, I did not, as I had done before, record which objects he found or did not find but, rather, made a list of those objects which he chose (not those requested) and noted how often he chose each one. The objects remained in the same positions and were requested with equal frequency. The results were: (1) that he reached particularly often for prominent objects, for example, a bottle; (2) that he reached for objects which lay in his line of sight; (3) that he perseverated on occasion, selecting the object which he had chosen immediately before. This last-mentioned feature, which was shown by Pick to be the cause of all faulty responses in a case of "pseudoapraxia," was present here as well but did not dominate the clinical picture as in Pick's case and in other cerebral cases; (4) In a large number of incorrect responses the wrong object was located immediately in front of, behind, or beside the object requested; (5) No single object was chosen correctly in all or in most cases.

The importance of number (2) was confirmed in the following manner: A certain object, for example, a change purse, was placed in the patient's line of vision. Each of the other objects was then requested three times, the change purse not at all. Yet he picked up the change purse seven times. The next most frequently selected incorrect object was picked up only three times.

Number (4), relatively the most common error (he picked up an object in the immediate vicinity of the object requested), suggested faulty projection [sic].

This suspicion was countered by the following experiment: After removing all of the other objects, a coin was placed in different spots on the table. Each time it was picked up on the first attempt. Nor did the patient err when the examiner pointed to various spots on the table and told him to "Reach here." Finally, when I picked up one of a number of objects lying in front of him and said "Take this," he succeeded effortlessly. Thus, as long as no choice was involved, as long as there was no competition between different objects, there was no trace whatever of faulty projection.

Ability to write and draw: One gap yet remains to be filled in the discussion of speech function. We have seen that the patient was completely unable to speak, repeat spoken words, or read aloud. Speech and reading comprehension, on the other hand, were preserved, although the latter was limited. As for writing, I have so far only provided a hint. He is almost completely agraphic with his right hand. In addition to well-formed up and down strokes (he usually holds the pen correctly) his writing contains a number of correctly formed letters, but not those intended. When asked to write his name, he usually scribbles something that begins with a well-formed Roman M, a letter which his name does not contain at all. Lower case m, too, appears frequently in his attempts to write. When single letters are dictated, he writes "m" instead of "r" and "i"; instead of "A" he produces a word that begins with a correctly formed Gothic B followed, perhaps, by "m" and "F."

The result is no better when he is asked to copy letters: He writes "m" for "B," "m" or "an" for "a," and something like "wia" for "m." His attempts to copy entire words usually have nothing in common with the original. Only lately did he succeed once in writing a word which remotely resembled the original, "Bismarck." But the copy contained a Gothic B whereas the original began with a Roman B. The following handwritten specimens will serve as illustrations.

With his left hand he usually—but not always—correctly composed words to command, using the letters from a letter game; words composed with his right hand were usually incorrect.

I should add that just as he is unable to copy letters and words with his right hand, he is also completely unable to copy simple designs. He is not even able to copy short horizontal or vertical strokes. Copies of designs made with his left hand are, as some of the specimens indicate, rather clumsy, but the shape of the model is recognizable throughout. He can draw a cross and a circle with his left hand from memory, but not with his right hand.

Writing produced by his left hand appeared at first to be senseless scribbling. Closer analysis, however, revealed that he employed a mirror script. The letters, though very clumsy, large, and, sometimes, incorrect, are always recognizable as the ones intended. At times, one cannot decipher something he has written with his left hand, but as soon as one knows what it is meant to signify, then one succeeds in recognizing the intention in every stroke. This is not at all the case with the writing

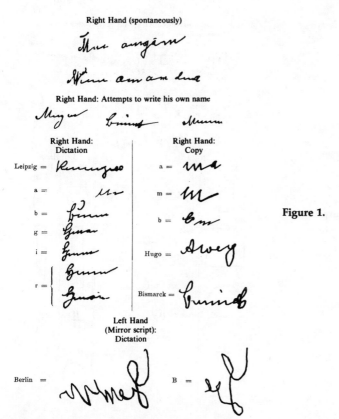

Right Hand (spontaneously)

Right Hand: Attempts to write his own name

Right Hand: Dictation | Right Hand: Copy

Leipzig =

a =

b =

g =

i =

r =

a =

m =

b =

Hugo =

Bismarck =

Figure 1.

Left Hand
(Mirror script):
Dictation

Berlin =

B =

produced by his right hand, as clearly demonstrated by the specimens. Compare, for example, how he writes the name of his superior (Renius) with his left and right hands. It is noteworthy that often, after producing a word to command with his left hand, he does not cease writing but appends a number of strokes and flourishes.

PERFORMANCE ON SIMPLE AND RELATIVELY COMPLEX RIGHT-HANDED AND TWO-HANDED TASKS

We must first mention a number of purposeful movements which were always performed correctly during the period of observation. As regards the lower extremities, I have already stated that the patient's gait was entirely normal.

He also succeeded in a number of simple tasks with his right hand. He was able to use a spoon with his right hand and to transfer food from a bowl to his mouth. Chewing and swallowing were normal. Furthermore—and this point is of great importance—the patient was

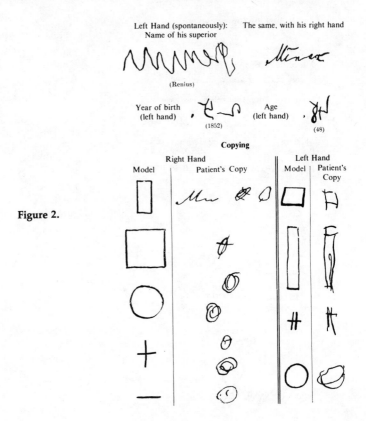

Figure 2.

always able to button and unbutton with his right hand, though he virtually never performed these tasks after the first request. Considerable persuasion was often required, but once his finger touched the button, the remaining sequence of movements was performed with reasonable dexterity. He did this even with his eyes closed, frequently, also, spontaneously. The patient can point out a spot indicated to him; he can pick up objects from the floor and can point to a larger object in the room. When told, "Point to the window, to the stove, to the lamp," he walks towards the object and often raises his hand to it. He usually succeeds in smoking a cigar if it has been lit for him. Sometimes, however, he puts it into his mouth the wrong way around. But once he holds the cigar correctly in his right hand, he is able to go through the sequence of motions: bringing the cigar to his mouth, drawing in the smoke, exhaling, etc. When he sets the cigar down, however, he frequently puts the lit end in the middle of the table. Moreover, the patient is able to place his fingers and hands in the proper position for playing the piano. He depresses the keys in the correct manner and can play simple melodies in a recognizable if somewhat faulty fashion. He is usually able to shake hands. From time to time he spontaneously twists his moustache for a moment or touches his eye. In contrast to the above, dressing and undressing are flawed if no help is provided. He succeeds, after a fashion, in putting on his trousers, but does so in such a manner as to bring the suspenders between his legs. On the other hand, he is unable to put on his socks. The following record was made of one such attempt: Right foot. After holding up his sock the wrong way around, he dons it correctly, as in this act the left hand leads. However, he struggles in vain to pull the other sock over his left foot (here the right hand leads); he pushes the right hand and arm into the sock and is then, of course, unable to don the sock. He puts it back onto the bed with some bewilderment, picks it up again and attempts to pull it over the right foot, which is already dressed. When he notices a large hole in the sock, he tries to hide it, and his facial expression conveys embarrassment.

The patient is handed a comb and asked to comb his hair. He does not obey this command but, instead, draws himself up into a stiff posture. Next he is asked to comb his hair with his left hand, and he does so without difficulty. "I am sure you will be able to do the same thing with your right hand." He picks the comb up properly and raises it to his hair; he turns the back of the comb towards his head, moves it backwards through the air twice and ends up in the supra-auricular region, finally putting the comb behind his ear like a pen, where he leaves it, satisfied with his performance. Combing is one of the tasks at which the patient is occasionally successful. Another such task is putting on and taking off his hat. He is often unable to perform many similar tasks on command, whereas they are sometimes accomplished spontaneously. Once the patient removed a blindfold with his right hand. On April 9, on being handed a toothbrush at a time when he was not accustomed to brush his teeth, he nevertheless employed it correctly with his left hand; with his right hand he used it as if it were a pen. On another occasion he put the handle into his mouth. On a third attempt he laughed in embarrassment, used the brush as if it were a spoon, shoveled with it, and put it into his mouth. Nor was he successful in using a trumpet or a harmonica.

He wants to dip his pen. He looks around for the inkwell. Having found it he moves his hand toward it, puts down the pen, picks up the inkwell, puts it down again, picks up the pen, puts it down again, picks up the lid, closes the inkwell and then says "Alas." With his left hand he succeeds immediately.

He is asked to put a number of building blocks into a box. He picks up the blocks and puts them down over and over again. Nor does he succeed in putting the lid on the box with his right hand. He places it over the box the wrong way around and puts it down next to the box. After having put all the blocks into the box and, on command, taken them out again with his left hand, he succeeded in performing both tasks with his right hand as well.

His behavior when faced with bimanual tasks is exceedingly interesting. Very simple tasks are not successfully accomplished because the purposeful activity of the left hand is thwarted by the faulty interaction of the right hand. For example, he is asked to brush the examiner's coat. He grasps its lower corner properly with his left hand and picks up the brush correctly with his right hand, but he lifts it repeatedly in rhythmic movements upwards and backwards above his right ear (see Fig. 3).

He is asked to pour water from a jug into a glass. His left hand takes the jug and wants to pour, but, simultaneously, his right hand lifts the empty glass to his mouth (Fig. 4). When the glass is held by another person the left hand succeeds in pouring without any difficulty.

He is asked to light a match. After several unsuccessful attempts he succeeds with his left hand in taking a match out of the box, which is held by his right hand. While the left hand is preparing to strike the match, the right hand puts the box down and, after further encouragement, raises it to his lips. When the examiner holds on to the box, the patient promptly strikes the match with his left hand. Handling a key, he often tries to insert the wrong end into the keyhole or inserts it with the notches upside down. Once the key is in the keyhole, locking and unlocking are accomplished most of the time.

On another occasion when attempting to light a match he picked up the match box with his right hand, turned it over and back, pushed the box half way out of the case, took out a match with his left hand, and prepared to strike it. In the meantime, however, perplexed, he put the

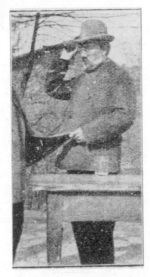

Figure 3.

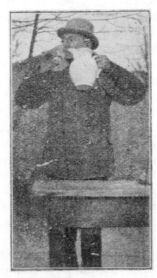

Figure 4.

box down with his right hand, picked it up, and put it down again. With his right hand he took out a second match, put the heads of both matches together and smiled, giving vent to a sigh of confusion. His behavior is altogether grotesque when he attempts to make a telephone call: with his left hand he raises one of the two receivers to his ear, while continually turning the crank with his right hand, first forwards, then backwards. He then seizes the other receiver with his right hand, places it against his forehead, nods, blows, lifts the receiver up to his eyes, looks into it and puts it next to his mouth and, finally, behind his ear.

He is unable to butter bread, knot a scarf, etc.

These examples suffice, though further examples might be given. After a means of communication with the patient had been established, it became possible to examine sensation and motility.

SENSATION

Vision: The patient was moderately myopic; visual acuity was adequate, as demonstrated by his ability to read. He could count fingers up to a distance of at least seven meters.

The ophthalmoscopic examination was entirely normal. Determination of the visual fields was extremely important. It could be established that there was no hemianopia. By tapping with his left hand the patient signified that he saw the test object (20 mm). The outer limits on the left side were 80° temporally and 50° nasally, on the right side 75° temporally and 55° nasally. Thus, the theoretically important question regarding unilateral cerebral blindness was also resolved. The patient had to fix on the midpoint. Test objects were then brought in from the side, and the patient was asked to tap with his left hand when he first saw them. He did so correctly when the objects were 30–50° from the point of fixation. The test objects were the size of a change purse, a key, and a toothbrush. The patient's performance could not have been significantly improved upon by a normal person. He did not look at the test objects. On one occasion three objects were placed on a table in front of him. From a second collection of similar objects one object at a time was exposed for a very short time at 40–50° while the patient was looking at the central point of the perimeter. At the end of the viewing period he never failed to point with his left hand to the corresponding object on the table.

His sense of color is preserved. He sorts out wool samples correctly and correctly correlates color names with color perceptions. Asked to indicate specific colors, he always succeeds with his left hand (his right hand reacts as usual when he is faced with a choice).

Hearing, taste, and smell were found to be intact. He always points correctly to the words "sour," "sweet," etc. and to the names of scents.

The results of testing cutaneous and (so-called) muscle sensation are of the greatest importance. In this respect I was able to establish the following: The left side of the patient's body was normal except for indifference to pinpricks over the left hand. However, forceful thrusts elicited withdrawal of the hand and exclamations.

Whatever is concluded about cutaneous sensation on the right side applies most rigorously to the extremities, to a lesser extent to the face and least of all to the trunk. Painful pinpricks and firm pressure are appreciated everywhere. In response to the former the patient exclaims and withdraws slightly. Pinpricks of moderate intensity are also appreciated, as indicated by the patient's signaling with his left hand and, sometimes, by movement of the parts stimulated—for example, the fingers. However, these stimuli are not painful and elicit even less reaction than on the left side. Moderately strong pressure on the arm and leg provokes no reaction whatever, nor does light pressure on the right side of the face.

The localization of pinprick and light touch is very poor indeed on the right side of his body. On the left side he accurately points to the spot stimulated with his left hand; on the right side of the face and neck he succeeds fairly well but becomes uncertain in the right infraclavicular region. He is totally inaccurate, however, as regards the right arm and leg. Frequently, he searches for the pinprick on the upper arm instead of in the hand. (Naturally the left hand was used in all these tests for indicating the spot stimulated). He never localizes pinpricks to the right hand however forcefully he is stuck, even when his right hand moves a little, which obviously represents withdrawal. This fact—namely, that the patient moves his right middle finger when it is stuck but nevertheless searches for the pinprick on his forearm with the left hand—is extraordinary and will be discussed further. When he is stuck in the right leg he often points half a meter away from the spot stimulated. On the trunk localization is less accurate on the right side than on the left side but is still fair. Distal to the inguinal ligament the patient is unable to localize at all.

Large differences in temperature are always appreciated, but the difference must be significantly greater on the right side than on the left side to be perceived. The patient is most uncertain when tested on the hand and the dorsal surface of the forearm.

The experiments were carried out in two ways: Either the patient had to squeeze the examiner's hand to signify "warm"; or, after fingering two test tubes which stood before him with his right hand, he had to point with his left hand to the warmer of the two. In this way mistakes which might have been caused by faulty right-hand responses were eliminated.

Differences in weight were recognized with the right hand. This was tested by filling one of two similar match boxes with sand while emptying the other one. When the patient weighed the two match boxes with his right hand, he regularly pointed to the heavier one with his left hand. Also, when he weighed one box with his left hand and the other box with his right hand, comparing the right- and left-hand weights, he knew whether the left one was heavier or lighter, provided that the difference in weight was substantial. More sophisticated examinations were not feasible. When equal weights were placed in both hands, he always thought the right one was lighter. With unequal weights, too, he tended to underestimate the weight in the right hand, so that the weight in the left [sic] hand had to be more than half again as heavy to be declared the heavier. This reflected a relative underestimation of the weight in the apractic hand.

Sense of position and movement: With his eyes open the patient could imitate the position of his right arm with his left arm reasonably well, though not perfectly; blindfolded he could not. At best the left arm was held in a position roughly similar to that of the right arm; often, however, it assumed a rather dissimilar posture. He was just as unable to make his left extremities imitate, even approximately, passive movements of his right arm and hand made by the examiner. To determine whether he understood the task, I asked the patient to imitate the position of his left leg with his left arm. This was carried out as accurately as it can be done. Small excursions of the fingers of the right hand were not appreciated at all. Nor was the patient able to imitate with his right arm the position of his left arm or passive movements of the same. This requires special mention, even though it may appear self-evident after what has been said about the inability of the right arm to imitate movements. Three very remarkable patients of Anton's, who appeared to be unilaterally paralyzed owing to a disorder of muscle sensation, were nevertheless able to perform movements on the diseased side which they were otherwise unable to perform—as soon as these movements were also made by the normal side. It seems to me essential to point out, therefore, that my patient's behavior was different. During all of these examinations the patient's performance was interrupted by various active contractions and accompanying (though not corresponding) movements of his right arm.

The obvious conclusion from these observations seems to be that as soon as the patient closes his eyes he has no knowledge of the position or movement of his right extremities. Whether or not this conclusion is valid shall be discussed in the following theoretical section.

The examination of tactile sensation, i.e., the ability to recognize objects by touch, was especially difficult. This ability is often infelicitously termed stereognosis, for what is involved is not only the recognition of form but, also, the appreciation of other properties such as soft-hard, smooth-rough, moist-dry, cold-warm, etc. In the complicated act of touching, all of the modalities of skin and muscle sensation are involved. The major role would seem to be played by the sense of position and motion. As Wernicke has shown, tactile paralysis—the inability to identify objects by touch—may occur even when some of these sensory modalities are reasonably well preserved, e.g., if the tactile conception of an object cannot be aroused because of a cortical lesion.

As regards my patient, it should be noted at the outset that object handling was not impaired; he handled the test objects as any normal person would. Thus, he rolled a ball back and forth between his finger tips.

It was impracticable to test him blindfolded as he did not persevere with a task and performed various faulty manipulations [sic] with the test objects. Consequently, I assembled two collections of similar objects, placed one set in front of him on the table and put one object at a time from the second set into a bag behind his back. He then examined the object inside the bag with his right hand and was asked to indicate the corresponding object on the table with his left hand. He failed in fourteen out of seventeen attempts. When he used his left hand to examine an object in the bag, he always pointed afterwards to the correct object on the table with his left hand, often with his right hand.

He was unable to indicate by tapping with his left hand whether the object he found in the bag was the one requested.

For reasons to be discussed below, this result did not completely convince me that I was dealing with a case of tactile paralysis. Strictly speaking, it proved only that tactile impressions received by the right hand, i.e., by the left hemisphere, could not be transmitted to the right hemisphere, the left hand, and the visual centers, respectively. I wished, therefore, to obtain some indication from the left side of the patient's brain as to whether he could recognize an object by touch with the right hand. Having him tap with his right hand to signify "yes" was not satisfactory; asking him to select one from a series of objects placed in front of him was also unreliable, because, as we know, he was not always able to pick out the intended object with his right hand. But the fact that the patient made many more mistakes when tested in this fashion than when he was told "Point to such and such an object" argues in favor of faulty tactile recognition being partly responsible for his mistakes. Next, I put three different objects into the bag and asked him to take out one of them. He chanced upon the correct object only now and then. Here, again, apraxia was hindering him; owing to various nonpurposeful movements the task of removing an object from the bag was obviously a most difficult one. Visual compensation (of little use to him) was nonexistent. He repeatedly took all three objects out together or took out none at all. In order to eliminate choice and, thus, to minimize patient error, I ultimately modified the test situation as follows: I had the patient feel a small bottle inside the bag; then I put the same bottle or a change purse back into the bag (so that at any given moment only one object was inside the bag) and told him to remove the object if it was the one he had felt initially; if not, to leave it in the bag. Again he made many incorrect responses.

That he really understood the task at hand was evident from the way he behaved during the tests of tactile sensation; he was visibly disappointed whenever he looked at an object he had felt before. His facial expression was repeatedly that of anger, even despair; one cannot but assume, therefore, that touching objects with his right hand did not result in any touch perceptions and that a right-sided tactile paralysis was present.

In summary, one must conclude that the sensitivity of the right side of the body was significantly decreased to touch and considerably decreased to pain and temperature. Tactile localization and the sensation of position and movement seemed to have been lost. The ability to distinguish large differences in weight was preserved. Tactile recognition was severely impaired.

Motility: There is a left lower facial paralysis. Electrical stimulation of the lower branch of the facial nerve is normal. No other paralyses are present. The tongue is not paretic, as indicated by the fact that chewing and swallowing are normal. This was also demonstrated directly; pricking the tongue with a pin results in its being pulled back or to the side. On May 4 I pulled his tongue forward after the patient had tried in vain to protrude it. Once his tongue was pulled out, he moved it several times to the right and left, pulled it back into his mouth, and stuck it out again. When I asked him two minutes later to protrude his tongue once again, he was unable to do so. The apparent weakness of his right hand vanished when we learned to deal with his apraxia. His muscle strength was diminished throughout and was not commensurate with that of a very strong man, but no actual paresis was found anywhere. When asked to flex his right knee in the prone position, he either does not move the leg at all, making, instead, snapping movements with his mouth, or else he strongly contracts the extensors or actually flexes the knee. When he flexes the knee it is apparent that flexion is performed with good strength. This applies, also, to extension. As regards the reflexes, it may be noted that the knee-jerks and the upper extremity reflexes have been very weak of late, especially the reflexes in the right arm, which are hardly elicitable. There are no contractures. Passive motion is normal. No dysfunction of bladder and bowel.

The above-mentioned forceful movements of the right upper extremity, which accompanied movements of the left hand during the early period of observation and which were so violent that it was often difficult to restrain the right arm, have decreased considerably of late.

OTHER PSYCHIC FUNCTIONS

I conclude the description of the clinical findings with an amplification of the psychic findings.

Musical ability and games: I mentioned before that the patient was able to play recognizable versions of some well-known melodies on the piano, though rather primitively, considering that he is said to have been an accomplished pianist. He is able to sing melodies without mistakes when accompanying others. During the rendering of a patriotic song he produced sounds that faintly resembled a few vowels of the text, a finding which has been described repeatedly in aphasic patients. After he had gone through several other songs in this way, the Marseillaise was sung to him. He joined in but stopped singing suddenly, undoubtedly because he considered it unseemly for someone in his position to be singing this particular song. He is no longer able to play checkers.

He is fairly well oriented in time; on April 18 of this year he stated that it was May 1900. He also knows where he is and makes his way about the ward. He understands his situation and recognizes doctor and orderly as such.

He is conscious of his personality. He knows his occupation and position and is well informed about his family and his previous life.

All of these conclusions were reached as follows: Various different numbers were read to him, and he was asked to tap with his left hand when his age was mentioned. Recognition of the right word was usually accompanied by lively reactions—nodding of the head, bowing, or saying "yes,yes." However, these responses were reliable only if he was admonished to reply in the affirmative; when forced to choose between yes and no he frequently failed to hit upon the right answer, as was noted above. A second method was to ask him to select the correct number from among various numbers written on a blackboard. A third—but very laborious and often unsuccessful—method was to have him write with his left hand.

Recall: 1. Visual impressions (April 16, 1900): The number 817 is written down for him; he finds the number at once among eight others shown to him three minutes later, and again ten minutes later. Having picked up two objects with his left hand, he can do so again five minutes later without their having been named a second time.

2. Auditory impressions: Having been told the number 1813, he finds it without delay ten minutes later among eight other written numbers. He recognizes objects palpated with his left hand several minutes afterwards; he is unable to do so with his right hand, as demonstrated by the touch test.

4. Passive movement: With the patient blindfolded, a pencil is put into his left hand and the hand guided in drawing a cross. He repeats the drawing one minute later. As expected, he does not succeed with his right hand.

In fine, his ability to recall, i.e., to reproduce fresh impressions, seems to be preserved with reference to all of the modalities tested, for the failures with his right hand cannot simply be written off as loss of recall.

The examination of memory in the strict sense—what the patient recollects from his previous healthy life—is extremely difficult. There do not appear to be any gaps as regards his personal experiences, as has been noted under "consciousness of personality." It can also be demonstrated that he is knowledgeable about many things.

The patient was fairly attentive during these investigations, although his attention flagged when he tired after fifteen minutes or half an hour.* In this patient as in other patients, it seemed useful to differentiate between a maximal and a habitual attentiveness, two quantities which are not at all proportional to one another. By maximal attentiveness I understand that degree of attention which can be achieved with the greatest exertion, with outside encouragement; habitual attentiveness refers to the amount of attention that a person accords to the events taking place around him. I saw a patient in the clinic in Breslau who reacted normally when he was being addressed, responding to everything he was shown or told, but who, when left to himself, sat still and comprehended hardly anything that was happening around him. A similar if less marked difference is demonstrated by my patient. He usually participates very little and is hardly aware of conversations which take place in his presence. When he was presented to the Society for Psychiatry and Nervous Diseases, he scarcely noticed the large audience, yet he invariably responded when spoken to directly and emphatically. To the weakness of his habitual or spontaneous attentiveness I also relate the fact that he frequently did not modify an incorrect response himself, although he made it clear that he realized his mistake when asked repeatedly whether the response had been correct.

Numerical concepts and arithmetic: He picks up the number of matches requested from a stack with his left hand but does not succeed in laying down eight minus five matches or two times three matches. It is apparent that he can solve these arithmetic tasks when asked to point with his left hand to the results of simple additions, subtractions, and multiplications on a blackboard full of numbers. Writing with his left hand in mirror script, he is able to add three-digit numbers. His inability, even with his left hand, to perform simple arithmetic operations

---

*I have not measured his attention span. These statements rely on impressions.

by selecting the correct number of matches proves that the left hand cannot, after all, be used in a completely normal fashion. It would seem to be too difficult a task to combine a simple arithmetic operation with the selection of the correct number of matches. As mentioned above, rudiments of left-sided apraxia were manifested by the rare occurrence of incorrect left-handed responses to choice.

Moods: The patient cried frequently at first, especially after receiving visits from his relatives. During the last few months he has usually been indifferent and carefree. A newspaper is often in front of him, but he indicated to me that he does not really understand it. On the other hand, he understands when the newspaper is read to him, which, of late, he requests frequently. He takes walks in the garden and in the corridor and enjoys smoking his cigar. When complimented on his little son, he laughs happily or is moved. The latter always occurs when his own state of health is mentioned; tears immediately come to his eyes, his face flushes, and he sobs. He is extremely willing to carry out all commands.

Some peculiarities of the patient and several occurrences during his stay on the ward are worthy of note.

When he attempts to use his right hand, this hand often grabs hold of the left hand instead and pulls it to the midline; then he clasps his hands.* When, on one occasion, the examiner told the patient that there was some milk on his moustache, the latter replied with an embarrassed smile, "Alas," raised his right hand to his neck, touched the right side of his chin and—only after repeated encouragement—his moustache, which, however, he let go of immediately.

He recognizes pictures instantly. He cheerfully points out photographs of himself and of me from among several others. A very curious fact should be commented upon. When the patient is asked to identify an object depicted on a picture-sheet, he makes proper pointing movements with his left hand, but with his right hand he frequently carries on as if he wanted to catch hold of the object in question. He tries, as it were, to remove it from the picture. It seems as if he is deceived into thinking that the pictured objects are three-dimensional. (I shall be able, I think, to provide a satisfactory explanation of this surprising behavior later on.)

Summarizing the actual findings: A man in his late forties, previously infected with syphilis, suddenly (after premonitory symptoms) loses the faculty of speech and the ability to write with his right hand; he is also unable to perform purposeful movements with this hand, to use objects appropriately, wherefrom results the semblance of imbecility.

Closer examination reveals that motility is preserved throughout,

---

*Cf. the patient's wife's statement that he frequently assists his left hand with his right.

whereas sensation on the right side of the body, especially as regards the sense of position and movement and the ability to touch, seems to be severely affected. The perversity of the patient's motor behavior is, on closer inspection, explained by apraxia confined to the right side of the body. Only the musculature of the head and neck is involved bilaterally. The functioning of the special senses is not impaired. The subsequent psychological elaboration of the impressions received by these senses and the patient's previously acquired store of knowledge are preserved.

A number of actions described above are not affected.

Epilogue

We, the two survivors of Hugo Liepmann's four children, are gratified by the posthumous honor paid to our father by the inclusion in this volume of the first of his apraxia papers, published in 1900.

Hugo Liepmann (1863–1925) was born in Berlin. As a youth he was possessed by a wide-ranging intellectual curiosity and inspired by high ideals. At school he was influenced by classical Greek and German literature; at university, he read linguistics, chemistry, psychology, and philosophy. His Ph.D. thesis dealt with the philosophy of ancient Greece. Later, he became a follower of Kant and Schopenhauer.

But in time he became dissatisfied with philosophy as the focus of his life's work. He yearned for something more concrete, for exact science. So, in his late twenties, he began to read medicine. Yet he always remained something of a philosopher, and in his own mind his special task related to the problem of body and soul.

After the medical *Staatsexamen*—there exists a witty letter to his family describing his examination by Virchow, the famous, hot-tempered pathologist—he worked for a short time at the Charité Hospital in Berlin and then, from 1895–99, as Wernicke's assistant in Breslau.

In his youth father was full of *joie de vivre*. He hiked and traveled with his friends and enjoyed good food. But even then he suffered periodically from despondency and self-doubt. These feelings were banished for many years when he met our mother. With his marriage and his association with Wernicke began the happiest and most productive period of his life. Yet the spirit of self-criticism, the fear of boring an audience, stage fright, remained. We well remember the heavy atmosphere at the midday meal on Wednesdays before father's weekly lectures; on other days these meals were particularly enjoyable for us children because father dined with us.

There seems to have been no reason for his diffidence; he was a successful lecturer. At Kraepelin's invitation he gave an annual course at a postgraduate seminar in Munich. Once, en route, he asked a railway porter to take especial care of one of his attaché cases as it contained fragile brain slides. The man replied, "You deal in brain slides? Can you make a living from that?" Recounting this episode to his wife father signed the letter: "Your commercial traveler in brain slides." He always saw the several sides of a situation, not least of all the humorous one.

In order to enlarge the scope of his investigations father would have liked to head up a university clinic and have research assistants. He was repeatedly nominated or short-listed for a chair, but, in the end, he was always passed over because he was Jewish. Once he was offered an appointment on condition that he explicitly renounce Judaism! Although his philosophical convictions prevented him from practicing any religion, his moral scruples precluded any, even a merely formal, connection between matters of religion and worldly success. The ensuing, continual disappointment threw a shadow over Hugo Liepmann's life.

Thus, his career was made in the municipal hospitals of Berlin rather than in the university, and after fifteen years at Dalldorf he became director of the large mental institute at Herzberge (1915–1920). However, administration was not his strong point. He was a perfectionist, and he could not treat small matters as small. He would ponder over any decision, whether it involved a question of style or the settlement of a dispute between members of his staff. On one such occasion a subordinate at the institute remarked, "Don't take offense, sir, but you really try too hard to be fair to everybody." Father took this criticism as a great compliment, for a sense of justice was one of his outstanding qualities.

Father was the proverbial absent-minded professor. In Breslau he once forgot, while examining an interesting new patient on the ward, that he had locked his bride in his office at the mental hospital, where she had come to visit him; it was several hours before he freed her. One of his children had the same experience some years later at Dalldorf.

When we children were small, father's personality was transmitted to us mainly by our mother; their marriage was a singularly happy and harmonious union. Father was absorbed by his thoughts and took little part in everyday life; but his ethical standards, his fanaticism for truth, and his utter integrity set the tone in our house—as did, also, his sense of humor.

He put questions to us, trying out tests he would subsequently administer to his patients. He told us fascinating stories about them, impressing us that he did not regard them merely as cases and that he took a human interest in them as persons. Many remained attached to him long after their stay on his wards.

Our father was not interested in practical things, nor did he have a close relationship to nature or the arts. He was a horseman and fond of dogs; he liked gymnastics, swimming, and bicycling and was proud of being strong (though he resented being short and stout). An enthusiastic chess player, he and his friends berated one another in good humor during their games, which provided him rare moments of relaxation.

Hugo Liepmann's was a complex nature. Dedicated to science and to philosophy, he was, nevertheless, a full-blooded man, good and wise.

Kate Liepmann (London)
Charlotte Hamburger-Liepmann (São Paulo)

PAIN AND SENSIBILITY

Introduction

Simeon Locke, M.D.
Neurological Unit
Boston State Hospital

THE KEY TO THE INTERPRETATION of the structure of the neopallium, wrote LeGros Clark, "lies in an intensive study of the thalamus" (1). He was citing Elliott Smith, whose Arris and Gale Lectures, published just four years after the article offered here in translation, emphasized the importance of the thalamus in a study of the history of the developing cortex (2). In subsequent years intensive study did occur. Aspects of thalamic anatomy and physiology were explored. The part played by the thalamus in speech and language was investigated (3–5), and the relation of its nuclei to movement and movement disorders was clarified (6). It is, however, its role in the perception of pain—perhaps the most dramatic symptom of the Dejerine-Roussy syndrome—that served as the focus of interest for many.

In 1905, at the time Dejerine and Roussy were analyzing the thalamic syndrome, Henry Head described the afferent nervous system "from a new aspect" (7). His views on protopathic and epicritic sensibility, summarized in 1920 (8), were sharply criticized more than twenty years later by Walshe (9), who wrote, "Head's protopathic and epicritic fibers... and the hypothetical dual system of pain fibers for the conducting of the different sensory qualities of pain, all come to grief when they make contact with the hard facts of anatomy." In the 1950s, some of the physiologic foundation for the duality of pain perception was worked out (10, 11), and the following decade brought better understanding of the anatomical alternatives. Pain fibers were found to distribute to the thalamic reticular nucleus, the intralaminar nuclei, and the centrum medianum, as well as to the more familiar specific sensory nuclei (12, 13). Stereotaxic thalamotomy disclosed that lesions in these specific nuclei produced profound sensory loss but little alteration of perception of pain. In contrast, lesions in the parafascicular

187

nucleus, the intralaminar nucleus, and the centrum medianum interfered with pain perception while causing little sensory loss (14). Indeed, the thalamic pain system was divided into a cortical conducting pathway via the ventral posterior nucleus and a subcortical system projecting to outer segment of pallidum via the thalamic intralaminar nucleus and, perhaps, centrum medianum (15).

The intensive study continues. The 1970s introduced new techniques. Study of anterograde and retrograde transport by the methods of autoradiography and horseradish peroxidase supplement the retrograde degeneration studies and silver methods of earlier investigators. Pain continues to be the symptom of outstanding concern to patient and physician. And the thalamus plays an important and still enigmatic role in its perception.

REFERENCES

1. Clark, W. E. L. "The structure and connections of the thalamus." *Brain* 55:406, 1932.

2. Smith, G. E. "The Arris and Gale Lectures." *Lancet* 1:1; 147; 221, 1910.

3. Ojemann, G. A., Fedio, P. E., and Van Buren, J. M. "Anomia from pulvinar and subcortical parietal stimulation." *Brain* 91:99, 1968.

4. Van Buren, J. M., and Borke, R. C. "Alterations in speech and the pulvinar." *Brain* 92:255, 1969.

5. Ojemann, G. A., and Ward, A. A. "Speech representation in ventrolateral thalamus." *Brain* 94:669, 1971.

6. Cooper, I. S. *Involuntary Movement Disorders.* New York: Harper and Row, Hoeber Medical Division, 1969.

7. Head, H., Rivers, W. H. R., and Sherren, J. "The afferent nervous system from a new aspect." *Brain* 28:99, 1905.

8. Head, H. *Studies in Neurology.* London: Oxford University Press, 1920.

9. Walshe, F. M. R. "The anatomy and physiology of cutaneous sensation." *Brain* 65:48, 1942.

10. Bishop, G. H. "The organization of cortex with respect to its afferent supply." *Ann. N.Y. Acad. Sci.* 94:559, 1961.

11. Sweet, W. H. "Pain." Chapt. 19 in *Handbook of Physiology Section 1: Neurophysiology Vol. 1.* Washington, D.C.: American Physiological Society, 1959.

12. Bowsher, D. "Termination of the central pain pathway in man: The conscious appreciation of pain." *Brain* 80:606, 1957.

13. Mehler, W. R., Feferman, M. E., and Nauta, W. J. H. "Ascending axon degeneration following anterolateral cordotomy: An experimental study in the monkey." *Brain* 83:718–750, 1960.

14. Mark, V. H., Ervin, F. R., and Yakovlev, P. I. "Stereotactic thalamotomy." *Arch. Neurol.* 8:528, 1963.

15. Hassler, R. "Die zentralen Systeme des Schmerzes." *Acta Neurochir.* 8:353, 1960.

The Thalamic Syndrome

J. DEJERINE AND G. ROUSSY

THREE YEARS AGO (on April 2, 1903) one of us presented the details of two individuals whose thalamic lesions were diagnosed during life and subsequently confirmed at autopsy. Since then two similar reports have appeared: Thomas and Chiray[1] described a woman who is still alive, and Dide and Durocher[2] (de Rennes)[3] presented a man whose illness was followed to autopsy. Somewhat later, two additional cases appeared—that of Long, which was presented to the Medical Society of Geneva in 1904, and Bourdon and Dide in 1905 (*l'Année psychologique*).[3]

These cases, which are clinically and anatomically similar, have led us to consider lesions of the thalamus and the role of these lesions in clinical illness. However, these published cases are insufficient in that they are either purely clinical or have only macroscopic pathologic details. We would like to fill this lacuna by presenting our observations on serially sectioned blocks from three cases with thalamic lesions. We will use these observations as well as information from several new clinical cases to illustrate the fact that there is a *characteristic clinical picture* which results from a *specific thalamic lesion* and represents a new clinical syndrome—the *thalamic syndrome*.

For the sake of brevity we will restrict ourselves to a short presentation. A more complete clinical and pathologic discussion will be presented by one of us in the future.[4]

The *thalamic syndrome*, as defined by our observations and those in the literature, is characterized by: (1) *a mild, rapidly improving hemiplegia*

NOTE: Translated by F. H. Hochberg from: Dejerine, J., and Roussy, G., "Le Syndrome thalamique," *Revue neurologique* 14 (1906), 521–32.

without contractures; (2) *a persistent superficial hemianesthesia (in some cases replaced by superficial hyperesthesia) always associated with obvious and unremitting difficulties with deep sensation;* (3) *mild hemiataxia and more or less complete astereognosis.*

In addition to these three main symptoms one may also find: (4) *sharp, enduring, paroxysmal, often intolerable pain on the hemiplegic side which does not respond to any analgesic treatment;* and (5) *choreo-athetotic movements of the extremities on the paralyzed side.*

These symptoms, appearing together, confirm the existence of a well-localized thalamic lesion which will be discussed in detail. Secondary symptoms of this disorder include: sphincter trouble (tenesmus of the bladder and rectal sphincters) and hemianopsia. These secondary symptoms are both rare and not, strictly speaking, part of the syndrome.

Frequency: Cases of the thalamic syndrome, as well as persistent hemianesthesia, are infrequent compared to the infinite number of hemiplegics seen in a clinic. However, the cases are not exceptionally rare. Since we first attracted attention to this syndrome we have been able to learn of eight cases, of which four were followed to autopsy. Five of these eight cases were seen by us. We have presented four of them to the Neurology Society. In addition, the literature may contain similar cases, reported as different entities, which might be included in the nosological group we wish to establish. Thus, during our incomplete review of the literature of hemiplegia with hemianesthesia we were able to confirm that the observations—those of Greiff[5] and Edinger[6]—represent examples of the thalamic syndrome. The instances of this syndrome are numerous enough for us to present a compilation and evaluation of this condition.

CLINICAL DETAILS

Most patients with the thalamic syndrome present with an unheralded hemiplegia similar to that associated with focal areas of softening. The patient notices the appearance of the hemiplegia after a period of dizziness or slight loss of consciousness of several hours duration. Sensory and motor difficulties appear coincidentally, but follow different courses. The motor problems tend to ameliorate and attenuate considerably while the sensory problems persist, often to the patient's death—which may occur several years later. At the onset, although not uniformly, the patient may greatly complain of urinary retention with tenesmus or incontinence.

In our analysis of the thalamic syndrome we will consider the signs that present several months, or even a year after the onset of hemiplegia. At this time the syndrome can be seen in its greatest clarity and is most easy to diagnose.

A. MOTOR DIFFICULTIES

Motor difficulties are those of mild hemiplegia or hemiparesis. *The face* is minimally involved. A slight facial asymmetry noted at rest may be more noticeable with mimetic motions, but we have never seen the paralysis of emotive mimicry that was noted by Bechterew and Nothnagel in association with lesions of the thalamus. Often patients do not even show facial paralysis or paresis. The tongue is not deviated, although it and the palate may have been involved at the onset. The pharyngeal reflex and movements of the superior face are intact. Several individuals have shown swallowing difficulties and must make several attempts to swallow liquid or solid food. Only one of our patients exhibited this rare symptom.

The arms and legs are minimally affected, and active movements are relatively preserved. There is mild hypotonia and diminished muscle strength, but no tremor. The hemiplegia is so mild and evanescent that it is useless to insist that it, or for that matter the movement disorder, becomes well-developed.

Of greater interest are the posthemiplegic motor phenomena—hemichorea and hemiathetosis—present in several patients. According to some authors, the thalamus plays a role in the genesis of these symptoms. We will return to this question later. The hemichorea seen here is not of the large variety. The movements of the extremities are small, usually involving the fingers and hands either with the disordered character of chorea or with the slow vermicular character of athetosis. None of our cases showed *hemitremor*.

Hemiataxia is one of the most interesting motor signs associated with the thalamic syndrome. The hemiplegic ataxia varies in intensity from case to case but always preserves certain features which distinguish it from medullary or peripheral ataxias. One of us has already drawn attention to this point[7]. The hemiataxia of cerebral origin is always mild, limited, and restrained, never attaining the severity of tabetic ataxia. The atactic nature of the patient's movements are reflected by their lack of smoothness and hesitation. However, the patients can coordinate a series of movements, such as opening fingers separately—an action impossible for a tabetic. When the patient is asked to place his index finger on his nose with his eyes closed, he mislocalizes and hesitates often, but as the finger approaches his nose the movements slow. Thus, although he may not be able to direct his finger to an exact point, he can at least regulate the amplitude and speed of its movement. He does not show the marked errors of the tabetic, such as touching his finger to his head or his shoulder. The slight degree of ataxia is thus not in keeping with the profound superficial and deep sensory difficulties, as will be seen. We will explain this apparent paradox by referring to a work previously published by one of us.

B. Reflexes

Reflexes are sometimes a little increased and sometimes normal as one might expect with an old mild hemiplegia. The cutaneous reflexes (cremasteric, abdominal, and epigastric), as well as the plantar reflex, are normal or absent. *The absence of Babinski's sign in all our cases,* despite the degeneration of the pyramidal tract in our sections, should be noted. This suggests either that the motor pathways play only a minimal role in the thalamic syndrome, or as we believe, that damage to the thalamus is not associated with the occurrence of Babinski's sign (the normal reaction to a pyramidal tract lesion).

C. Sensory Difficulties

Sensory difficulties dominate the thalamic syndrome by virtue of their intensity, constancy, character, and modality. The problem is one of impairment of both objective and subjective sensations, including pain on the hemiplegic side, which we will discuss later.

Objective sensations: The three modalities of superficial sensation (touch, pain, and temperature) are affected in the thalamic syndrome. These peripheral sensations are not abolished; rather the impressions of these sensations are modified, as is seen in typical cerebral anesthesia. The anesthesia is never absolute as in hysterical hemianesthesia, is most notable at the periphery, decreases as one moves from there to the more proximal areas, and may cross the trunk to involve one to two centimeters on the healthy side.

The absent or diminished sensation of touch (as tested with the bristles of a shaving brush) involves the skin and the mucous membranes. Pain and temperature are never completely abolished—a feature found in all forms of cerebral hemianesthesia.

The quantitative and qualitative sensory changes in organic hemianesthesia include: perverted perceptions of place and mode of sensation, dysesthesias, topoanesthesia, and topoanalgesia, with slowness in sensory perception and enlargement of Weber's circles. We have encountered the same order of superficial sensory difficulties in the thalamic syndrome, as have Long[8] and Brécy.[9]

As our patients did not show gross alterations of superficial sensation, we were obliged to evaluate them with great care. *Deep sensation* in all its components (joint, muscular, tendinous, osseus) was most affected. Several cases showed diminished or absent osseus sensation (as evaluated with a tuning fork) as well as muscle sensation.

Our patients showed diminished or abolished perceptions of active or passive motion, resistance, force, and weight on the abnormal side. The notion of position or attitude of the extremity (akinetic) was strongly affected. To varying degrees, "stereognosis" was always affected.

In summary, the objective sensory difficulties associated with the thalamic syndrome are: (1) a superficial hemianesthesia (tactile, pain, and temperature) which is persistant and characterized by dysesthesia and topoanesthesia; and (2) a marked alteration of deep sensation, lasting indefinitely, with dissociated difficulties of superficial and deep sensation.

Subjective sensations: The presence of pain on the hemiplegic side is a finding of some importance. Pains, associated with thalamic lesions, have been noted by other authors: Greiff, Henschen, Lauenstein, Biernacki, Reichenberg, Goldscheider, Edinger, and the Dejerines. We have found mention of these painful symptoms in most published or personally evaluated cases of the thalamic syndrome. These symptoms occur frequently enough for us to have related them to a thalamic lesion. More precisely they seem to be related to destruction and irritation of fibers which arborize in the ventral thalamus. As such, the sign (pain on the hemiplegic side) has great clinical importance as a means of localization, especially when seen in conjunction with the other symptoms of the thalamic syndrome. However, the sign is not constant, having been absent in one of our cases. As this is a subjective finding, the examiner must bear in mind that all patients react differently.

These pains are grouped with pains of "central origin" as was noted by Anton, Edinger, Goldscheider, etc. They appeared early in the illness, either at the start of the hemiplegia or several months thereafter, and affect the face and trunk as well as the hemiplegic areas. The brow, the cheek, the orbit (with a sensation of pulling of the eye), the chin, and the ear are involved. In the extremities the joints are not selectively involved; rather, the pains radiate from proximal areas into the toes or fingers. . . . It is difficult for the patient to indicate the exact location of the pains, or whether they are deep or superficial; but most patients note that they are rather superficial, involving the skin and the subcutaneous tissue. The pains continue with paroxysmal exacerbations which wrench cries from the patient, hinder his sleep, or wake him up brusquely. One of our patients continually said that arm and leg pains prevented her from moving her left hand and walking. These vivid pains impaired the function of her arm and leg causing a true *painful impotence.*

The pain is not exclusively spontaneous. It may be provoked by the touch of a finger, pin, contact, heat or cold, and pressure. The patients are thus sometimes quite hyperesthetic. They compare these pains to superficial or deep burns, shooting twinges of pain, violent sensations of painful pressure, or sensations similar to those of a knife cut. Between these paroxysms of pain the patient experiences pins and needles or sensations of numbness in the extremities or, sometimes, the face.

There is one additional feature: the aches respond to neither internal nor external treatment. Nothing offers solace to the patient whose sufferings are sometimes intolerable.

D. Sphincter Difficulties

Two of our cases showed significant sphincter disturbances perhaps related to the influence of the thalamus on sphincter functions noted by Bechterew, etc. We have noted instances of urinary frequency and impaired urination as late as several months after the debut of the illness. These difficulties are usually fleeting and are not noticed several years after the onset of the illness.

E. Special Sensations

1. Vision.   There are no abnormalities of the extraocular muscles and the pupils are normal and react to accommodation. One clinical case had a lateral homonymous hemianopsia suggesting involvement of the postero-inferior thalamus and the thalamic radiations.

2. Hearing, smell, and taste.   These are usually not involved in the thalamic syndrome. Two instances of slight, brief, special sensory involvement have been noted and will only be mentioned.

F. Vasomotor and trophic difficulties

Vasomotor difficulties may be seen in association with the hemiplegia of thalamic origin. One of our patients showed coolness and bluish discoloration of the extremities, cyanosis of the digits, and flushing and congestion of the cheek on the paralyzed side. This same patient showed trophic changes of the skin and subjacent tissue in the fingers of the right hand. However, these symptoms accompany hemiplegias of all causes and are not more frequent in the thalamic hemiplegias.

G. Secretory Difficulties

One of our cases had salivation difficulties, and presented with unilateral xerostomia (on the paralyzed side) with dryness of the mouth and difficulty with swallowing. As with the vasomotor difficulties, we are content to mention this without stating its relation to the thalamic lesion. We have never noted sweating difficulties, nor have other authors.

In summary, thalamic hemiplegias (whose topography we will spell out later) present as slight, transitory, rapidly improving motor hemiplegias occurring without an ictus, tremor, or Babinski's sign. The hemiplegia is accompanied by subjective and objective sensory disturbances. Subjectively, the patient experiences vivid and tenacious pains (on the paralyzed side) which are unresponsive to treatment and which serve as the basis for a real impotence (painful hemiplegia). Objectively, the patient may sometimes show hypesthesia to tactile, painful, and thermal stimuli or sometimes hyperesthesia with dysesthesia, paresthesia, and topoesthesia. In addition there may be persistant troubles with deep sensation, and loss of muscle sensation along with astereognosis and hemiataxia. Often there are choreoathetotic-like movements. Hemianopsia may occur when the lesion involves the posteroinferior thalamus.

DIAGNOSIS

The thalamic syndrome is associated with a clear-cut clinical picture distinct from that due to lesions of neighboring areas—in particular the subthalamic areas through which the thalamic fibers pass. A lesion of the pons or peduncle, involving these fibers but not greatly affecting the motor pathways, might produce a clinically similar picture, namely significant sensory impairment with only minimal hemiplegia. The addition of signs of cranial nerve abnormalities related to lesions at these levels would allow us to topographically localize this processes. The gaze palsies (conjugate bilateral ocular palsies) are the major findings associated with lesions of the *superior quadrigeminal bodies*. This relationship is still poorly understood and we will not dwell on it.

The presence of extraocular muscle paralyses allows one to distinguish between the thalamic syndrome and that due to a lesion of the dorsal portion of the upper pons (*the superior pontine syndrome*) as described by Raymond and Cestan[10]. In the latter condition one sees a mild hemiplegia with conserved muscle strength and spontaneous movements, preserved cutaneous and tendon reflexes, a superficial and deep hemianesthesia with pins-and-needles sensations and sometimes painful sensations in the affected extremity, a hemiataxia, and choreoathetoid movements. The differential diagnosis is facilitated by the findings, in the patients of Raymond and Cestan, of resting tremors, asynergia, dysarthria, and—most significantly—a paralysis of upward and downward conjugate ocular movements with nystagmoid jerks.

For the sake of completeness, we will mention in passing that one may rarely see hemianesthesia, hemiataxia, hemitremor (alternating sensory-motor hemiplegia) in the inferior peduncular and pontine syndromes. The associated paralyses of the third to seventh cranial nerves and the absence of signs on the face and trunk leave no doubt as to the differential diagnosis.

The occurrence of *persisting anesthesia with hemiplegia* due to a cortical or subcortical lesion has been shown [by Long, together with one of the authors (J.D.)] to be due to the extension of lesions into the thalamic corona radiata. The involvement of pyramidal fibers results in the marked hemiplegia with contracture, tremors, exaggerated reflexes, and a Babinski's sign usually without choreoathetoid movements. Pain is a rare symptom but may exist, although less vividly. In this last instance, where the problem is one of differentiating cortical or subcortical anesthesia from thalamic anesthesia, considerable importance is attached to the intensity and degree of paralysis.

Hysteria is easily diagnosed by the topography of the anesthesia, its centripetal diminution, and its less intense nature. In addition, the thalamic syndrome is associated with qualitative sensory abnormalities and other findings which are not usually seen in hysteria.

PATHOLOGY

The anatomic basis for the thalamic syndrome has not previously been well studied except in an elementary fashion on macroscopic sections hardened in bichromate. Our anatomic observations are based on the microscopic study of rigorously performed serial sections *from three cases.* Two cases were reported by one of us to the Neurology Society on April 2, 1903. The clinical description and pathologic blocks from the third case were provided by our colleague and friend, Dr. Long (of Geneva).

A complete and detailed description of these cases along with supporting pictures will be published in the future. Our limited presentation is designed to emphasize the location, topography, and extent of the lesions in our three thalamic syndrome cases.

In the first case (Joss) the original lesion occupied almost the entire extent of the posterior thalamus. In the superior thalamus the destruction occupied a great part of the posterior third of the internal [medial] and external [lateral] nuclei. The lesion diminishes inferiorly but involves the external nucleus and encroaches medially on the internal and medial nuclei and on the pulvinar posteriorly. In the inferior thalamus the lesion is represented by a track which traverses the external nucleus. At its highest point the lesion involves the posterior portion of the posterior limb of the internal capsule. In the posterior portion of the putamen it is seen as a small secondary foyer, a lacuna of disintegration.

The second case (Hud) showed an equally large area of destruction occupying the two inferior tiers of the thalamus (Fig. 2) stopping at the

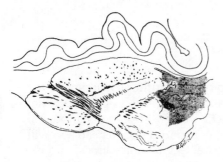

Figure 1. The Joss case.

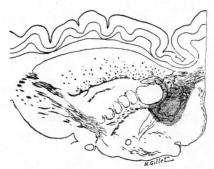

Figure 2. The Hud case.

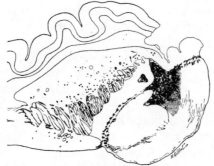

Figure 3. The Thal case.

superior edge of the subthalamus. The destruction involved most of the external nucleus and portions of the internal nucleus, medial nucleus, and the pulvinar. Leaving the thalamus, the destruction involved the posterior and retrolenticular segments of the internal capsule as well as the posterior putamen.

The third case (Thal) serial sections showed involvement of the same regions but to a much lesser extent. Of some interest is the fact that the clinical signs, although evident, were less intense than in the first two cases. The destruction occupied the midthalamus, principally the posterior portion of the external nucleus (Fig. 3), and medially, the internal and medial nuclei, while sparing the pulvinar. Laterally, the posterior limb of the internal capsule as well as a small segment of the posterior lenticular nucleus were involved. The capsular lesion was visible only on the superior sections. There was no involvement below the thalamus.

As a result we feel that:

1. there is a lesion of the thalamus, involving the posterolateral portion of the external nucleus, a portion of the medial and internal nuclei, as well as the corresponding portion of the internal capsule which produces a characteristic clinical picture.
2. this clinical picture, with its characteristic symptoms and signs, represents a new syndrome which is best identified as the *thalamic syndrome*.

PATHOLOGIC PHYSIOLOGY

To complete our work we will explore the pathophysiology of the thalamic syndrome and attempt to resolve the question of the part that the thalamic lesion plays in the production of the observed symptoms. This discussion would oblige us to extend ourselves. Instead we will delay this, allowing one of us, using in-depth anatomic-clinical and experimental methods to base his thesis on this subject. We will restrict ourselves to two principal points which stand out from our anatomic and clinical description: (1) the dissociation of motor and sensory phenomena; and (2) the physiologic interpretation of motor and sensory troubles.

1. *The dissociation of the motor and sensory phenomena,* in the hemiplegia of cerebral origin, is the most salient and pathognomonic indicator of a thalamic lesion. In cases of classical organic hemiplegia, sensory troubles are less pronounced and regress more rapidly than the motor difficulties. Usually, the hemiplegic initially experiences marked sensory difficulties, which return to normal well before the disappearance, or attenuation, of his paralysis. A cerebral lesion might approximate the thalamic syndrome if the lesion involved the central sensory pathways but only grazed the motor pathways. This could occur only at a point where the motor and sensory conduction fibers are well separated. One of us, in collaboration with Mrs. Dejerine and Dr. Long, has shown that the motor and sensory pathways are, for the most part, intermingled in the cortex (sensory-motor area)[11], and in their subcortical and central paths (corona radiata and internal capsule). From the internal capsule the motor tract passes into the pes pedunculi, while the ascending fibers of the sensory pathways, leaving the dorsal pons, have a way-station in the ventral thalamus. Only at this level could a lesion involve sensory fibers while only minimally affecting the motor projections. As we have seen on serial sections from the three cases studied, there was indeed a lesion at this level. We have really only viewed the supra-peduncular diencephalic portion of the motor and sensory fibers, because this is the area of involvement.

The ascending and descending tracts in the peduncle, pons, and bulb are distinct enough to be selectively involved. In these instances the realization that we are not dealing with a cortical process, along with the appearance of other previously mentioned symptoms, would allow us to distinguish these processes from the thalamic syndrome.

2. *What is the cause of the paralytic and sensory difficulties?* The cause of the paralysis is obvious. It is due to a lesion in the posterior portion of the internal capsule (present in our three cases) which has resulted in a descending degeneration of the pyramidal tract. We do not believe that

the thalamic lesion plays a role in the production of the motor difficulties.

The following anatomic-clinical data support this belief:

a. The motor difficulties are proportionate to the extent of the capsular lesion. When the latter are marked, the former are more notable and vice versa.
b. The motor difficulties are not proportionate to the extent of the thalamic lesion.
c. As a result of experiments on monkeys, one of us has found that a localized destructive lesion in the thalamus, which does not involve the internal capsule, does not produce paralysis.

It is clear that the sensory difficulties are dependant on thalamic lesions. One of us, with Long[12] in a study of the location of capsular hemianesthesia, showed that abnormalities of general sensation are seen in central lesions of the hemispheres in two conditions:

1. In thalamic lesions destroying the terminal sensory fibers from the peduncle as well as the thalamo-cortical fibers.
2. In cases where the connections between the thalamus and the sensory-motor cortex are more or less destroyed but the thalamus is intact. In this instance the lesion is always widespread.

The cases that we have studied and reported allow us to add that when the lesion involves the external nucleus of the thalamus (lateral and posterior portions especially), encroaches on the internal and median nucleus of the thalamus, and only involves a portion of the posterior segment of the internal capsule, one sees the thalamic syndrome. Such a lesion involves the centripetal ascending neurons and the general sensory central pathways which end in the thalamus. We cannot state the actual representation of the different pathways. Along with Long, we feel that the medial lemniscus (Ribbon of Reil) only represents an important part of the sensory pathway along which is transmitted all the superficial sensory impressions (touch, pain, and temperature) as well as the deep sensory impressions which are altered to varying degrees in our cases. The former appear to be quantitatively altered; the latter, qualitatively.

REFERENCES

1. Contribution to the study of pathological physiology of motor incoordination. Messrs. Dejerine and Egger, Société de Neurologie, April 1903, in *Revue neurologique*, n. 8, 1903.
2. *Société de Neurologie*, July 1904, in *Revue neurologique.*
3 *Société médicale de Genève*, November 24, 1904.

4. See Roussy, "Les coches optiques: étude anatomique, physiologique et clinique." *Thèses de Paris*, 1906.

5. *Archiv für Psychiatrie*, vol. 14, p. 598.

6. *Deutsche Zeitsch. f. Nervenheilk.*, 1881, p. 266.

7. *Revue neurologique* no. 8, 1903 (cited above).

8. *Thèses de Paris*, 1899.

9. *Thèses de Paris*, 1902.

10. *Gaz. des Hôpitaux*, 1903, no. 82.

11. Following the recent work of Sherrington and of Campbell, it seems that the ascending frontal circonvolution is uniquely motor and that the ascending parietal circonvolution is uniquely sensory. These interesting facts have not yet been confirmed in a study of localizing cerebral lesions.

12. J. Dejerine and Long, *Comptes rendus des séances et Mém. de la Société de Biologie*, December 24, 1898.

SPINOCEREBELLAR DEGENERATIONS

Introduction I

Raymond D. Adams, M.D.
Chief, Neurology Service
Massachusetts General Hospital
and
Bullard Professor of Neuropathology
Harvard Medical School

IT IS THE FATE OF THOSE who toil in what might be called the lesser employments of literary effort, such as the translation of the works of famous people, to be exposed to censure with little prospect of praise, to be accused of misinterpretation where correct interpretation would have received no applause.

Yet translations we must have, in a quasi-literate world where large professional groups speak no language but their own. And such translations are likely to be undertaken only by self-abnegating scholars. It is thoughts like these that lead me to commend Drs. Rottenberg and Hochberg for their achievement in translating from the original French three important articles on the cerebellar and sensory ataxias, articles to which reference is being made continually by English-speaking neurologists.

As every neurologist knows, the ataxias caused by heredo-degenerative diseases are rather frequent and always raise questions about Friedreich's ataxia and Charcot-Marie-Tooth peroneal muscular atrophy. However, since most of the observed cases of these types obviously do not seem to conform to either of these two diseases, an endless amount of time is spent in trying to decide where they do fit nosologically. It is then that the possibilities of Marie's cerebellar ataxia, Dejerine-Thomas's olivopontocerebellar atrophy, or the Roussy-Lévy sensory ataxia are raised. These valuable translations will surely facilitate such comparisons.

This brings to mind that neurologists are a curious breed. Confronted with an almost infinite number of diseases, mostly of unknown cause and pathogenesis, they attach great importance to naturalistic description and classification. Often diseases stand to be identified solely on this basis, graced thereafter with the names of the neurologists who reported the first case. Disappointingly, one may discover that the original description was so imprecise that even when accurately reproduced or translated it is impossible to decide what was being described. Sometimes, as the reader will note in Marie's paper, there are probably included a number of diseases presenting a similar syndrome. Or, as in the Roussy-Lévy syndrome, the data are inadequate by modern standards to permit its placement among the hereditary polyneuropathies. But one has to start someplace, and perhaps it is better to have inadequate descriptions of neurological phenomena and diseases than no descriptions at all.

The reader, instead of being dismayed by these inadequacies, should be prepared to examine the diseases critically, and, if they cannot be reconciled with present-day classifications, to view them as interesting historical landmarks.

Introduction II

Robert R. Young, M.D.
Associate Professor of Neurology
Harvard Medical School

THE TRANSLATION of these papers into English brings these syndromes more clearly to life for those who read English but not French. Unfortunately, the diagnosis of these conditions remains now, as it was when they were originally described, an entirely clinical affair. No specific biochemical, pharmacological, physiological, pathological, or other laboratory hallmark of any one of these illnesses has yet been found. Therefore, knowledge of the fine clinical details of the originally described cases remains of utmost importance. Furthermore, many of the clinical issues raised fifty to seventy-five years ago are still current.

For reasons unclear (perhaps because of its rather euphonious title or because of the recondite nature of neurologists), the Roussy-Lévy syndrome has always excited more interest than its rather infrequent incidence would appear to warrant. In 1965, Dr. Peter Dyck and his colleagues[1] attempted, for example, to simplify the nosology of the Roussy-Lévy syndrome by suggesting that the term be used to refer to patients and families where both a Charcot-Marie-Tooth-type, chronic, slowly progressive, distal, largely motor polyneuropathy and a typical familial-essential tremor coexist. The existence and nature of tremor in the Roussy-Lévy syndrome have long been debated, and careful reading of this translation suggests that tremor, in fact, was *not* a prominent or essential feature of the original patients.

Lapresle and Salisachs, in 1973,[2] have contributed immensely both to our understanding of the Roussy-Lévy syndrome and its peripheral neuropathology (a musculocutaneous nerve biopsy revealed the "onion-bulb" changes of a hypertrophic neuropathy) and to our historical edification by describing one of Roussy and Lévy's original patients in whom a

205

typical senile-essential action tremor developed more than forty years *after* she had initially been described. Her motor conduction velocities were markedly reduced (15 meters/sec). The nature of this illness and the pathophysiology of the symptoms still elude us, in part because of our difficulty in understanding and objectifying disorders of motor control and gait, especially those unassociated with clear-cut weakness, spasticity, cerebellar ataxia, or posterior column signs.

The same comments apply also to the nature of those several differing illnesses grouped together by Marie under the title "Hereditary Cerebellar Ataxia," though some of the disability from which those patients suffered is a bit more clearly definable. Marie very precisely differentiated those extremely rare diseases with true progressive degeneration of the cerebellum from the less rare spinocerebellar degenerations, such as Friedreich's ataxia, though, of course, it was not done in so many words, and he did not use the term "spinocerebellar degeneration." Even today, students of neurology must be reminded that the very clear-cut classical "cerebellar signs" demonstrated by patients with Friedreich's ataxia are not caused by anatomical lesions of the cerebellum; most likely, those are due to functional disorders of the cerebellum, since that structure—which is usually anatomically intact in these patients with spinocerebellar degeneration—is cut off from its usual input. The point was very clearly made by Marie that the cerebellum in Friedreich's ataxia is usually intact, and that "hereditary cerebellar atrophy" is quite another illness. Dejerine and Thomas, not entirely satisfied with Marie's differentiation, later defined yet another clearly different illness in this general group. Their "olivopontocerebellar atrophy" is an example of a classical advance in neurology-neuropathology, though the paper itself is rather long, overly detailed, and clinically imprecise. The authors also gloss over, all too briefly, the major point of Marie's which was mentioned above.

One of the difficulties faced by medical translators is exemplified by the term "clubfoot" in the paper by Roussy and Lévy and the one by Marie. Though the translation is literally correct, the foreshortened, high-arched, atrophic foot described in both these papers is not, in English, referred to as a clubfoot. It is best described as *pes cavus* or, perhaps, as "Friedreich's foot."

While reading these papers again, one is struck with how little progress we have made in the past seventy-five years. Dejerine and Thomas, for example, report very detailed observations on vestibular function as tested by rotating patients in a chair. Though electronic monitoring devices are now available in certain very specialized otoneurological laboratories, today's neurologists would do well to emulate the purely clinical studies carried out by Dejerine and Thomas. Another striking feature is the difficulty, present now as then, resulting from the use of nonobjective clinical descriptions, which underscores the need for quantitative methods for recording tremor and other movement disorders. It is difficult enough, even when the patient is at hand, to be certain of the nature and extent of the elemental abnormalities without objective tests and may very well be impossible retrospectively, no matter how precise the description.

NOTES

1. Yudell, A., Dyck, P. J., and Lambert, E. H. "A kinship with the Roussy-Lévy syndrome." *Arch Neurol* 13:432–440, 1965.
2. Lapresle, J., and Salisachs, P. "Onion bulbs in a nerve biopsy specimen from an original case of Roussy-Lévy disease." *Arch Neurol* 29:346–348, 1973.

Hereditary Cerebellar Ataxia

P. MARIE

It is well known that hereditary ataxia is appropriately named after Friedreich, who first described it. Although his first observations date from 1861, the illness has been recognized as a nosologic entity only during the past ten years. Since then, the name "Friedreich's malady" has been generally adopted and substituted for the term hereditary ataxia. Hereditary ataxia is a generic name for a group of clinical cases distinct from Friedreich's ataxia, but sharing two features in common with it: an identical movement disorder and a hereditary origin. I will restrict my presentation to the facts which define hereditary ataxia as an entity separate from Friedreich's ataxia. The addition of the term "of cerebellar origin" when discussing hereditary ataxia will become clearer when I discuss the pathology of this condition.

Before proceeding further, I would like to restate the characteristics of Friedreich's ataxia. This will point out the differences between Friedreich's ataxia and hereditary cerebellar ataxia.

The motor disorder in Friedreich's ataxia consists of marked disturbances in both gait and position initially resembling titubation more than ataxia; Romberg's sign is absent or rarely present. Movements are accompanied by a series of oscillations of the extremities, even of the head or trunk, similar to the intention tremor of multiple sclerosis. The movements also have a choreic quality. Sensory difficulties are minimal, lightning pains are rare, and anesthesia or analgesia either absent or

NOTE: Translated by F.H. Hochberg from Marie, P., "Sur l'hérédo-ataxie cérébelleuse," *La Semaine médicale* 13 (1893), 444–47.

infrequently noted. Cutaneous reflexes are usually preserved, but the patellar reflexes are absent. The most frequently noted and most important eye sign is nystagmus, which is especially marked with fixation (in the anatomic position) or on lateral gaze. In most instances diplopia and ocular muscle paralysis are absent. Visual functions and the optic nerve are spared. Pupillary reactions to both light and accommodation are normal. Taste, hearing, and smell are preserved. Vertigo is rather frequently observed and may be permanent. Intelligence is not affected, although sometimes poorly developed. In the average case, speech is quite altered; it is slow, uncertain, a little scanning (arhythmic), and explosive. There are no genito-urinary difficulties except delayed puberty. Although there are no cutaneous manifestations, there are very characteristic bony deformities: a sort of clubfoot with shortened antero-posterior axis, a clawlike deformity (position) of the toes with notable retraction of the great toes. Sometimes, rather marked spinal scoliosis is present. Infrequently, selected muscular atrophy is seen. The illness is progressive, the first findings often being retraction of the great toe or disappearance of the patellar reflexes. Friedreich's is a familial illness involving several members of a family, especially in a single generation. In most cases the illness appears before age fourteen.

These are the classical clinical features of Friedreich's ataxia. Variants exist, but they do not significantly differ from the above. On the other hand, there are other cases (referred to as hereditary cerebellar ataxia) which share some features in common with Friedreich's ataxia (heredity, disturbances, movement disorders, etc.) but show a number of atypical features. Today I wish to discuss these special cases.

The cases in order of date are: Fraser's[1], Nonne's[2], Sanger Brown's[3], and Klippel and Durante's[4]. Later I shall cite other more or less analogous observations.

I would like to discuss the characteristics of this group of cases and, in doing so, emphasize how they differ from Friedreich's ataxia. With respect to etiology, all cases are clearly familial in character—in Sanger Brown's family there were no less than twenty-three persons affected. It should be noted that in the cases described by Sanger Brown, Nonne, and Klippel and Durante, the influence of heredity is immediately apparent. For example, in Sanger Brown's report, the great-grandmother presented with symptoms of this illness, as did her daughter, granddaughter, and great-granddaughter. In typical Friedreich's ataxia, on the other hand, it is rare to find affected ancestors; most often several children of one generation are involved. This is not an absolute rule. The slight differences between the two illnesses might be due to the fact that Friedreich's ataxia typically starts in childhood or at the onset of puberty. Those afflicted rarely marry and have progeny. On the other hand, patients with hereditary cerebellar ataxia become symptomatic between twenty and twenty-three years of age—making them more likely to marry and procreate.

From Sanger Brown's observations, it would seem that women are more often affected than men—of thirty-three men in the family, twelve were affected, whereas eleven of the nineteen women were affected. In one branch of the family only the single girl was affected—her four brothers remained healthy.

It is not rare for hereditary ataxia to skip one or even two generations; thus, an affected grandmother with a healthy son and a healthy granddaughter might have several affected and several unaffected great-grandchildren.

Hereditary cerebellar ataxia seems to be passed by the female line. In Sanger Brown's family, there were three instances in which the father was the origin of the children's involvement, but nine instances in which the mother was the origin.

Families with individuals "affected" by hereditary cerebellar ataxia show "unaffected" individuals with neuropathies. In Nonne's family, individuals not suffering from hereditary cerebellar ataxia had many and varied neuropathies.

As to the age of onset of hereditary cerebellar ataxia, it must be noted that although some individuals are afflicted in childhood, most are afflicted later—after the twentieth year, often (as in the cases of Sanger Brown, Klippel and Durante) after age thirty and in two cases (of Sanger Brown) at the advanced age of forty-five years.

In the typical Friedreich's ataxia the age of onset is generally much earlier; it appears most often in childhood, very rarely after sixteen years of age.

I shall now discuss in a general way the mode of onset of hereditary cerebellar ataxia, its presenting symptoms, and its course.

The illness first appears as a slow and progressive lower extremity instability noted while standing or walking. Lightning pains in the legs and lumbar region have also been noted as first signs. The motion instability involves the hands within one to three years (Sanger Brown has seen hand involvement as a first sign but this is quite unusual). At about the same time speech and vision become involved. The patellar reflexes are preserved and rather often exaggerated. Sometimes muscle spasms are seen. Several cases have shown altered cutaneous sensation. Dementia may occur. Swallowing and urinary spincter troubles are rarely seen. The illness is essentially progressive but may remit, and is not in itself fatal. Death often in older age usually follows an intercurrent, often pulmonary, illness.

Having described the clinical features and the progress of this illness, I will now deal with its symptoms, signaling the principal aspects of each. The impairment of lower extremity function is similar to that seen in Friedreich's ataxia. Both illnesses show titubating gait resulting more from disequilibrium than from true muscular incoordination. The legs are spread, the steps irregular; the feet fall heavily on the ground but without the excessive, useless, and antagonistic movements which gives the tabetic gait its unique stamp.

The patients (with hereditary cerebellar ataxia) walk with their torso thrown back and their lower back curved. Initially they are able to move without too much pain, but, little by little, as their disability increases, they are obliged to use a cane. Soon the cane is no longer satisfactory. Then they must be supported by the arms. When alone, they support themselves on walls or furniture. In certain cases, standing upright is also difficult. The patient, body bent forward, supports himself against a wall by shifting his weight slightly. His head is thrown back and swings as if it were too heavy for his neck to hold it steady. The head is thrown back to counterbalance the forward bend of the body. These descriptions apply to cases of long standing. Early on, patients have difficulty with lower-extremity function notable only after great fatigue or after a long walk. Sometimes, the patient is initially unaware of the gait disturbance—which is obvious to his friends. It is not unusual for the initial titubation to be taken for inebriation. Closure of the eyes produces little change in equilibrium; unlike in Tabes, Romberg's sign is absent. Romberg's sign is commonly absent in typical Friedreich's ataxia. Some patients complain of vertigo which increases their standing and walking difficulties.

Arm motility is more slowly and less obviously affected than that of the legs. As in Friedreich's ataxia, the motor disorder is a sort of *pseudo-trembling* occurring during voluntary motion. Initially, delicate motions such as writing, picking up a pin, and buttoning clothes are the most altered. As the illness progresses, grosser movements are affected. The patients eat and lift a full drinking glass with great difficulty. The motor disturbance is seen during voluntary movements and ceases when the movements are completed. For example, the ataxic movements which appear when the patient attempts to grasp a pencil cease when his hand has reached it. He then holds the pencil firmly and without tremor. Eye closure has only a slight effect. During various activities the head and torso oscillate together with the extremities, but this oscillation ceases when the movement is completed and the patient is sufficiently "im-mobilized." There is no weakness of the upper or lower extremities.

Apart from the disorders of motility, I wish to emphasize the occur-rence of *muscular tremors*. Several authors call these "fibrillary trem-blings," but they are not similar to the almost continuous fine fibrillary contractions seen in the various amyotrophies. These tremors are seen in many torso and limb muscles (back, thigh, and thenar eminence) according to Klippel and Durant. Exaggerated contractions of the facial muscle often accompany changes in facial expression, speech, or limb movements. Sometimes, sudden contractions of the extremities are seen. These various muscular findings are also seen in typical Friedreich's ataxia.

The occurrence of *spastic phenomena* is particularly interesting. This sign is one of the bases for the diagnosis of hereditary cerebellar ataxia. There is general agreement that the patellar reflexes are increased, although not greatly. Only in the case of Klippel and Durante (François H.) were the patellar reflexes decreased. These reflex changes are distinctly different from those of Friedreich's ataxia, in which the patellar reflexes are abolished. Early in the illness they may be present. On the other hand, the patellar reflexes are increased after more than fifteen years of hereditary cerebellar ataxia. As Sanger Brown noted, the hyperactivity of the patellar reflexes often preceeds other symptoms and thus serves as an indicator of future illness in family members. Ankle clonus is very rarely observed (three cases of Sanger Brown).

Most authors speak of a more or less permanent *spasticity* of the extremities—especially the legs. One of Sanger Brown's patients had "the thighs flexed almost at a right angle—the contracture being partially overcome by pulling with slow and continuous force on the extremities." In the same vein, Klippel and Durante noted that in "Miss X, it was difficult to determine the state of the reflexes because of the rigidity which occurred when one examined them." Nonne, describing his three cases, notes that "there was a difficulty in relaxing the voluntary muscles during passive motion."

With regard to sensation, sharp pains occur in the legs and loins, especially at the onset of the illness. Objective sensory disturbances are rare. Klippel and Durante observed them in their three patients, especially in Miss H., who was *anesthetic* to all sensory modalities on the inner aspect of the legs and along the tibial crests; *sensory perception* was diminished in other areas as well. Patient Louis H. was anesthetic in the legs and feet and had markedly diminished sensation in the forearms and hands, slightly diminished sensation over the face, and preserved sensation over the arms and torso. Pinprick was absent in the same distribution but was most notable over the knees and elbows. The face was spared. Heat was perceived throughout; cold was not felt at all. Two points applied simultaneously 8 cm apart could be appreciated on the extremities. These sensory findings are not typical of Friedreich's ataxia and thus support the diagnosis of hereditary cerebellar ataxia.

There is a difference of opinion regarding proprioception (we have already pointed out the complete or partial absence of Romberg's sign). Most authors feel that it is either intact or minimally affected, but Klippel and Durante considered that proprioception was significantly altered in their three patients. It is also difficult to explain the motor disturbances in classical Friedreich's ataxia.

The plantar reflex is most often conserved, rarely increased, and sometimes abolished.

The special senses, other than vision, are not noteworthy. In Klippel and Durante's cases there were three instances of decreased *auditory acuity,* one patient with decreased olfactory perception on the left, and one patient with minimally abnormal taste. The visual apparatus is quite another story, and I shall consider the extraocular musculature, the pupillary reactions, and formal visual function in detail.

Cases 9 and 18 of Sanger Brown had pronounced but incomplete ptosis with the eyes in the primary position. The latter patient could still lift his lids and uncover the sclera above the cornea. This incomplete ptosis gave the patient's gaze a unique appearance similar to that produced by intense emotion. In Klippel and Durante's cases, in which ptosis was absent, the eyes were wide open but the face had an "astonished appearance."

In most patients true nystagmus is absent, in contrast to patients with multiple sclerosis. However, nystagmuslike tremors are observed at the extremes of gaze. This is also a finding in typical Friedreich's ataxia.

Many patients exhibit varying degrees of *paralysis of the external rectus muscle.* This appears as a fixation of the gaze in one direction (up and to the left—Fraser); as *internal strabismus,* or as transitory diplopia. Convergence is frequently weak.

The pupils are usually equal, neither dilatated or constricted. However, their reactions leave something to be desired. The *light reflex* is slow or even abolished (Sanger Brown) while accommodation is preserved. The *Argyll-Robertson sign* is present in these cases as in Tabes. Two of Klippel and Durante's cases (Louis H. and François H.) had total pupillary immobility resulting from either weak or absent *accommodation reflexes.*

I wish to emphasize the disturbances of *visual function* which have diagnostic significance. The visual fields are bilaterally constricted in many cases. This constriction is pronounced in some patients and less in others. Less often *dyschromatopsia,* especially for green, is noted; visual acuity is frequently, but not always, diminished. One of Nonne's patients (Fritz) had an acuity of 1/9 on the right, 1/6 on the left; the acuity of one of Heinrich's patients was 5/10 bilaterally. In Sanger Brown's cases 10 and 18 the acuity was 20/200 bilaterally; the patients were able to read line 5 on Snellen's chart at a distance of 8 inches with difficulty. Case 19 of the same author read Snellen's line 3 at 10 inches. Others have noted greater diminution in visual acuity: Klippel and Durante speak of amaurosis in two of their cases; Botkine's patient was blind in the left eye,[5] and Sanger Brown's case 9 was almost completely blind. Many of Sanger Brown's patients with only slightly diminished visual acuity were able to read better in feeble than in ordinary light.

Although it is hard to be precise as to the course of the diminished visual acuity, certain points are worthy of note: the phenomenon shows itself many years after the onset of disease, at a time when the lower extremity motor difficulties are already accentuated.

Case 9 of Sanger Brown showed diminished vision twenty-two years after the onset of hereditary cerebellar ataxia. However, this is not always the situation; case 7 of the same author suffered a diminution eight years after the onset of illness. Mr. Louis H. (described by Klippel and Durante) showed diminished vision four years after the onset of illness. The visual troubles usually start in one eye. The other eye is involved after an interval of one, two, or three years. The visual difficulties are slowly progressive.

Klippel and Durante noted no abnormalities of the optic fundus of patients with visual troubles; but Fraser, Sanger Brown, and Nonne observed obvious changes. These consist of a whitish discoloration of the discs and a decreased caliber of disc vessels. The disc rim is well preserved. Similarly, atrophic lesions of the choroid and retina are seen.

The visual system involvement serves to distinguish hereditary cerebellar ataxia from typical Friedreich's ataxia. It is true that nystagmuslike tremors are seen in both illnesses. In Friedreich's ataxia, ocular muscle palsies are absent or extremely rare[6], the pupillary reactions are normal, there is no narrowing of the visual field (aside from the cases with concomitant hysteria as noted by Charcot), there is no dyschromatopsia, and the visual acuity and optic fundus are without abnormalities.

Speech function is similar in both hereditary cerebellar ataxia and Friedreich's ataxia. The speech is slow, gutteral, hesitant, nearly explosive—approaching that of individuals with multiple sclerosis, but less scanning. As Klippel and Durante noted, the integrity of the patients' intelligence is questioned as a result of the exaggerated movements of his tongue, lip and facial muscles during speech. This is especially true for polysyllabic words which are pronounced without skipping a syllable. As we shall see in most of the cases, this (suspicion of altered intelligence) is in error.

In general, the mental faculties are not affected. At most, a *diminution of memory* and a *melancholic* appearance are noted. Sometimes patients have more accentuated mental troubles. Sanger Brown's case 12 appeared bewildered, and Nonne's patients showed a *foolishness*, a veritable morbid insouciance. Nonne, in addition, remarked that these patients had particularly small skulls.

As regards the *digestive organs*, there is nothing of note. Sanger Brown's cases 5, 15, and 17 had difficulty with swallowing—the patients choked when they drank without precaution. Botkine's case experienced excessive salivation.

The only notable *genito-urinary* difficulty is the delayed onset of menstruation in women with hereditary cerebellar ataxia (generally at age eighteen)—a phenomenon found also in typical Friedreich's ataxia. Otherwise, the periods seem normal in frequency and quantity. The sexual functions of male patients are not obviously altered.

Sanger Brown's case 10 had difficulty retaining urine. Fearing an accident, the patient was obliged to urinate following the first urge to do so. Aside from this, the *sphincters* always functioned normally.

Trophic disturbances are usually absent in hereditary cerebellar ataxia; although patient François H. (of Klippel and Durante) experienced nail loss. Sanger Brown's case 5 developed amyotrophy and the authors noted loss of weight among patients. With the exception of Botkine's case (with a mild kyphoscoliosis), patients with hereditary cerebellar ataxia show no trace of the scoliosis that is so frequent in typical Friedreich's ataxia. Moreover, in hereditary cerebellar ataxia one doesn't find the unique clubfoot of Friedreich's ataxia. This clubfoot appears in such a precocious fashion in certain families that it constitutes one of the best signs of the onset of the latter illness.

I have come to the end of my clinical presentation. I have emphasized those symptoms which differentiate hereditary cerebellar ataxia from typical Friedreich's ataxia. Rather than reiterate these differences, I will rapidly enumerate the principal and distinctive characteristics of hereditary cerebellar ataxia: age more advanced at the onset of illness, preserved or exaggerated patellar reflexes, frequent spastic phenomena, visual troubles (diminished visual fields, dyschromatopsia, diminished visual acuity), and absent kyphoscoliosis and clubfoot.

Comparison of the symptoms of the two processes causes one to realize the necessity of differentiating them.

I must now determine whether the same separation can be made from a pathologic point of view. Unhappily, there are few documents on the pathologic anatomy of hereditary cerebellar ataxia. In reality, only two autopsy reports—Fraser's and Nonne's—are available; but their data are in agreement. In both, one aspect is striking: the *cerebellar atrophy.* The weight of this organ had been reduced by one quarter. It weighed 81 grams in Fraser's case and 120 grams in Nonne's, normal weight being 150 to 170 grams. On the contrary, the brain, which seemed normal in Fraser's and in Nonne's cases, had only suffered a loss of 1/9 of its normal weight. Nonne did not notice any microscope cerebellar change. Fraser reported that while the cerebellar cortical grey matter was especially reduced in volume, the white matter was scarcely involved. Fraser even noted the disappearance of a great number of Purkinje cells and the alteration of the remainder. In summary, one fact seems well established—the cerebellar atrophy. One other chief fact springs from the two autopsies—the spinal cord, examined microscopically, presents no changes. Only decreased volume of the cord was noted (Nonne).

I would like to compare these pathologic facts to those that we have about typical Friedreich's ataxia. Although there are symptomatic and pathologic[7] similarities between the two afflictions, their differences are marked. In Friedreich's ataxia, which shows a similarly diminished spinal cord, microscopic examination of all autopsies reveals interesting, extensive degenerative lesions in the tract of Burdach (fasciculus cuneatus), the tract of Goll (fasciculus gracilis), the direct cerebellar tract (dorsal spinocerebellar tract), the crossed pyramidal tract (lateral corticospinal tract), and the cells of Clarke. This is a marked difference from hereditary cerebellar ataxia, which is not accompanied by any spinal-cord degeneration.

These facts seem to legitimize the group, hereditary cerebellar ataxia. In order to be most clear and to present the picture of this illness in sufficient relief in this brief account, I have described only those cases with rather clear-cut pathologic or clinical features. Before closing, I would like to present certain reservations concerning this question.

There are many cases with less well-defined symptoms or more complex pathologic lesions which do not easily fall either into this new morbid group or into that of typical Friedreich's ataxia. Sharing features of both illnesses, they fall between the two and represent transition forms which are difficult to rationally classify.

The two cases of Steegmüller[8] had their onset after puberty, had exaggerated patellar reflexes, and differed from typical cases of Friedreich's ataxia. As visual troubles were absent or appeared to be absent, these cases could only be classified as being related to hereditary cerebellar atrophy.

In the first report of Rouffinet, the patient's age and visual troubles suggested the possibility of hereditary cerebellar ataxia. However, the report is so abridged that a decision cannot be made.

The case of Menzel[9] is certainly the most embarrassing of all. The patient had almost all the classic symptoms of typical Friedreich's ataxia, but exhibited exaggerated patellar reflexes and other spastic phenomena (clawlike hands, legs contracted in flexion). Only the absence of visual troubles prevented me from including the case within the group hereditary cerebellar ataxia. It seemed that the autopsy would permit an easy resolution of the difficulty; but the lesions, as well as the symptoms, shared characteristics of hereditary cerebellar ataxia and typical Friedreich's ataxia. As in the latter, the spinal cord showed multiple pronounced degenerative changes (posterior columns, lateral corticospinal tracts, dorsal spinocerebellar tracts, columns of Clarke, etc.) and, as in the former, there was evident cerebellar atrophy with loss of Purkinje cells and fibers.

One such case is enough to inspire the reservations that I mentioned previously. Until we are better informed, given the information at hand, I wonder whether the pathologic changes of hereditary cerebellar ataxia and typical Friedreich's ataxia are not closer than was apparent at first glance. The divergences between them are more a product of differences in symptoms than pathology. It is possible that both are parts of the same morbid process. This hereditary degenerative process as represented in the two conditions might initially affect similarly functioning but anatomically distinct nervous centers, or in Friedreich's ataxia might affect a number of other systems in addition to those affected in hereditary cerebellar ataxia.[10]

NOTES

1. Fraser. "Defect in the cerebellum occurring in a brother and sister." *Glasgow Medical Journal*, 1880, fasc. 1.
2. "Über eine eigentümliche familiare Erkrankungsform des Centralnervensystems." *Arch. f. Psychiatrie* 22:283 (1891).
3. Sanger Brown. "On hereditary ataxy with a series of twenty-one cases." *Brain*, 58 (1892).
4. Klippel and Durante. "Contribution a l'étude des affections nerveuses familiales et héréditaires" [Contribution to the study of famial & hereditary nervous diseases]. *Revue de med.*, October 1892, p. 745 and *Semaine Medicale*, 1892, p. 467.
5. Botkine. "Un cas de maladie de Friedreich" [A case of Friedreich's ataxia]. *Revue Médicale*, Moscow, 1885, no. 1. I only know of this case through a brief abstract, but I have every reason to believe that it is really hereditary cerebellar ataxia.
6. Rouffinet. "Essai clinique sur les troubles oculaires dans la maladie de Friedreich et sur le rétrécissement du champ visuel dans la syringomyélie et la maladie de Morvan." [Clinical essay on the ocular problems in Friedreich's ataxia and on visual field constriction in syringomyelia and Morvan's syndrome (distal phalangeal analgesia, often with necrosis, of multiple etiologies)]. *Théses de Paris*, 1891.
7. I recall that Senator (*Berl. Klin. Wochenschr.*, 22 May 1893) recently hypothesized that the initial lesion in Friedreich's ataxia was in the cerebellum. However, this hypothesis is based on the cases of Nonne and of Menzel, which were not really patients with typical Friedreich's ataxia. On the one hand, in a recent autopsy of a patient with very atypical Friedreich's ataxia, E. Auscher (*Arch. de physiol.*, April 1893) noted that the cerebellum was infinitely less atrophic than the brain and the brain stem. It seems, therefore, that although cerebellar lesions play an important role in Friedreich's ataxia, they are less pronounced than in hereditary cerebellar ataxia.

8. Seeligmüller. "Hereditäre Ataxia mit Nystagmus." *Arch. f. Psychiatrie* 10:222 (1879).

9. P. Menzel. "Beiträge zur Kenntniss der hereditären Ataxie und Kleinhirnatrophie." *Arch. f. Psychiatrie* 22:160 (1891).

10. It should prove rather interesting to compare cases of hereditary cerebellar ataxia and the cases of *familial cerebral diplegia* reported by several authors, especially by S. Freud (*Neurol. Centr.-Bl.*, 1893). Spastic phenomena are more pronounced in the latter. Some features are shared by both illnesses: slow speech, nystagmus, and optic nerve atrophy. Although both are quite similar, they differ in that spastic phenomena are more exaggerated in familial cerebral diplegia. This is so much the case that the patient's gait has a frankly spastic quality. In addition, patients with familial deplegia show no pseudo-tremors or pseudo-incoordination, which are so obvious in hereditary cerebellar ataxia. Thus we see how the differences between these separate illnesses result from the hereditary degenerative process coincidentally involving many organic systems—some similar and some distinct.

Olivopontocerebellar Atrophy

J. DEJERINE AND A. THOMAS

THE MEDICAL LITERATURE contains similar clinical cases of cerebellar atrophy which are pathologically distinct. We shall try to classify these atrophies with reference to two personal cases, one of which was autopsied. In doing so we hope to emphasize a particular anatomic type, one instance of which has already been reported (Thomas, *Le Cervelet Obs.* 4:207, Th. Doctorate, 1897).

We will discuss the symptomatology of the cerebellar atrophies, the diagnosis and pertinent aspects of cerebellar anatomy and pathophysiology.

CASE 1

D.V., a fifty-three-year-old female newspaper dealer, was hospitalized at the Sâlpetrière Hospital on April 29, 1896. Her parents had been healthy: her father died at seventy-three year of age, her mother at eighty-three. She was the youngest of eight healthy children. There was no history of hereditary diseases, and the patient knew of no other relative with a malady similar to hers.

The patient had eight full-term infants, of which all but one (now thirty years old) had died in childhood of poorly described illnesses. Her husband died at sixty-four years of age. The patient did not know the nature of his terminal illness. She reached menopause uneventfully in 1894 at age fifty-one. Her past history included generalized joint pains

NOTE: Translated by F.H. Hochberg from Dejerine, J., and Thomas, A., "L'Atrophie olivo-ponto-cérébelleuse," *Nouvelle Iconographie de la Salpêtrière* 13 (1900), 330–70.

for twenty years, but it was impossible to determine if this was actually rheumatoid arthritis.

The patient presented with an insidious illness of eight months duration. She walked with difficulty, and became quickly fatigued. Although she trembled and her equilibrium seemed to be disturbed, she recalled no falls. She had neither vertigo nor the illusion of objects revolving around her. Sometimes, while standing, she felt drawn forward and, fearing a fall, would clutch nearby objects. Later, she became less and less sure of herself while walking, and fatigued sooner. Her speech became slower and somewhat saccadic, her arms clumsier, her writing increasingly illegible and marked by tremulousness and poorly formed letters. Her personality changed little by little. Whereas formerly she had been extremely gay, often singing, she became quiet and withdrawn, and constantly tormented herself about her illness. Her memory was intact, and her vision was not affected. During the three months prior to admission she complained of constant dribbling of urine. There was no fecal incontinence, and she was rather constipated.

Examination of May 7, 1896:   The patient was strikingly immobile in bed. Her head was fixed and her face expressed astonishment. The rest of her body was immobile. She lay with her hands crossed over her chest. Her lips were slightly elevated on the left; on the right they were slightly lowered. She could close her eyes without much force and could not knit her brows. Pupillary reactions were intact. Extraocular movements were normal with the exception of upward gaze, which was performed in a jerky nystagmoid fashion. This was not true nystagmus. Vision was intact without diplopia. Ophthalmoscopic examination failed to reveal any funduscopic lesions. Color vision was intact, but formal visual fields were not obtained. Unfortunately, an examination in the rotating chair, a technique used to test the intactness of compensatory movements and nystagmus, was not performed. (At the time of the above-mentioned examination we were not familiar with the apparatus and were unaware of its usefulness in the diagnosis of this illness. We were able to perform this examination on our second patient.) Lip movements (lip elevation, mouth opening, and pouting) were intact but slow and listless, especially on the right. The tongue protruded in all directions, and the palate moved with good strength. There were no difficulties with swallowing or chewing; the masticatory muscles functioned normally. Speech was slow with a slight drawl and a scanning quality. Feeble lip and mimetic movements resulted in dysarthria. Flexion, extension, inclination, and rotation of the head and neck were normal, even against resistance. These movements, as all of her movements, were slow. Facial sensation was intact; touch, pain, temperature, and the special sensations (vision, smell, and taste) were normal.

There was no arm weakness, but passive motion revealed greatly increased flexor and extensor tone. There were no oscillations or digital tremors of the outstretched, vertically extended arms. There was no intention tremor. When the patient brought an object to her mouth, the moving extremity had no more tremor at the start than at the end of the motion. Nevertheless, voluntary movements were hesitant and slow, and those involving a heavy object or dexterous manipulation were clumsily performed. She spilled liquid when attempting to fill a glass because the hand holding the bottle trembled. Her handwriting was also altered: her arm trembled while holding a pen. The muscles of the thenar eminence had fibrillary contractions. Her writing clearly showed the extent of this tremulousness. Written characters were irregular, unequally spaced, and often unrecognizable, though they were written slowly and with considerable care (Fig. 1).

Position sense and proprioception were intact. She could use her right hand to imitate postures that had been imparted to her left hand. This could be done with her eyes open or closed. She could touch her finger to her nose or ear. Touch, pain, and temperature sensation were normal in the upper extremities. The triceps and radial-periosteal reflexes were increased. There was no wrist clonus.

Movements of the lower extremities were perfect, including extension, abduction, and flexion. There was no muscle atrophy. However, considerable resistance to passive motion was encountered. Position sense and proprioception were intact. The tendon reflexes were exaggerated bilaterally, but there was no patellar or ankle clonus.

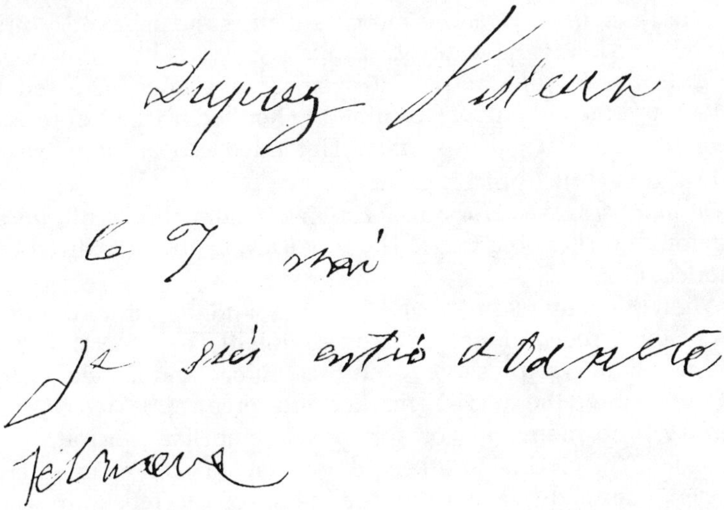

Figure 1.

Equilibrium and gait problems: The patient could not arise from a sitting position without support because of severe trunkal ataxia. She stood with a wide base, her legs separated, elbows abducted, and body titubating in both antero-posterior and side-to- side directions. We were obliged to support her, as she feared she was about to fall forwards. Pro- and retropulsion made her quite unstable. Despite all this, she could stand unsupported for several seconds with her legs abducted. When she was helped to bring her heels together, she was obliged to separate them once again to maintain her balance. As a result, she was fearful and needed someone to support and escort her while working. She walked with legs spread. She slowly lifted each foot and paused after each step. After several hesitations she took a short step by brusquely lifting and brusquely replacing her foot. These movements were accompanied by whole body oscillations.

In summary, her gait lacked any trace of normal rhythm, cadence, and measure. She did not titubate like a drunkard; rather she advanced uncertainly. She could almost walk a straight line without swinging her legs in an ataxic fashion; but each step was performed hesitantly and with considerable effort.

While standing or walking with her eyes closed she developed trunkal ataxia. There was no Romberg's sign; eye closure only minimally worsened the gait ataxia and hesitation.

Treatment consisted of small doses of sodium iodide. The general examination showed no organic abnormalities. In the hospital, the patient's clinical state grew perceptibly worse—her speech was slower (the syllables more saccadic and enunciated with greater difficulty), her gait more hesitant, the oscillations more numerous and of greater amplitude. She could no longer move forward unless supported on someone's arm. The difficulties with station and balance were now increased by eye closure, and the patient was confined to her bed because of progressive disequilibrium and gait disability. Her intellect was diminished. She died suddenly on April 11, 1898.

The autopsy was performed forty-eight hours after death because of the family's earlier objections. The thoracic and abdominal viscera were excluded.

When the brain was removed from the skull the extraordinary smallness of the cerebellum and pons were noted. The general structure of the cerebellum was preserved, but the laminae and lamellae [sic] were quite narrow and the sulci less marked—the organ appeared compressed. There was no meningitis or superficial cerebellar, cortical, or bulbar adhesions. The cerebral arteries did not show thickening or atheromata. Meynert's cut allowed us to fix the bulb, pons, cerebellum, midbrain, and basal ganglia in one block. The medulla seemed smaller than normal and was fixed and hardened in the same way. After fixing in Müller's fixative, and embedding in celloidin, the block was serially sectioned on Gudden's microtome. Transverse sections were stained using the Weigert-Pal and carmine methods. Prior to this, small pieces of cerebellar cortex were set apart to be carmine-stained en bloc or by Forel's method and sectioned after inclusion in paraffin. This would allow for a complete and detailed examination of the histologic changes. Small segments of the medulla, taken at various levels, were set aside and examined after similar staining.

The pathologic findings will be presented in the following sequence:

1. Cerebellum
2. Cerebellar peduncles: their nuclei of origin and their medullary, bulbar, pontine, and cortical pathways
3. The cerebellar peduncles at their entrance into the cerebellum

EXAMINATION OF THE CEREBELLUM

A. Cortex: There was diffuse atrophy of the cortical laminae which was not uniform, being less pronounced in the vermis than in the hemispheres. The molecular and granular layers, as well as the white matter, were also atrophic. High-power examinations of the Weigert-Pal–stained whole brain sections revealed hardly any myelinated fibers in the white matter of the laminae.

The central vermal regions showed varying degrees of atrophy: the pyramid of the inferior vermis and the culmen of the superior vermis were the least involved, followed by the uvula, nodulus, lingula, and central lobule, and the most severely affected declive and posterior tubercle of the vermis.

The extremely reduced tonsil and flocculus approached the vermis, rather than the hemispheres, in their degree of alteration. The peduncles of the flocculus were still discernible. The atrophy was maximal in the cerebellar hemispheres—especially in the lobes and lobules of the inferior surface of the cerebellum. The laminae bordering the superior vermis, namely, those most medially located in the *superior semilunar lobule*, were relatively less affected, but the difference was not considerable.

Histologic examination of cortical segments at the level of the semilunar lobules (a region which had been set aside to be stained en bloc with carmine) showed:

1. Medullary layer: This layer [superficial molecular layer: subpial] was made up of a reticular glial meshwork in which some neuroglial nuclei can be seen at the intersection of fibrils. There were no Deiters' cells in the middle of the meshwork. Several rare axis cylinders were seen.

The vessels appeared normal, without evidence of proliferation, thickening, or hemorrhage. Normally the medullary layer is a loose glial network composed of myelinated fibers; in the present case this layer has been stripped of most of its nerve fibers and reduced to a glial reticulum. In certain areas this meshwork appeared thickened—more as a result of compression than of glial hyperplasia.

2. Purkinje cells: Most of the cells had disappeared, but in an irregular fashion. Portions of a lamina contained no Purkinje cells, or rare, isolated cells, while on the opposite surface or on the rim there might be six or more cells. These cells were appropriately distant from each other but irregular, shriveled, and deeply stained with carmine. At higher magnification the nucleus and nucleolus appeared deformed and irregular, occasionally spiral rather than round or oval. The cell body was irregular and scalloped. Other cells showed more obvious and more advanced changes: the nucleus might be difficult to discern, yet appear to give rise to radiating protoplasmic filaments which partitioned the cell and gave it a vacuolized appearance. Elsewhere the nucleus had disappeared leaving a vacuole-filled cell or only protoplasmic debris. No vascular lesions or glial proliferation were appreciated.

3. Granular layer: With carmine stain the granule cells appeared pale rose-colored, grey, or yellow, rather than the customary red. They were irregular, oval, crenated, or polygonal rather than round, and had granular cytoplasm. Other cells were rounder with a more prominent grainy cytoplasm. The cells were not compressed; the intercellular spaces were often large and without a glial feltwork. Myelinated fibers, axis cylinders and glial fibers were rare in this layer. The vessels were not increased or abnormal.

4. Molecular layer: Normally this is composed of: (1) Purkinje-cell processes, (2) the stellate basket cells whose processes surround Purkinje cells, and (3) the T-shaped divisions of the granular fibers.

The Purkinje-cell processes were almost completely absent, and basket cells were lacking in certain areas. Elsewhere, the latter were atrophied with indistinct processes and irregular or discolored nuclei. There was no glial hyperplasia, meningeal thickening, or vascular alterations. The meningeal vessels had thickened walls without perivascular cuffing [accumulated embryonal elements indicating mesenchymal reaction]. Amyloid bodies were common. In view of these lesions we were not surprised by the atrophy of the lobes, lobules, laminae, and lamellae.

B. *Central nuclei (Figs. 2 and 3D)**: These were smaller than normal but were less atrophic than the cortex. The dentate nuclei were relatively

*Figures 2–4 in this translation were called plates XLVII–XLIX in the original article—EDS.

well preserved, but overall were reduced in size. Their festoons and infoldings were small, and the nucleus appeared retracted, especially its posterior inferior folds [festoons]. The fibers of the dentate hilum and those surrounding the dentate [toison] stood out by their intense staining for myelin. At higher magnification the medullary fibers and cells appeared normal in number.

The roof nuclei were small and were only visible in selected sections. The fibers surrounding them were even more attenuated than those surrounding the dentate. The emboliform and globose nuclei were atrophic, but the thickness of the section prevented a detailed examination. However, nerve cells were present.

C. *Cerebellar white matter (Figs. 2 and 3):*

1. Cortical: Deeply stained fibers were seen in the vermal cortex, the internal laminae of the tonsil, the pedicle of the flocculus, and especially in the pyramis and the culmen. For the most part these were projection fibers but some were [intrinsic] association fibers or fibers with a wreath-like pattern [the garland of Stilling—see Dejerine, *Anatomie des Centres Nervaux*, p. 507–586, 1901, vol.2]. The remainder of the preserved cortical fibers were association fibers; a few fibers could be traced to the border of the granular and molecular layers, but very few entered the hemispheric white matter.

2. Central nuclei: The intense staining of the fibers surrounding the dentate nucleus and of the fibers of the central (hilar) white matter has already been mentioned. The latter are continuous with the superior cerebellar peduncle. The fibers surrounding the fastigial, emboliform, and globose nuclei were less numerous. The usually beautiful fascicles of fibers emanating from these nuclei to form the internal semicircular fibers of the cerebellum could not be seen.

3. Central vermian white matter (arbor vitae): In contrast to the above atrophy the middle third of the central vermian white matter contained well-myelinated fibers. The anterior and posterior thirds appeared partially degenerated and contained poorly stained fibers. Converging fibers along the internal border of the dentate and/or along the posterior medullary velum [valvule de tarin] to the tonsil terminate anteriorly in the middle third of the vermis. This confluence, which is formed principally by vermian fibers, is partially continuous with a prominent bundle (the restiform body) which outlines the dentate nucleus posteriorly and then penetrates the hemispheric white matter (Fig. 2D,E). The fibers of the restiform body were easily followed from there because the white-matter fibers of the hemisphere had disappeared. Thus, we could distinguish fibers leaving the restiform body to enter the lobules of the superior semilunar lobe [Crus I lobuli ansiformis of Larsell] near the midline. These fibers pass in the layer below the restiform

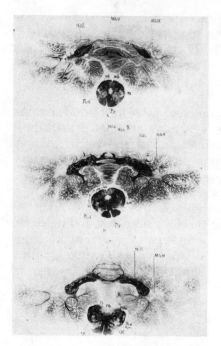

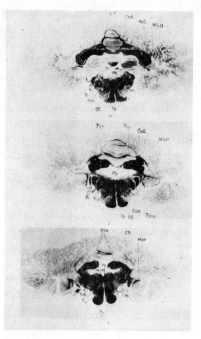

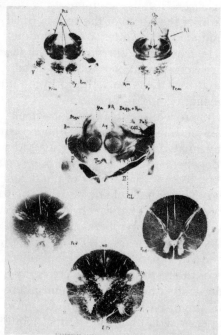

Figures 2, 3, and 4.

A.	Tonsil	Ndl	Dentate nucleus
Aq.	Aqueduct of sylvius	NG	Nucleus of Goll (gracile
B.	Nucleus emboliformis		nucleus)
Brqp.	Inferior quadrigeminal	Nr	Red nucleus
	brachium	Nsp	Nucleus globosus
CGl	Medial geniculate body	NT	Roof nucleus (of cerebellum)–
CL	Nucleus of Luys (subthalamic		fastigial nucleus
	nucleus)	NVI	Sixth nerve nucleus
CR and Crst	Restiform body	OL	Inferior olive
EPy	Pyramidal decussation	P	Cerebral peduncle
Fcc	Central tegmental tract	Pcm	Middle cerebellar peduncle
Fcd	Zone of degeneration	Pes	Superior cerebellar peduncle
	corresponding to the descend-	PVI	Pulvinar
	ing cerebellar tract.	Py	Pyramid
FcV	Cerebello–vestibular fasciculus	Qa	Superior colliculus
Floc	Flocculus	Qp	Inferior colliculus
Flp	Posterior longitudinal	Re	Lateral ribbon of Reil (lateral
	fasciculus (medial longitudinal		lemniscus)
	fasciculus)	Rm	Medial ribbon of Reil (medial
Fs	Solitary tract		leminiscus)
Ln	Substantia nigra	Tm	Mammillary body
MbH	Central cerebellar hemispheric	II	Optic tract
	white matter	V	Trigeminal nerve
MbV	White matter of the vermis	Vs	Trigeminal nerve–descending
NB	Nucleus of Burdach (cuneate		tract
	nucleus)	VII	Facial nerve
NBe	External nucleus of Burdach or	VIII	Acoustic nerve
	of Monakow (accessory		
	cuneate nucleus)		

body, and could be recognized by their circular trajectory and segmented appearance. The vermian decussation was reduced in its transverse and longitudinal aspects.

D. Central hemispheric white matter (Figs. 2 and 3): Everything had disappeared with the exception of isolated, residual fibers of the restiform body. As was already noted, the majority of internal semicircular fibers (of the cerebellum) were absent. The remainder in the shrunken cerebellum could not be distinguished from the intermingled fibers of the superior cerebellar peduncle. The external semicircular fibers had also vanished. They could not be separated from the white-matter fibers surrounding the dentate nucleus. A certain number of the semicircular fibers blended with those of the restiform body.

The superior cerebellar peduncles, leaving the cerebellum, were intensely stained and not degenerated. They were twisted by a slender horizontal/oblique fiber band belonging, probably, to Gowers tract [ventral spinocerebellar tract].

THE CEREBELLAR PEDUNCLES AND THEIR NUCLEI OF ORIGIN

A. Inferior cerebellar peduncle, restiform body (Fig. 3D,E,F); cord (Fig. 4K,L,M); medulla (Fig. 2A,B,C).

1. *Cord:* The thoracic and lumbar sections—examined using Pal or carmine en bloc techniques—showed no degeneration. The tracts, roots, central grey, and columns of Clarke were not atrophied. Examination of the dorsal spinal cord at twelve levels confirmed the lack of changes in Clarke's column. The cervical cord was unusual in two respects: a) There was a heterotopia of the central grey. The anterior horn on one side sent a prolongation into the anterior fasciculus at the level of the C5 and C6 roots. At certain levels this prolongation was detached from the anterior horn; b) Above the level of the C3 root (Fig. 4L) there was a small symmetric peripheral zone of degeneration (olivo-spinal tract). This zone lay between the anterior and lateral fasciculi, was located in front of the anterior edge of Gowers tract, and was approximated by a line connecting the anterior limits of the anterior horns. This area of degeneration was enlarged at the C1—C2 level (Fig. 4K,M).

2. *Medulla:* There was no degeneration of the spinal tracts as they entered the medulla; the dorsal and ventral spinocerebellar tracts (Pal stained) were not pale. The bilateral degeneration became more notable in the medulla than it had been in the upper cervical cord (Fig. 2A,8). It was located posterior and slightly external to the olives (Fig. 2C,D) but was hard to follow beneath the olives. The nuclei of the posterior tracts (the nuclei of Gall, Burdach, and Monakow), the internal arcuate fibers, and the medial lemniscus were normal. The pyramids and their decussation were well stained. The inferior olives and juxta-olivary nuclei were extremely atrophic, but the atrophy was asymmetric and more pronounced in the inferior portions. The hilum, including the most internal layer of the medullary peri-olivary white matter, was almost totally decolorized. The cells of the inferior olive and juxta-olivary nuclei were sparse, small, shrunken, and atrophied.

The supero-external segment of the internal arcuate fibers (retrotrigeminal, intertrigeminal cerebello-olivary fibers of Mingazzini) and the external arcuate fibers (zonal cerebello-olivary fibers of Mingazzini) were completely absent. Rostral to the olive, the lateral and posterior myelinated fibers began to reappear. These fibers belong to the central tegmental bundle and form the external layer of the peri-olivary white matter. This central tegmental bundle emerged gradually; it was relatively well preserved but less compact than normal. This relative integrity explains why the white matter of the superior olive was better seen than that of the inferior olive. On the other hand, the central bundle was smaller on one side and the ipsilateral olive less well developed. The diminution in the size of the central bundle was perhaps due to atrophy of the pontine reticular substance.

The arcuate nuclei of the prepyramidal medulla were lacking and the bulbar reticular substance and nuclei seemed atrophied. The restiform body forms at the superior end of the cuneate nucleus (nucleus of Monakow). The olives were not visible at this level, and there was no abnormality seen. Just prior to entering the cerebellum, the central portion of the restiform body was composed of healthy medullary fibers, from the cuneate nucleus, and, perhaps, lateral medulla. As the olives appeared, a decolorized zone could be seen on their internal border. This decolorized zone increased in size towards the superior end of the olive (Fig. 3D,E), where it involved the external olivary border, the cochlear nucleus, and the acoustic stria. The fibers on the medial border of the cuneate nucleus, which form the internal portion of the restiform body or the cerebello-vestibular tract, were atrophied. This atrophy could be followed rostrally to the level of Deiters' and Bechterew's nuclei.

B. *Middle cerebellar peduncle, pons, tegmental reticular substance (Fig. 4H,I)*:   The pons, especially anteriorly, was atrophied. The pontine nuclei were severely depleted. The nerve cells were replaced by spider cells (microglia) as well as glial fibrils. (The gliosis was not dense). The vessels were not altered. All the transverse fibers of the anterior pons were missing. The middle cerebellar peduncle was totally degenerated. As a result, the fibers of the peduncle were no longer fasciculated and were grouped as a single round tract on each side.

The cells of the tegmental reticular substance were asymmetrically decreased in number. The corresponding central tegmental tract was also smaller in size.

The atrophy of the pons and middle cerebellar peduncle made it easier to follow the fibers of the trapezoid body, which are usually indistinguishable. The entire acoustic system—trapezoid body, superior olives, juxta-olivary nuclei, lateral leminiscus (and its nucleus)—was intact. The acoustic stria, normally bordering the floor of the fourth ventricle, was not apparent.

The vestibular roots, although thinner and scantier than normal, were well seen on picrocarmine stained sections. The cells of Deiters' and Bechterew's nuclei and the triangular acoustic nucleus (which connects with the vestibular portion of the eighth cranial nerve and the cerebellum) appeared numerous, but the nuclei were small. Most of the cerebello-vestibulary fibers were continuous with the vestibular root.

The fifth, sixth, and seventh cranial nerve nuclei were preserved.

The fascicle of the descending tract of the trigeminal nerve was clearly discernible, as the inter- and retrotrigeminal fibers of the restiform body were degenerated.

The medial longitudinal fasciculus and the medial leminscus were normal.

C. *Superior Cerebellar Peduncle and Midbrain (Figs. 3E and F, 4H,I,J):* The superior cerebellar peduncle and its decussation were well stained and not degenerated, though not as large as normal. The cells of the red nuclei were preserved, but the nuclei were small. The thalamus (including tegmental radiations, the fields of Forel, the thalamic radiations, the external medullary lamina, the lateral nuclei, the centrum medianum, and the medial nuclei) were proportionately smaller than normal but without degeneration.

The third and fourth cranial nerve nuclei and the superior and inferior quadrigeminal bodies were unaffected. On Pal-stained sections the cerebral peduncles were well stained and small. The internal capsules were asymmetrically atrophied.

EXAMINATION OF THE PEDUNCLES ENTERING INTO THE CEREBELLUM—ANATOMIC CONSIDERATIONS OF THE CEREBELLAR-PEDUNCULAR CONNECTIONS

The complete atrophy of the anterior pons (pontine nuclei), the middle cerebellar peduncle, and the cerebellar hemispheres confirms the connections between these three areas—connections established by experimental physiology and remarked above.

The preserved fibers of the restiform body—namely, the direct cerebellar tract and fibers from the gracile, cuneate, and lateral column nuclei—all connect with the vermis. Some connect with areas adjacent to the superior semilumar lobe [Crus I lobuli ansiformis of Larsell] (a region which receives more myelinated fibers than the other lobes). Entering the cerebellum they occupy the center of the restiform body. The degenerated fibers, mostly of olivary origin, occupied the periphery of the restiform body and (probably) terminated in the vermian cortex and the region adjacent to the cerebellar hemispheres. It is impossible to precisely determine where these fibers terminated, as they have disappeared along with the projection fibers from the cerebellar cortex to the nuclei.

The restiform body also projects to the flocculus.

The atrophy of the medial portion of the restiform body (or cerebello-vestibular fibers) was explained by the scarcity of internal and external arcuate fibers. The loss of these fibers probably also explained the degeneration of the retro-olivary fibers and absence of the small fascicle in the antero-lateral column of the high cervical cord (which may correspond to the descending cerebellar fascicle that Thomas has noted in animals). It was impossible to follow the degeneration of these antero-lateral fibers up to the cerebellum, as the fibers are not grouped in the pons.

The atrophy of the internal semicircular fibers and the vermian decussation resulted from the atrophy of the central nuclei, i.e., the fastigial, emboliform, and globose nuclei.

The flocculus and tonsil must be considered vermal appendages, as they had degenerated to a lesser extent, and they are known to have fibers linking them to the vermis.

The relative integrity of the dentate nucleus explained the preservation of the superior cerebellar peduncle. The small dentate was in proportion to the small red nucleus and thalamus.

RESUME

The neuraxis was small. There was cerebellar cortical atrophy, more marked in the hemispheres than in the vermis. There was degeneration and disappearance of most afferent and efferent cerebellar hemispheric and projection fibers. The nuclei which give rise to afferents—the bulbar olives, pontine nuclei, and, to a lesser extent, the central cerebellar nuclei (dentate, fastigial, external emboilform, globose) were atrophied. These changes were due to a simple cellular atrophy, as there were no vascular changes, hemorrhages, areas of softening, or sclerosis. The smallness of the neuraxis and the cervical cord heterotopia seemed to indicate incomplete or abnormal neural development. However, olivoponto cerebellar degeneration, as I have described it, with its late appearance and characteristic degeneration, is not to be attributed to abnormal neural development.

CASE 2

P. Albert, a forty-four-year-old farmer from Malesherbes, was seen by Dr. Dejerine on May 17, 1899. The patient's family history was poorly recorded: his father died of an unknown illness at forty-six years of age and his mother died of apoplexy at age seventy. One sister died at an early age of an illness unknown to the patient. On repeated questioning he stated, in a categorical fashion, that no direct or collateral ancestor had difficulty with gait or equilibrium.

His only child had been stillborn—his wife having had no other miscarriages. He enjoyed good health and denied venereal diseases (syphilis or gonorrhea) and alcoholic excess.

His illness began four years ago when he had suffered precordial pain, palpitations, digestive troubles, and lost 10 or 12 lbs. over a short period. Following this, he suffered from neurasthenia, becoming mentally and physically depressed. A possible explanation was found— three years previously he had been forced to separate from his wife because of philandering. For many months following this he had been depressed and developed insomnia. However, even during this depression and neurasthenia, his gait and his equilibrium remained normal.

Two years ago his friends began to joke with him about his titubating gait. This difficulty appeared acutely. The first manifestations coincided with an attack of vertigo upon awakening. The vertigo was intense enough to cause him to absent himself from that days preparations for his village's festival.

From that time on the difficulty standing and walking grew worse. He suffered from continual dizziness, although he couldn't define this symptom precisely. He also could not identify the position (sitting, lying, standing, or walking) in which it occurred, but it was apparently not increased by standing and walking. Awaking at night he felt as if he had a heavy head, felt drowsy, as if in a fog, but was not vertiginous. We frequently questioned him about sensations of spinning, propulsion, or descension. He denied having had any of these symptoms and had never seen spinning or displaced objects.

He fatigued easily. Whereas three months before he had been a good walker, capable of hiking three or four kilometers; he could now no longer advance and had not worked for a year. For the past two years he had felt clumsy, "less in control." During the past few months he had fallen rather frequently while walking, washing himself, or bending over.

Examination of May 18, 1899:   The examination was performed so as to precisely define the patient's equilibrium difficulties. We observed him performing movements while seated and standing. Next, we studied his difficulties with gait and station following passive motion, such as pro- and retropulsion.

Seated: Seated on a footstool, feet on the floor and back unsupported, the patient titubated slightly in the antero-posterior direction. He had some difficulty bringing his feet and knees together. Keeping them together was even more troublesome. Despite his efforts, and although he tried hard to maintain this position, his thighs began to shake, and his knees strayed, spread apart, and turned outwards. When the patient was asked to cross one thigh over the other, he had scarcely done this when they began to slide apart slowly. He was no more able to maintain this position than to keep his knees together.

During this last maneuver, if he tried to rapidly move one thigh over the other, his trunk began to oscillate and he felt unsteady.

We asked him to simultaneously raise both feet off the floor. Since he was afraid of falling, he performed this while seated in a chair and did not lose his balance. He was able to collect objects placed between, in front of, in back of, or to either side of his legs. All these movements were characterized by slowness, uncertainty, and hesitation. When he lifted his extended or adducted legs, large amplitude oscillations appeared in his trunk and extremities. He found it easier to maintain a seated position on a stool with his eyes open than with his eyes closed. With his feet together he was unable to stand from a sitting position—he fell backward or sideways. On the other hand, it was extremely difficult for him to stand unsupported with his feet spread apart.

Standing: with feet spread apart, his base was quite wide—his ankles were 33 cm apart. He experienced low-amplitude trunkal oscillations. He seemed to have to pay careful attention to his balance and made adequate attempts to maintain his position. Sometimes the oscillations were of increased amplitude, and the upper trunk swayed to and fro (but minimally sideways) four or five times consecutively. On these occasions he had to make an extreme effort to avoid falling forwards or backwards.

He could stand with his feet together but he had more frequent oscillations of larger amplitude which spread from the trunk to the legs. These oscillations were more marked with eye closure and were associated with flexion and extension movements during which the skin was elevated by muscular contractions.

He was able to bow with difficulty. When he stood up again his upper trunk swayed forward and backward through an axis which passed transversely through his antero-superior iliac spines.

While erect, his arms were held out from his body. He could maintain equilibrium by throwing his shoulders forward and bending his ankles and knees slightly. He could not, of course, stand on one foot.

He sat down and lay down without assistance—but slowly and awkwardly. In doing so, his body fell brusquely, oscillated two or three times about the longitudinal axis, and then came to rest. When he attempted to sit or to hold both of his hands on one side of his body he became unstable and tremulous. Following this, after a series of rather slow and hesitant hand motions he could work himself into a sitting position. During this activity his body did not lurch to one side or the other.

Gait: was significantly affected. The lower extremities were not ataxic, and were not being thrown about.

The patient walked with feet and arms spread wide. After several hesitant movements each foot was quickly lifted and replaced. When his weight was supported on one foot and he feared that he was about to fall he quickly advanced his other foot. Consequently, he did not take a step unless one foot was completely in contact with the ground. These irregularly spaced steps might occur at intervals of several seconds. He appeared ill-at-ease and said he didn't feel stable. Although he stood erect and held his head steady he was unable to walk a straight line—the oscillations forced him to diverge. His gait undulations were slow but he did not have the sinusoidal, rapidly undulating gait of a drunkard. The patient's slowness and uncertainty was quite striking. It appeared as if he were planning all of his movements in advance. Despite his tremors his attitude gave his body a rigid, unsupple appearance. In order to walk, he required as many precautions as a tightrope walker on the wire. Both share the same fear, careful attention, and uncertainty.

If he stopped short, his trunk underwent two or three large-amplitude anteroposterior oscillations before coming to rest. He was not thrown forward or backward, however.

He could turn around but was awkward. Although he did not actually fall it appeared as if he were about to fall at any moment because of increasing trunkal ataxia and uncertainty. After saying he was unable to do it, he walked backward, with great difficulty: with his body bent backward, he moved each foot backward several centimeters. As he began to oscillate he started to overstep himself, but regained his balance with difficulty.

We noted earlier that eye closure slightly increased his instability. Strictly speaking, however, Romberg's sign was absent. He could walk with his eyes closed but was slightly unsteady and quite anxious. His gait was more irregular, lateral trunk deviations greater; but coordination of the lower extremities was unaffected.

Ordinarily he didn't look at his feet while walking. A screen placed under his eyes to prevent him from looking at his feet did not alter his gait. On the other hand, he said that staring at an object made walking more difficult. We verified this ourselves.

Even with support he had great difficulty walking up and down stairs. Without support he risked falling forward or backward with each step.

When he exercised, or after a slightly prolonged walk, he felt fatigued—especially in the calf muscles.

Passive motion: Propulsion brought about large-amplitude oscillations of the trunk. This was especially true for rapid flexion, extension, or balancing movements. Retropulsion and lateral pulsion were less likely to produce oscillations. He was able to detect movement when he was placed on a very slowly rotating apparatus. When I stood behind him and gently touched his upper lids with my index finger, I could feel horizontal ocular oscillations.

Compensatory movements were normal. During rotation to the right his head inclined to the left. A sudden stop caused his head to return to the midline then turn slightly to the right. During the period of post-rotatory vertigo his head and body were inclined markedly to the right but he could not define the sensation that preceeded the vertigo. In sum, his responses were normal for both right and leftward rotation. On the other hand, his difficulty standing and walking was not greatly increased when he held his head to either side or backward. Although this examination was not very sophisticated we concluded that his vestibular apparatus was normal.

Arm motility: There was no paralysis or muscular atrophy. The right hand registered 40 on the dynamometer; the left, 50. There was no incoordination. He performed the finger-to-nose test with his eyes open. With his eyes closed he performed less well. This was not true ataxia or intention tremor; more precisely, there was a slight hesitation. His hand movements were awkward. When he reached for an object such as a glass he grabbed for it. There was no tremor, but he hesitated when he lifted a glass and seemed unsure of himself; small-amplitude lateral movements deflected his hand, and he missed his mouth. In addition, he noted that his hands had been less skillful for some time and that he frequently overturned objects which he held or carried.

He had experienced a great deal of difficulty writing for the past several months. Written characters were formed deliberately, and his hand trembled. The attached specimen, which took him ten minutes to execute, convincingly demonstrates his disability (Fig. 5). The upper-extremity deep-tendon reflexes (wrist, triceps) were exaggerated.

Leg motility: There was no atrophy or paralysis. With the eyes open or closed there was no incoordination. Crossing the left leg over the right was slightly more difficult than vice versa. The deep-tendon reflexes (ankle and patella) were exaggerated, but the cutaneous plantar reflexes (Babinski's sign) were normal. (As in a normal individual, scratching the plantar surface of the foot produced flexion of the great toe.) Resistance to passive movement of the arms and legs persisted for several seconds. There was no hypotonia in the arms or legs.

Head and face: There was no tremor of the head at rest or with head, neck, or trunk motion. The patient appeared foolish, and held a fixed gaze. Facial mimicry was poorly developed. His speech was profoundly altered and at times difficult to understand—drawling, hesitant, inter-rupted, and slightly nasal. He spoke through his teeth in a scanning fashion, without the explosive quality of a patient with multiple sclerosis. The ends of words and sentences were pronounced with more force than the beginnings. He elevated and depressed his tongue readily; he moved it easily to the right but less strongly to the left. The

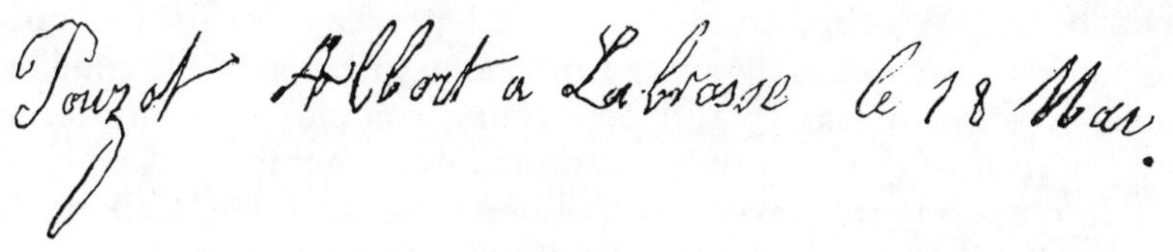

Figure 5.

soft palate was slightly prolapsed to the right and, when contracted, pulled better to the left.

He could pout his lips easily but could not whistle. His facial muscles seemed to contract normally. Electrical examination of the nerves and muscles was not performed. Position sense, proprioception, and stereognosis were intact.

Special sensation: *Vision*—the pupils were equal and reacted equally during convergence and accommodation. Dr. Rodnan-Durigneaud's ophthalmoscopic examination was normal, but the visual fields were not tested. There was no dyschromatopsia. Small nystagmoid jerks, slightly more prominent than those observed in a normal individual, were present on extreme lateral gaze.

Hearing and *smell* were intact, and taste was not significantly affected. He recognized the *taste* of quinine sulfate, salt, and sugar but remarked that his taste was less acute than before. Dr. Nattier's laryngoscopic examination was unremarkable.

Sphincters: he was sometimes incontinent and had urinary hesitancy.

Notes of reexamination in July 1899: He appeared worse—with greater disequilibrium. His arms were slightly tremulous, and he was noticeably more hesitant, slower, and uncertain when he grasped an object or brought something to his mouth.

Notes from the last examination performed August 8, 1899: He had new symptoms: diplopia without obvious oculomotor paralysis, and vertigo. Objects seemed to turn, then stop, but he had no sensation of spinning. Balance was worse. The legs were spread apart wider than before (the intermalleolar distance was 37 cm). He walked with small steps consisting of a series of quick foot movements. After being erect for several seconds with his eyes open, he experienced large-amplitude antero-posterior oscillations and was forced to clutch nearby objects. He fatigued more rapidly than before. The effect of eye closure was best observed when he stood with ankles together. This produced large-amplitude oscillations. His intelligence seemed less acute and his speech more altered and nasal.

It serves no useful purpose to note the similarities between both cases; having seen the first case it was easier to diagnose the second. The diagnosis in each case depended on the association of disequilibrium while standing, walking, and performing complex body movements, and the relative integrity of isolated limb movements.

All complex body movements (while sitting, standing, walking, lying down, standing up) were profoundly affected—slowed, hesitant, uncertain, and awkward. Falls resulted from this imbalance.

In general, the patients stand on a wide base, their feet spread out.

Minimal tilting of the body forward or backward results in varying degrees of titubation, disequilibrium, and falls. Standing unsupported on one foot, he becomes immediately unstable, and falls.

He walks as if uncertain of his balance: legs spread apart and arms abducted. His steps are short, irregular, and wandering, and he tires easily. After hesitating, he quickly moves his feet. Bending of his body produced titubation.

Isolated movements of the extremities are well performed when the patient is seated or lying down; but when he is erect, upper-extremity movements affect his balance. He is awkward when he picks up or lays down objects, and his writing is tremulous. Atonia, paralyses, changes in muscle strength, Romberg's sign, and sensory disturbance are not observed.

Speech is slow, scanning, or drawling. The cerebellar syndrome, as described by one of us, is completed by nystagmoid movements and hyperactive reflexes.

Neither patient showed the discoordination or the gait disorder of the drunkard. Head oscillations were not significant. It appeared that the patient *fears* losing his balance more than he actually loses it.

The topography of the pathologic lesions in our first patient was unique: (1) *symmetrical cerebellar cortical atrophy*, greater in the hemispheres than in the vermis, with relative preservation of the dentate, fastigial, globose, and emboliform nuclei; (2) *total atrophy of the pontine grey and middle cerebellar peduncle* with relative preservation of the superior cerebellar peduncle, which originates in the dentate nucleus; (3) *pronounced atrophy of the inferior olives and justx-olivary and arcuate unclei and degeneration of the external arcuate fibers of the restiform body.* The pyramids and cerebral peduncles appeared small but had not degenerated.

The lesions in the cerebellar cortex, pontine grey, and inferior olives appeared to be of the same age. The Purkinje cells were almost totally absent—the remaining ones were altered. The neurons of the pontine grey were completely absent and those of the inferior olives were atrophied or absent. Secondary degeneration occurred as a consequence of these cellular lesions: loss of the cells of the pontine grey resulted in degeneration of the middle cerebellar peduncle. The loss of inferior olivary cells was associated with partial degeneration of the restiform body, the Purkinje cell atrophy resulted in degeneration of cerebellar projection fibers. The net effect was cerebellar cortical and white matter atrophy. The cerebellar atrophy may be thought of as primary—without perivascular inflammation or neuroglial proliferation.

We have divided the previously published cases of cerebellar atrophy into those with complete or partial, symmetric or asymmetric, sclerotic or degenerative parenchymatous atrophy.

Partial and asymmetric atrophy is usually secondary to a zone of softening or hemorrhage. Sclerosis is usually present but rarely may it occur without inflammation or necrosis of the cerebellar grey matter (granule and Purkinje cells). In the case of Lannois and Paviot (1) there were no vascular lesions; there was cerebellar agenesis in that of Neuburger and Edinger (2).

Complete and symmetric atrophy may be *sclerotic and vasculo-inflammatory* as noted by Spiller (3); *simple and congenital* as in Nonne's report (4)—in which the cerebellum was small but proportionately developed, suggesting an *in utero* or neonatal developmental arrest, unlike the complete cerebellar agenesis noted by Combettes [not referenced]; or *degenerative parenchymatous*—in which Purkinje-cell and cerebellar cortical atrophy results in medullary fiber degeneration and a decrease in cerebellar size without sufficient gliosis and vascular *inflammation* to explain the degenerative changes.

Our cases represent a degenerative atrophy with one unique feature—the pontine grey and the inferior olives are both involved by the same process. We designate this process as *olivopontocerebellar atrophy* by virtue of the systematic involvement of the cerebellar cortex, bulbar olives, and pontine nuclei. This variety of cerebellar atrophy reported above represents a rare form of a rare entity. There is only one comparable observation in the literature—Case IV in the thesis of one of the authors (Thomas, 1897). This patient exhibited slight ataxia of the lower extremities, atrophy of the muscles of the hands, and anterior horn cell atrophy in the eighth cervical segment, in addition to similar cerebellar, bulbar, and pontine lesions. The cord was otherwise unremarkable; the periphery of the lateral columns was slightly pale. We believe this represents the same entity. The onset was delayed in both cases, and in neither case was there a family history of neurologic disease.

The cases of Pierret (5), Menzel (6), Rojet and Collet (7), Arndt (8), and Thomas—Case V (9) are clinically (cerebellar syndrome) and pathologically (involvement of the olivary, pontine, and cerebellar grey matter without cerebellar nuclear involvement) similar to the preceeding cases but differ in certain respects.

Menzel's patient presented with ataxia of the upper extremities, a positive Romberg's sign, increased muscle tone in the arms and legs, and muscle contractures. Muscle contractures were also observed in the case of Rojet and Collet. The legs of Arndt's patient wavered and oscillated in a fashion which seemed to have been ataxia and tremors. In Pierret's case, sensation was decreased in the hands, and the patient convulsed, suffered tetanic spasms in the jaw and legs, and vomited frequently. Thomas's Case V was complicated by coincident hysteria and anesthesia of skin and mucous membranes.

The anatomic differences are equally striking: cerebellar cortical atrophy was accompanied by varying degrees of sclerosis. (Pierret, Menzel, Rojet and Collet, Arndt). Other authors have regarded the case of Rojet and Collet as an example of multiple sclerosis localized to the cerebellum, although the cerebellum was not examined histologically. Other cases (Menzel, Arndt, Thomas's Case V) were characterized by degeneration of the cerebellar afferents: (Clarke's column, dorsal and ventral spinocerebellar tracts). In some cases, (Menzel, Arndt, Thomas's Case V) there were changes in the noncerebellar tracts (pallor of the pyramidal tracts and partial degeneration of the posterior columns). The atrophy of the olives in Thomas's Case V was less marked than that observed in either Thomas's Case IV or in our case.

Pierret's patient became symptomatic at age four following a fall on the head. All of the other cases became symptomatic after age thirty.

Two cases (Menzel, and Thomas's Case V) had a family history of neurologic illness. Menzel's patient had three brothers and three sisters. The eldest brother was normal, another had a tremor, and the youngest was mentally retarded but not tremulous and had a normal gait. An older sister developed a hesitating gait at thirty years of age. She was unable to fix the position of her head, which fell to the side. Subsequently she became delirious and committed suicide. A second sister had an uncertain gait, and a third, who was constitutionally weak, was neurologically normal. The mother, in her later years, developed a head tremor and an uncertain gait.

Thomas's Case V had a hysterical mother who became insane and died in an asylum, a first cousin who was a lunatic since the age of twenty, five children who died at an early age, and a sixth child with recurrent seizures. Thus, only Menzel's case, with its poorly detailed family history, shows a hereditary pattern.

The cases of Menzel and Thomas most closely resemble our own case, but the previously noted anatomic, clinical, and etiologic differences prevent us from grouping their cases with ours. The case of Rojet and Collet differs by virtue of the scirrhous consistency of the cerebellum, which was not examined histologically. Pierret's case differs from ours by virtue of its evolution, the early onset, and the histologic changes.

Arndt's case is analogous to ours, but he considered the cerebellar atrophy to be sclerotic. Possibly the sclerosis is a secondary phenomenon, as it is not sufficiently marked to be the primary pathologic process and the cause of the atrophy. Nevertheless, the case is similar to ours, especially in view of the late occurrence of trauma.

The preceeding cases have attracted our attention. Cases like that of Schultze (10), with cerebellar nuclear and cortical injury, differ from ours, which was characterized by systematic anatomic change.

Symptomatically, the illness we studied is analogous to that described by Marie (11) as hereditary cerebellar ataxia and also by Londe (12). Marie based his description of hereditary cerebellar ataxia on the observations of Fraser (13), Nonne (4), Sanger Brown (15), and Klippel and Durante (16). Hereditary cerebellar ataxia is clinically characterized by a *drunkard's gait, incoordination of the lower extremities, choreiform movements of the arms, and legs, head tremor, truncal titubation while erect, and the absence of Romberg's sign.* Londe said the patients seem to be trying to regain the balance they are constantly about to lose. Their legs are spread apart to widen the base of support. As the illness advances the arms become involved, the hands hover and hesitate while grasping, an intention tremor develops, writing become tremulous, and muscle tone becomes exaggerated. Muscle contractions become prolonged but are of normal strength. Position sense is normal. Sometimes there are choreiform jerks of the arms and lateral instability of the fingers. The patient appears astonished as a consequence of exaggerated muscle contractions and mimetic difficulties. Speech is irregularly slow or explosive, saccadic, indistinct, gutteral, and monotonous. The head tremor is increased by movement, emotional strain, and standing, but dizziness is inconstant. The patellar reflexes are normal or increased. Additional findings include headaches, back pains, fatigue, neurasthenia, and mild intellectual impairment. Smell is preserved, but optic atrophy with restricted visual fields has been observed, and most patients have nystagmus; paralysis of the extraocular muscles is common. Sanger Brown's patients had slow or abolished pupillary light reflexes.

Together with Marie's fundamental observations, Londe mentioned the reports of Brissaud and Londe (17) and two personal cases (12) which he observed while working with Prof. Robin. It was Londe's view that the cases of Seeligmüller (19), Erb (20), and Hervouet (21) represent hereditary cerebellar ataxia, and Menzel's case represents an illness with features of both hereditary cerebellar ataxia and Friedreich's ataxia.

Since Marie's report, only two autopsied cases have been reported: Fraser's (22) and Nonne's (4). Fraser's pathological notes are sparse—the cortex was reduced to half its normal size, the lamellae were narrowed and condensed, the Purkinje cells were decreased in number and clearly altered, and the white matter stained poorly yet was dense in comparison to the grey matter. Sorrowfully, a more detailed examination of the cortex, white matter, medulla, and pons was not made.

Nonne's notes are quite complete. The cerebellar atrophy seemed to be due to a developmental arrest. The brain was small, and although the cerebellar folia appeared macroscopically and microscopically normal, they were fewer than normal. There was no evidence of degeneration or cellular lesions. If one uses the term atrophy to denote destruction and regression, the cerebellum was not atrophic, only small. The author noted, furthermore, that there was an increased number of small fibers in the anterior and posterior roots of the cervical and lumbar spinal cord with fewer large fibers. The peripheral nerves were similarly involved.

Despite qualifications regarding the pathologic examination in Fraser's case, it is quite similar to Nonne's—a fact appreciated by Marie when he applied the term hereditary cerebellar ataxia to both of them, noting that brothers and sisters, but not parents, were affected in both instances. In addition, there was an extensive neurological history in Nonne's family.

Sanger Brown, and Klippel and Durante do not provide autopsy confirmation of the illness described by Marie along with Fraser and Nonne. Meyer's (23) autopsy examination of Sanger Brown's sixth patient failed to reveal unequivocal cerebellar atrophy, but the spinal cord was small and contained lesions throughout its extent. In the cervical regions the cells of Clarke's column were diminished, as were the fasciculus gracilis and the dorsal spinocerebellar tract. Thus Sanger Brown's cases, unlike those of Fraser and Nonne, are not examples of hereditary cerebellar atrophy. It is more difficult to classify Klippel and Durante's report because of the lack of autopsy data.

Spiller reported a brother and sister with confirmed sclerotic cerebellar atrophy at autopsy. Even in the absence of an established hereditary pattern he considered these to be examples of hereditary cerebellar ataxia because of their familial occurrence. Spiller hypothesized that an infectious illness (diphtheria or scarlatina) had activated the illness in genetically predisposed individuals. Spiller's cases represent a familial sclerosing cerebellar process and, thus, cannot be linked with those of Nonne or Fraser, despite similar symptoms and evolution. Spiller's pathologic findings were not the same as Nonne's nor as clearly systematized as ours; the distribution of the sclerotic lesions differed. The clinical and anatomic details of these various reports have been evaluated by one of us (Thomas's thesis).

Miura (24) provided an interesting report of two brothers with hereditary cerebellar ataxia. Their mother, the son of their mother's cousin, and one of their own cousins had a similar illness characterized by an unsteady gait, dysarthric speech, visual problems, and uncertain, tremulous upper-extremity movements. Two sisters had eye problems. The one autopsied case, who had had measles in childhood and abdominal typhus at age eighteen, developed gait instability at age twenty-five. At age thirty his gait had become ever more unsteady; his body reeled and his hand movements were less adept. He improved for a short time, but his disability increased following a febrile illness at age thirty-three. His speech and vision became impaired at thirty-five years of age, and as a result he was forced to stop working one year later. In retrospect, he recalled having noticed a veil in front of his eyes at age twenty-two.

On examination, his body swayed whenever he walked, his extremities were ataxic, and his speech and vision were impaired. His speech was explosive, poorly articulated, scanning, difficult to understand, and provoked abundant salivation. He had a stupid expression on his face. The visual fields were irregularly and asymmetrically constricted, the visual acuity 6/6 (left) and 6/9 (right); the pupillary response to light and accommodation was slow, and mild horizontal nystagmus was present. A test of visual acuity revealed that the largest numbers appeared blurred to him. The optic fundi were injected, poorly defined, and lightly shaded. The patient had a mild dorsal kyphoscoliosis convex to the left. He moved towards his bed or seat with knees bent and body unsteady. He could not touch his forefingers together with his arms spread apart whether his eyes were open or closed; he wrote awkwardly with obvious ataxia although his hands were not tremulous. Biceps, wrist, knee, and ankle tendon reflexes were normal; the cremasteric reflex was easier to elicit on the left, and the cutaneous plantar reflexes were normal. When he was erect his trunk titubated, his legs spread apart, and his great toes hyperextended. Eye closure had little effect on the oscillations. He was unable to walk without his cane and without looking at the ground. He drifted to the right, left, or backward, could not follow a straight line, and was always about to fall. Sensation, including position and muscle sense, was intact, as was sphincter function. Later, his equilibrium worsened, the patellar reflexes disappeared, his legs became mildly hypesthetic, and sphincter functions were altered. He died of cardiac insufficiency following a bout of vomiting and edema.

At autopsy, the spinal cord was small, and its posterior meninges were injected. On cut section the thoracic cord appeared sunken between the anterior and lateral columns, and the anterior horns were atrophic. The smallness of the cord, especially on the right side, was most notable in the mid-dorsal segments. In the lower dorsal segments the central canal was dilated and became double in the lumbar region.

The pia mater over the cerebral hemisphere was edematous, opaque, and thickened in places. The right central and frontal gyri were atrophic with enlarged sulci. At the base of the brain the pia mater was thickened, but the major arteries and the Sylvian fissure were without adhesions.

The cerebellum was small and flat, its meninges thickened and injected, its white matter firm. In addition to the cerebellum, the cord and pons were small. The transverse pontine fibers of the middle cerebellar peduncle seemed decreased in number, but the pyramidal fibers were unaffected. The medullary origin of the restiform body was less obvious than usual but histologically normal, and the olivary neurons and fibers were spared.

The cerebellum weighed 80 grams, and there was increased space between the laminae and lamellae. The gray and white matter were equally and proportionately underdeveloped; the number of laminar connections was normal, and the cortical and nuclear structure was not altered. The white matter was unaffected and was not sclerotic. Examination of the flattened cord revealed neither cellular alterations nor tract degeneration. There was no increase in the number of small fibers in the sixth thoracic or right third lumbar posterior roots. Since the patient also had beriberi (Kakke), the degenerated fibers in peripheral nerves of the leg were of no interest to us.

The bilateral mid-retinal fields stained red or deep blue with carmine or nigrosine, while the peripheral fields were paler. The red spots were both more frequent and more peripheral in sections of the left eye.

The patient's brother had almost the same symptoms beginning at age thirty-three. Although we will not consider him in detail, he had absent patellar reflexes, weak ankle jerks, and complete loss of all sensory modalities over the lateral face, legs, and sides. In addition, one sister had marked visual loss with restricted visual fields and optic fundus changes.

Miura's report seems clinically and pathologically similar to Nonne's and illustrates a clear hereditary propensity and familial character. However, Nonne's patient had exaggerated patellar reflexes, whereas these reflexes were absent in Miura's patient. Their absence, as well as the sensory disturbances, were attributed to a beriberi peripheral neuritis. The cerebellum of Miura's patient was smaller than that of Nonne's, weighing 96 grams to the latter's 120 grams, and the brain in Miura's case weighed 1185 grams (normal) vs. 1020 grams (less than Schwalbe's normal of 1150 to 1170 grams). Both of these cases seem to be prototypical examples of hereditary cerebellar ataxia (perhaps more appropriately called hereditary cerebellar atrophy) by virtue of the cerebellar atrophy, the cerebellar signs, and the familial character. This statement rests more on the pathologic findings than on the inherited predisposition, familial pattern, or cerebellar symptoms.

The pathologic changes allowed us to distinguish our patients from those of Miura and Nonne. Our cases had well-developed cerebellar symptoms but no hereditary predisposition or familial pattern. The sporadic nature of our cases does not exclude a hereditary disease. Sporadic cases of muscular dystrophy and Friedreich's ataxia do exist. However, the older age of our patients makes a hereditary illness less likely. Finally, the abnormally small cerebellum which we described was the product of regressive changes, slow cellular destruction and atrophy, as well as secondary nervous system degeneration, whereas the healthy small cerebellum of hereditary cerebellar ataxia results from arrested development. Our case is similar to Nonne's only by virtue of the small size of the nervous system (even though this change is less distinct in our material).

Londe tried, from both clinical and pathological viewpoints, to separate hereditary cerebellar ataxia from the nonfamilial cerebellar atrophies, but his arguments are specious rather than decisive. He proposed that hereditary ataxia had a familial character, was often related to trauma or infection, was associated with intellectual changes and epilepsy, and was often accompanied by asymmetric ataxia. We have already noted the familial character of hereditary ataxia but consider that trauma or infection may also play an etiologic role. We did not observe asymmetric incoordination in our case and conclude that it is an inconstant finding in hereditary cerebellar ataxia, though sometimes seen in nonfamilial cerebellar atrophy.

Londe is of the opinion that the pathologic picture of nonfamilial cerebellar atrophy is more straightforward than that of hereditary ataxia: "In order to avoid confusion, the case of nonfamilial atrophy that we reviewed should be called cerebellar sclerosis or atrophic sclerosis." However, our observations indicate that nonfamilial atrophic cases may not have cerebellar sclerosis. Moreover, there are familial cases with cerebellar symptoms and pathologic cerebellar sclerosis in which infection has played an important role (Spiller's report). In effect, the differential clinical diagnosis of the cerebellar atrophies is subtle and difficult. They all present with the same cerebellar syndrome, follow a more or less rapid course, and demonstrate pathologic changes in various sites. The nature and severity of symptoms may vary from patient to patient, but the symptoms are always the same. Thus, the pathologic substrate, rather than the nuances of the cerebellar syndrome or the etiology, provides the only basis for the classification of the cerebellar atrophies. However, one may suspect hereditary cerebellar ataxia if several family members present with a cerebellar syndrome. This is justifiable as long as one realizes that the lesion may be of various types: *a diminutive cerebellum* (Nonne, Miura), *sclerotic atrophy* (Spiller), *degenerative atrophy with spinal cord lesions* (Menzel), and *spinal-cord sclerosis* (Meyer).

The nature of the anatomic lesions may serve as a basis for a new classification of the hereditary cerebellar ataxias. The atrophic cerebellar changes are not always the same; rather there may be involvement of either the cerebellum itself or its afferent or efferent tracts. Thus, the nature and sites of lesions may vary in hereditary cerebellar ataxia. On the other hand, the hereditary propensity to develop a similar or dissimilar neurologic illness, the familial pattern, and the coexistence of acquired or congenital malformations of the nervous system in the hereditary cerebellar atrophies are only curiosities. If one subscribes to this point of view, then Friedreich's ataxia may be considered as a hereditary cerebellar ataxia.

If the illness in question followed an infection, then we would suspect a vascular etiology and would expect inflammatory and sclerotic cerebellar atrophy. This is not always the case, however.

Thus, our first patient's illness was not hereditary cerebellar atrophy. The illness began at an older age, and there was nothing to suggest a heredofamilial process. Moreover, the history, the clinical picture, and the pathologic findings seem inconsistent with a cerebellar atrophy of inflammatory origin.

As in another simple neuronal atrophy (the anterior horn cell atrophy of the Duchenne-Aran illness), the pathogenesis of hereditary cerebellar atrophy is obscure. We can only restate the conclusions previously recorded by one of us.

It is difficult to establish a definite link between our Cases I and II. This is especially true in the absence of an autopsy in Case II and in view of the considerations mentioned above. We were impressed enough by the symptomatic similarities and various clinical features to report Case I here.

In summary, we have divided the cerebellar atrophies into: sclerotic atrophies, degenerative atrophies, and simple atrophies. This anatomic classification includes all of the cases reported and seems most useful, since they are all related by common clinical and etiologic factors. The generalized atrophies are most often systematized—either grouped with our system degenerations or, as in the case of olivopontocerebellar degeneration, remaining unassociated.

We encounter some difficulty in dealing with pseudocerebellar disorders of balance, the result of noncerebellar causes. These cases make the diagnosis of cerebellar atrophy (and olivopontocerebellar atrophy in particular) even more difficult. In most instances, however, a methodical and thorough examination allows one to isolate instances of true cerebellar atrophy. The differential diagnosis of other cerebellar processes, such as tumor or abscess, is usually not difficult.

Duchenne of Boulogne (25) was the first to attempt to distinguish between the cerebellar and locomotor ataxic disorders. Patients with locomotor ataxia have typical symptoms as well as symptoms (such as titubation) in common with cerebellar disease. Duchenne considered that cerebellar titubation is due to vertigo rather than to incoordination. He stated, "that is why I refer to it as vertiginous titubation." He assumed that the titubation of locomotor ataxia was due to a loss of motor coordination and stated, "that is why I refer to it (locomotor ataxia) as asynergic titubation."

This distinction is appropriate for the material that Duchenne studied, namely, the cerebellar processes associated with irritation and compression, such as tumors, meningitis, and abscesses. In these conditions vertigo is a significant symptom but is not necessarily the sole cause of titubation. Indeed, it is not certain that the cerebellar lesion is the sole cause of the vertigo. If one studies the somewhat scanty cases of autopsy-confirmed cerebellar atrophy or sclerosis, the absence or rarity of vertigo is striking. Whether or not vertigo plays a secondary role or no role at all in the origin of cerebellar titubation, the term vertiginous titubation should not be used. Dejerine's concept of the pathologic physiology of cerebellar titubation, at least insofar as it concerns cerebellar atrophy, is no longer of value.

Common findings in cerebellar tumors, abscesses, or meningitis—in addition to vertigo and the extreme character of the titubation—include asymmetric signs, coexisting eye problems (especially papilledema), vomiting, and headache. This list does not include sensory and motor symptoms due to extension of the cerebellar tumor to the medulla or pons, nor does it include those signs due to hydrocephalus and the specific cerebellar location of the tumor.

Tabes is so well known that confusion with cerebellar atrophy is rare. The diagnosis of tabes (Duchenne's disease) is based on the findings of Westphal's sign (loss of patellar reflex), Argyll Robertson's sign (myotic pupils responding to accommodation but not to light), and Romberg's sign. The latter is not observed in cerebellar atrophy.

Friedreich's ataxia has a number of features in common with cerebellar atrophy: titubation, instability and swaying while standing, scanning speech, and nystagmus. Friedreich's ataxia begins earlier, at puberty, and progresses more slowly. In addition, there is limb ataxia, and marked skeletal deformities such as scoliosis and clubfoot. With the exception of Botkin's and Londe's cases (both with autopsies), scoliosis is rare in cerebellar atrophy. Londe observed it in three out of five cases of hereditary cerebellar ataxia. Nonne and Miura also noted mild kyphosis or scoliosis. Marie noted additional inconstant signs in hereditary cerebellar atrophy such as optic atrophy, constriction of the visual fields, and Argyll Robertson pupils—signs which are extremely rare in Friedreich's ataxia.

Reflexes are abolished in Friedreich's ataxia but increased in most cases of cerebellar atrophy. Londe has observed cases of Friedreich's ataxia with features of hereditary cerebellar ataxia. These differ from hereditary cerebellar ataxia only in the diminution of the patellar reflexes. In cases with pathologic confirmation the diagnosis turns out to be Friedreich's ataxia.

The ataxia of Friedreich's disease is more like that of cerebellar disease than that of tabes. In Friedreich's ataxia the dorsal spinal cerebellar tracts and Clarke's columns are profoundly altered, but the posterior roots and columns are less diseased than is the case in tabes. The pathological changes explain the cerebellar character of the titubation in Friedreich's ataxia. This titubation is absent in tabes, which is characterized by generalized peripheral ataxia. In pernicious anemia, symptoms similar to cerebellar titubation are often observed, possibly as a result of lesions involving the cells of Clarke's column and the dorsal spinocerebellar tracts [Dejerine and Thomas (26)]. However, the rapid evolution of pernicious anemia, the less severe titubation, and the presence of different neurologic symptoms and signs make the differential diagnosis easier. We should point out that we have not emphasized the role of cerebellar lesions in the causation of ataxia in Friedreich's illness and in pernicious anemia. Cerebellar atrophy was observed in a single case of Friedreich's ataxia (that of Auscher). It would be desirable to examine serial sections of future cases to resolve all doubts.

Based on Menzel's case (in which cerebellar atrophy was associated with medullary lesions topographically similar to those of Friedreich's ataxia), Londe discerned a relationship between hereditary cerebellar ataxia and Friedreich's ataxia. He compared the two illnesses both clinically and pathologically and argued that the disturbed equilibrium characteristic of both illnesses was the result of degeneration in a poorly understood cerebello-medullary system. "In Friedreich's the cerebello-medullary system is involved either exclusively or principally in its medullary portion, whereas in early hereditary cerebellar ataxia the same system is involved in its cerebellar portion." This seductive concept does not survive close scrutiny. One must take into account both the anatomic location as well as the nature of the lesions.

The differential diagnosis of multiple sclerosis is sometimes difficult. As Charcot pointed out, patients with multiple sclerosis may exhibit various disorders of gait. Three principal types of gait have been noted: spastic, cerebellar, and spastic-cerebellar. Scanning speech, intention tremor, and nystagmus are observed both in cerebellar atrophy and in multiple sclerosis. In cerebellar atrophy the intention tremor is less constant and less marked, the speech is less explosive, and the nystagmus less quick and of less amplitude. Paresis, spasticity of the upper and lower extremities, and contractures are constant findings in multiple sclerosis; they are rarely observed in cerebellar atrophy. Reflex hyperactivity is more marked in multiple sclerosis. Babinski (27) correctly noted that intention tremor, scanning speech, and nystagmus are not characteristic of multiple sclerosis. They are, in his view, the signs of a cerebellar lesion. Pontine plaques involving cerebellar connections must cause the symptoms so common in multiple sclerosis. When the plaques are restricted to the spinal cord these symptoms are absent. Without making a definite statement regarding the role of lesions of cerebellar afferents and efferents in the pathogenesis of symptoms of multiple sclerosis, we wish to observe that these symptoms are less severe when the lesions are restricted to the cerebellar cortex rather than the internal or external cerebellar connections (as is the case in multiple sclerosis).

Patients with pseudo-bulbar palsy walk with small steps, exhibit disequilibrium, awkwardness, tremors of the extremities, and symptoms suggestive of a cerebellar lesion. They may have softenings in the pons involving cerebellar connections. These patients clearly differ from patients with cerebellar atrophy by virtue of their facial diplegia, limb paresis, and spastic laughing and crying.

Voltolini has noted that some deaf patients may have a difficulty standing and walking which closely resembles cerebellar titubation. They must stand with feet spread apart on a wide base, and they cannot stand on one leg. Their gait is awkward with unequal, irregularly spaced steps. The patient's body is tilted too far to the left or right. Endurance is decreased and the patients fatigue quickly. Several signs—in addition to bilateral and very severe, if not complete, deafness—make the diagnosis an easy one.

Romberg's sign is always present in labyrinthitis, and the disequilibrium is worsened by changes in head position. Muscle weakness is more pronounced. The patient is not able to orient himself to passive rotational or position-changing movements. In addition, post rotatory nystagmus and vertigo are absent, as are the nystagmus and vertigo evoked by galvanic current across the ears. In addition, disequilibrium is less prominent in deaf-mutes. James (28) pointed out that they become disoriented in the water and will drown if left to themselves. This has also been the experience of Ewald (29) and of one of us (30) who noted that labyrinthectomized animals are similarly disoriented in the water. Animals deprived of their cerebellum can still swim [Luciani (31) and Thomas (30)]. In the future we should evaluate patients with cerebellar disease in this way.

In some patients the aforementioned signs are not present. Egger (32) reported a case with dissociated dysfunction of the static and semicircular canals. The patient, who was completely deaf, had cerebellarlike disequilibrium but normal perception of the direction of motion as well as intact compensatory eye movements during passive rotation. On the other hand, he had a markedly positive Romberg's sign and exhibited severe disequilibrium when his head was tilted.

Astasia-abasia, neurasthenia, and hystero-neurasthenia sometimes exhibit features of cerebellar atrophy, but the differential diagnosis is usually simple. As regards the neuroses, the onset is more rapid, the evolution more bizarre, the severity of symptoms may vary, and nystagmus and dysarthria are rare. The patient is susceptible to suggestion and sometimes takes on affectations.

Our observations are in accord with the theory derived from experimental physiology that the cerebellum is an equilibratory center

(Fluorens, Thomas). This would explain disequilibrium and locomotor difficulties in the face of preservation of isolated limb movements.

The asthenia, fatigability, and decreased tone in certain muscles (thigh adducters, for example) supports Luciani's theory. Luciani considers that the cerebellum augments the energy potential of the neuromuscular apparatus [sthenic action]. Through its tonic action it amplifies the degree of resting muscle tension. During activity it accelerates the rhythm of single impulses and assures the synergy and continuity of muscular movement.

The difference between these two theories is that the first relates the cerebellum to the maintenance of equilibrium, whereas the second allows the cerebellum a more general role. Luciani demonstrated that destruction of the cerebellum in an experimental animal did not affect its equilibrium; in fact, there are data which suggest that this function was normal. One of us has already discussed the relative merits of each theory, and it is not necessary to repeat the discussion. However, it is difficult to deny that the cerebellum is concerned with the maintenance of equilibrium in view of the symptoms associated with cerebellar atrophy. The fact that the sense of balance is not completely abolished in cerebellar atrophy means either that portions of the central nuclei or cerebellar cortex are preserved or that the labyrinth is a secondary equilibration center. This has been experimentally demonstrated (33).

The role of the cerebellum in the maintenance of equilibrium is nicely illustrated by our second patient. Towards the end of his illness he suffered from abnormal movements, which Babinski (34) referred to as "cerebellar asynergis."

Patients with cerebellar atrophy also exhibit other signs and symptoms; mild tremors of the arms, nystagmoid jerks, and altered speech. The arm tremors, absent at rest, are related to voluntary movement and are weak and often absent. Tremulousness in our patients was more reminiscent of awkwardness than of the tremors. These findings result, perhaps, from the loss of the fibers of the descending cerebellar tract.

One of us suggested that the speech disorder is related to poor head fixation. The speech of Menzel's patient was affected to a lesser extent when he lay on a bed and did not have to support his head and body. The nystagmus is related to interruption or involvement of fibers connecting the cerebellum to Deiters' and Bechterew's nuclei or to the oculomotor nuclei.

It should be noted that in most cases of cerebellar atrophy there is accompanying olivary, pontine, and cortical atrophy, all of which may contribute to the production of the clinical syndrome.

In summary, it is difficult to explain either the physiology or the cause of the tremor, nystagmus, and speech alteration. We have described a cerebellar syndrome characterized by atrophy of the cerebellar cortex, bulbar olives, and pontine grey; degeneration of the middle cerebellar peduncle, partial degeneration of the restiform body, and by relative preservation of the cerebellar nuclei. This is a systematic degenerative atrophy without sclerosis or inflammation. The clinical picture is less well defined but includes the cerebellar symptoms and signs common to all of the cerebellar atrophies. There is no hereditary, familial, or congenital pattern, and the disease begins late in life. The etiology is obscure, but it falls into the group of primary cellular atrophies. We have named it olivopontocerebellar atrophy.

REFERENCES

1. Lannois and Paviot. "Sur un cas d'atrophie unilatérale du cervelet." *Revue neurologique*, 15 Octobre 1898.

2. Neuburger and Edinger. "Einseitiger fast totaler Manzel des Cerebellums." *Berlin. Klin. Wochenschrift*, 1898, no. 4.

3. Spiller. "Four cases of cerebellar disease (one autopsy) with reference to cerebellar ataxia." *Brain*, Winter, 1896.

4. Nonne. "Über eine eigentümlich familiare Erkrankungsform des Centralnervensystems." *Arch. für Psychiatrie*, 1891.

5. Pierret. "Note sur un cas d'atrophie périphérique du cervelet avec lésion concomitante des olives bulbaires."

6. Menzel. "Beitrag zur Kenntniss der hereditären Ataxie und Kleinhirnsatrophie." *Arch. für Psychiatrie*, 1891.

7. Rojet and Collet. "Sur une lésion systématisée du cervelet et de ses dépendances bulbo-protubérantielles." *Arch. de Neurologie*, 1893.

8. Arndt. "Zur Pathologie des Kleinhirns." *Arch. für Psychiatrie*, 1894.

9. Thomas. Th. Doctorale, 1897.

10. Schultze. "Über einen Fall von Kleinhirnschwund mit Degenerationen im verlängerten Marke und Rückenmarke warscheinlich in Folge von Alkoolismus." *Virchow Archiv*, 1887.

11. Marie. "Sur L'hérédo-ataxie cérébelleuse." *Semaine médicale*, 1893.

12. Londe. "Hérédo-ataxie cérébelleuse." Th. doctorale, 1895.

13. Fraser. "Defect of cerebellum occurring in brother and sister." *Glasgow Medical Journal*, 1880, fasc. 1.

15. Sanger Brown. "On hereditary ataxy with a series of twenty-one cases." *Brain*, 1892.

16. Klippel and Durante. "Contribution à l'étude des affections nerveuses familiales et héréditaires." *Revue de médicine*, 1892.

17. Brissaud et Londe. *Revue neurologique*, 1894.

19. Seeligmüller. "Hereditäre Ataxie mit Nystagmus." *Arch. f. Psychiatrie* 10:222.

20. Erb. "Über hereditäre Ataxie mit Krankenvorstellung." *Neur. Centralblatt*, 1890.

21. Hervouet. *Gazette médicale de Toulouse.* 1893.

22. Fraser. "Defect of cerebellum occurring in brother and sister." *Glasgow Medical Journal,* 1880, fasc. 1.

23. Meyer. "The morbid anatomy of a case of hereditary ataxy, with introduction by Dr. Sanger-Brown." *Brain* 79:276, 1897.

24. Miura. *Mitteilungen der med. Faultät der Kaiserlich-Japanischen Universität zu Tokio,* Bd.IV, Heft. I, 1898.

25. Duchenne de Boulogne. De l'Electrisation localisée, 1872.

26. Dejerine and Thomas. "Étude clinique et anatomique des accidents nerveux développés au cours de l'anémie pernicieuse." *Cinquantenaire de la Société de Biologie,* 1899.

27. Babinski. Société de Neurologie de Paris, 1er février, 1900.

28. James. "The sense of dizziness in deaf-mutes." *Americ. Journ. of Otology,* 1882.

29. Ewald. *Physiologische Untersuchungen über das Endorgan des nervus octavus.* Wiesbaden, 1892.

30. Thomas. "Étude expérimentelle sur les fonctions du labyrinthe." *Revue intern. de Rhin. Otol. Laring.,* 1899.

31. Luciani. "Il cervelleto. Nuovi studi di fisiologia normale e pathologica." Firenze, 1891.

32. Egger. "Troubles vestibulaires. Étude physiologique et clinique." *Revue internationale de Rhin. Otol. Laryngol,* 1899.

33. Lange. "Inwieweit sind die Symptome, welche nach Zerstörung des Kleinhirns beobachtet werden, auf Verletzungen des Acusticus zurückzuführen?" *Pflüger Archiv* 50:115.

34. Babinski. "De L'asynergie cérébelleuse." *Revue neurologique,* 1899, no.22.

Seven Cases of a Unique Familial Illness: Gait Disorder, Clubfoot, Generalized Areflexia, and Clumsiness of the Hands

G. ROUSSY AND G. LÉVY

WE HAVE OBSERVED seven individuals with a familial illness characterized by unique and previously undescribed symptoms. Despite certain similarities, this illness does not belong to any of the previously classified familial maladies. The clubfoot and deep tendon reflex changes are similar to those of Friedreich's ataxia and, perhaps, Charcot-Marie-Tooth disease (although amyotrophy is uncommon in our patients).

In this report we shall examine this rare clinical illness and discuss some of its nosologic and pathogenetic features.

Mrs. Berthe Pli., twenty-five years old, and her two children were evaluated at the Paul-Brousse Hospital in September, 1925, because of a gait disorder. Mrs. Pli.'s mother, maternal grandfather, several brothers and sisters, and other relatives had had a similar disorder. Almost all of the seventeen children of the patient's twice-married paternal grandfather were also affected. In addition, the descendents of four of the female children were known and are included in the following table. One of these children is the mother of our three adult patients as well as the grandmother of four children.

NOTE: Translated by F.H. Hochberg from: Roussy, G., and Levy, G., "Sept Cas d'une maladie familiale particulière: Troubles de la marche, pieds bots et aréflexie tendineuse généralisée, avec, accessoirement, légère maladresse des mains," *Revue neurologique* 1,4 (1926), 427–50.

CASE 1

Mrs. Berthe Pli. "always had weak legs." She was a late walker: "I was at least two years old at the time and fell while walking. At school I walked downstairs like an invalid." Her legs always gave way. She had lost her job in a chocolate factory because her legs bent when she carried anything heavy. She was aware of extreme awkwardness of finger movements while sewing or peeling vegetables. Her past history was unremarkable. She was intelligent and had never been sick. At seventeen years of age she married an alcoholic, but the details of this marriage are not known. She was pregnant three times and had three children, of which two are living and reported here. The third died at age twenty-six months of whooping cough complicated by pneumonia.

On examination she was of slight stature but well proportioned and without scoliosis or atrophy. She was 1 meter, 44 cm tall and weighed 39.5 kg. Her only deformity was clubfeet which were anteroposteriorly compressed, markedly arched, and had hollowed plantar surfaces. These changes were accentuated in her right foot. The right leg seemed slightly turned out but was not deformed. She could not sustain an erect posture because of oscillations. These oscillations increased when she closed her eyes. When she attempted to stand on one leg, especially on the right, she lost her balance. Her gait was slightly unsteady but not ataxic. Movements of the right foot had a mild steppage quality. She ran with difficulty and recalled that when she tried to run as a child her legs bent and "got tangled up." Crouching was difficult but she easily arose from a prone position without any of the maneuvers employed by myopathic patients.

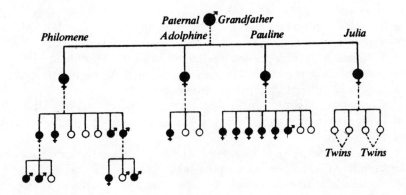

Figure 1. Partial family tree of the Bon. family. Affected individuals – ●; healthy individuals – O. The sex is indicated by an arrow or a cross.

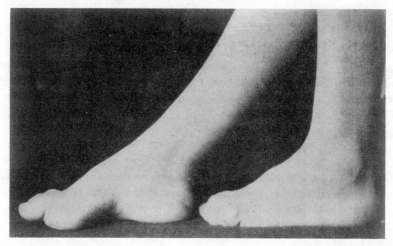

Figure 2. The two feet are deformed. The deformity is noticeable only on the medial border of the foot.

Muscle Strength: was equal and satisfactory in the upper extremities except, perhaps, for mild weakness of the fingers of the left hand. All movements were well performed. In threading a needle she had to steady one palm against the other; while sewing, she held the needle with all of her fingers, and tremulously pushed it into the material. This was accomplished with some difficulty. In order to peel a potato, she grasped it and the knife in her hand. While drinking she had a mild unusual tremor, which disappeared at rest. There was weakness of the right toe extensors and the left anterior compartment muscles; thigh extension was diminished bilaterally; flexion was normal, and all other leg muscles were of equal bulk and of normal strength. Head and trunk flexion and extension were weak—flexion more so. Lateral neck movements were intact.

Reflexes: including the abdominal reflexes were absent. The left plantar response was inconstantly extensor, the right flexor; but unequivocal extension of either toe was not observed.

Cerebellar testing: including finger-to-nose, rapid alternating movements, (marionettes), hell-to-knee, and heel-to-buttock maneuvers were intact.

Tone: was somewhat decreased. Postural reflexes were intact; but the left anterior tibial reflex was equivocal.

Facial exam: revealed mild asymmetry and enophthalmos. The right palpebral fissure was narrowed. The lids were lowered but not really ptotic. The left side of the face moved more than the right when the

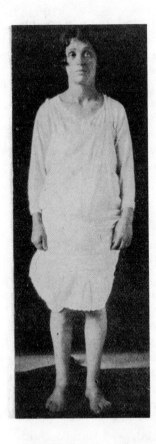

Figure 3.   General appearance, Case 1.

patient laughed. The cranial nerves were otherwise unremarkable. The masseters contracted equally well, the patient could purse her lips to blow or whistle with ease; the corneal reflexes were present but diminished; the palatal reflex was normal, but the pharyngeal reflex was absent.

Sensation: Subjective sensation was normal. There was no dysesthesia. Objective sensation was normal (touch, pin, heat, cold, position, stereognosis), and, except for atrophy of the thenar eminences (most marked on the right) there were no trophic abnormalities.

Electrical exam (Miss de Brancas): revealed slight faradic and galvanic hypoexcitability of the small muscles of the arms and legs as well as the muscles surrounding the popliteal fossa that are innervated by the sciatic nerve.

Ophthalmologic exam (Dr. Bollack): revealed normal pupils, normal ocular motility without nystagmus, and normal fundi. The visual fields were normal; visual acuity: Right 7/10–0.10, Left 5/10–0.10.

Hearing, speech, and writing were normal, and there were no sphincter disturbances. She had had enuresis until the age of twelve and thereafter continued to be incontinent when she laughed.

The serum Wassermann reaction was positive.

Summary: This twenty-five-year-old woman presented with "giving way" of her legs, awkwardness of hands, generalized areflexia, club-feet, and a mildly unsteady steppage gait. Except for mild intention tremors of her hands there were no cerebellar findings. The toes were flexor, and certain muscle groups were minimally weak. There were no sensory disturbances and no nystagmus; but the responses to electrical stimuli were abnormal.

CASE 2

Simone Pli., the seven-one-half-year-old daughter of Case 1, presented with a gait disorder. The disorder had improved but was still present. She was the product of a normal-term pregnancy, weighed 8 pounds at birth and cried immediately. She was breast-fed until one year of age, cut her first teeth at eight months, spoke at one-and-one-half years, but began walking at three years, at the same time as a younger brother. She had attempted to walk at two years of age but couldn't. She fell and continued to crawl on all fours. This condition improved slowly. She reached her current level of performance at about five years of age. Although she appeared to be very intelligent and could recite a fable perfectly, her school performance was poor. She had had whooping cough at age four and roseola recently.

On examination she was a 17-kg., pockmarked, well-formed child with genu varum but without scoliosis. Her feet were bent but normal in size. She easily stood, with both feet together and without disequilibrium, but had difficulty standing on one foot. Eye closure caused her body to oscillate. She wavered when she walked, supporting herself on her heels which she dragged along the floor. She fell easily. She lay down and stood up without difficulty. We observed that the patient had difficulty with fine finger movements. The patient's mother had not noticed this. There was no tremor, and muscle tone seemed normal; postural reflexes were intact. Her upper and lower extremities were very strong, although her thigh extensors and flexors were weak (the extensors more than the flexors). Head and trunk flexion were weak but extension was normal. Lateral head movements were also well performed. The deep tendon and upper abdominal reflexes were absent, whereas the lower abdominal reflexes were intact. Both plantar responses were inconstantly and equivocally flexor.

Finger-to-nose cerebellar testing was well performed with a mild tremor, more marked on the right. Rapid alternating hand movements such as pronation-supination of the hands on the thighs were poorly performed. These movements were difficult when performed rapidly. The heel-knee-shin test was done well but there was some difficulty, possibly due to inattention, in touching the knee. The heel-to-buttock test was well performed.

The face appeared normal and was symmetric. No cranial nerve abnormalities were observed. The facial nerve was normal; she blew well. The corneal responses were normal and the pupils equal and reactive to light. Sensation was subjectively and objectively normal, and no trophic abnormalities were noted. There were no sphincter disturbances, but the patient was enuretic and suffered from incontinence. Electrical examination revealed changes similar to those of her mother.

Ophthalmologic examination (Dr. Bollack) revealed normal pupils and motility with small horizontal nystagmoid jerks on right lateral gaze. The fundus was normal and acuity 7/10 bilaterally.

Speech and hearing were normal. She wrote slowly and tremulously with the pen grasped in her hand.

The blood Wassermann test was faintly positive.

Summary: This was a seven-and-one-half-year-old patient with a gait disturbance dating from the time she began walking at three years of age. During the ensuing years the gait difficulty had improved. The patient had a clubfoot, absent deep tendon reflexes, and a mild intention tremor; but despite these signs, there were no obvious cerebellar, sensory, or atrophic disturbances.

Case 3

Raymon Pli., the two-year-old brother of the preceding case presented with a tabeticlike gait, a right clubfoot deformity, and a tendency to fall when unsupported.

The patient's birth followed a full-term pregnancy and uncomplicated delivery. He cried immediately and weighed 9 pounds. He was breast-fed until thirteen months of age, cut his first teeth at seven months and spoke at a year. When he learned to walk at eighteen months, it was noted that his legs bent as soon as he stood on them. He had recently recovered from measles.

On examination he was a normal-appearing child with rachitic bulges on the wrists and malleoli, and flaccid, perhaps atrophic, calves. The lumbar lordosis was exaggerated, and the right foot was slightly flail. His gait was unsteady and quite abnormal: he dragged his heels, and threw out his feet as a tabetic would, after which he staggered and fell. He stood with his feet spread apart, swayed, and appeared un-

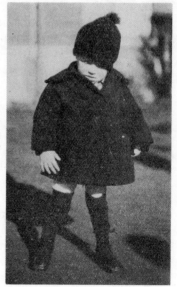

Figure 4. The patient (Case 3) could only stand for several seconds without support if his legs were spread widely apart.

stable. He easily arose from a prone to a standing position, which he maintained unsteadily. On arising he did not rest his hands on his thighs as a dystrophic might.

It was impossible to test muscle strength, but all movements—including those of the feet, toes, and legs—were well performed, and muscle tone seemed absolutely normal.

The deep tendon reflexes were absent, the superior and inferior abdominal reflexes were present bilaterally, and the plantar response was equivocal on the right and not elicited on the left.

The cerebellar examination was difficult because of the child's age but appeared normal with the possible exception of finger-to-nose testing on the left. Sensation could not be adequately evaluated. There was no atrophy or sphincter disturbance, but the child had been enuretic. The eyes and fundi, examined by Dr. Bollack, were normal. Extraocular movements were normal and without nystagmus. Speech was normal.

Summary: the patient had a clear-cut gait disorder and generalized areflexia without clubfoot or dorsiflexion of the great toe. There were no obvious cerebellar difficulties in this intelligent two-year-old with normal speech and without amyotrophy.

Case 4

Miss Julia Ur., a thirty-two-year-old factory worker and sister of Case 1 presented with bilateral painful clubfoot, which had resulted in a marked gait disturbance. She had always had foot deformities and a gait disorder and recalled falling often as a child. Her past medical history was otherwise unremarkable. Her birth was uneventful, and it was not known when she began to walk. She seemed of normal intelligence and attended school through age thirteen, after which she was employed. Her first husband was tuberculous. A normal-appearing child, the product of this marriage, died of asphyxia one hour after birth. Her second marriage to a healthy man produced no children, no miscarriages.

On examination her gait seemed normal at first, although complicated by her foot deformity (especially on the right). The foot appeared foreshortened, squared off with a marked plantar curvature. The toes appeared malpositioned. Their distal portion was on a level with the sole of the extraordinarily short foot. The patient wore a size (33) shoe.

Standing erect, the patient tended to hold her right leg abducted and externally rotated. No atrophy was observed. The calves were large. The right calf was slightly deformed. Its fleshiest portion lay antero-laterally and was located immediately under the knee.

The patient spoke and wrote well, and her face and hands were normal, although she complained that exercise brought on cramps in her hands. Her facial muscles contracted well on both sides. The pharyngeal, palatal, masseter, and corneal reflexes were normal. Hearing was intact.

Visual acuity had been impaired since the age of two. Dr. Bollack's ophthalmologic examination revealed acuity OU of 2/10 + 0.75 and nor-

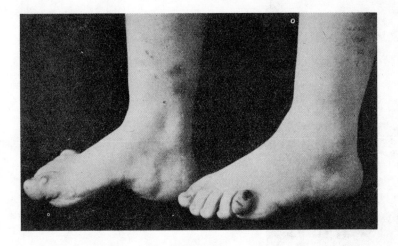

Figure 5a.   Case 4 showing marked foreshortening of the clubfoot (shoesize 33).

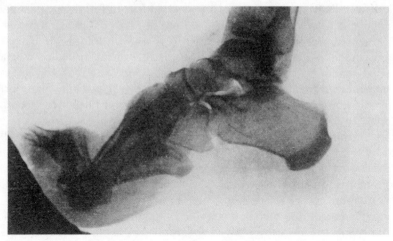

Figure 5b. X ray of the foreshortened clubfoot.

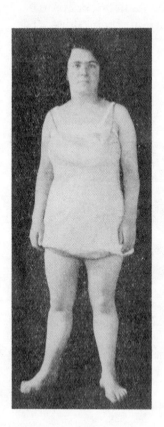

Figure 6.   The same patient. Note the appearance of the right leg.

mal fundi (with bilateral congenitally small, inferiorly placed discs). There was no nystagmus, and ocular motility was normal.

Muscle strength was normal and equal in all four extremities. Toe movements were limited by the malposition of the toe in the foot as previously noted; only the great toe moved normally. *There was generalized deep tendon areflexia,* and the cutaneous abdominal reflexes were abolished. The plantar reflexes were flexor bilaterally, and the sphincters were intact. Muscle tone and bulk seemed normal; no hypertonia or hypotonia was observed during passive momement. Cerebellar testing of the upper and lower extremities was normal. Although the patient complained of cramps while walking, sensation was intact to pin, temperature, position, and stereognosis.

Blood serology was slightly positive.

Summary: the patient had a marked clubfoot and generalized tendon areflexia but no cerebellar, pyramidal, or sensory disturbances. In addition, there was no nystagmus, speech disorder, or atrophy. Her difficulty walking was attributed to cramps and to her foot deformity. She also suffered from cramps in the hands after exertion.

Case 5

Summary: Mr. Bonne, a turner, refused to be examined. He was thirty-eight years old and the oldest brother of the two preceding cases. He stated he was normal and gave the appearance of a remarkably robust, muscular, and athletic man.

He had done his military service "without ever missing a march." His face was clearly abnormal—with mild bilateral exophthalmus and a flat nose (probably the result of old trauma). His feet were small and clubbed, similar to those of his most affected sister. He wore a size 39 shoe; was 1 meter, 20 cm. [sic] tall and weighed 75 kg. We were able to examine his deep tendon reflexes, which were all absent. He had been married twice. A daughter (Case 6) by his first wife, and one of his two sons by his second wife (Case 7) presented similar signs. He tended to sway when standing. This was especially true when his eyes were closed. He had no difficulties using his hands.

Case 6

Andrée B., the seventeen-year-old daughter of Case 5 and half-sister of Case 7, presented with a gait disorder and awkward hand movements (especially fine movements). Her birth and childhood history were not available. It is known that she walked at twenty-two months and had a right otitis. She could not read or write, having attended school for only fifteen days. If one took into account her cultural deprivation, her

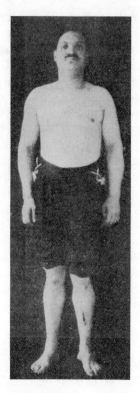

Figure 7. The brother of the two adult patients (Case 5).
Note his slender lower legs and foot deformities.

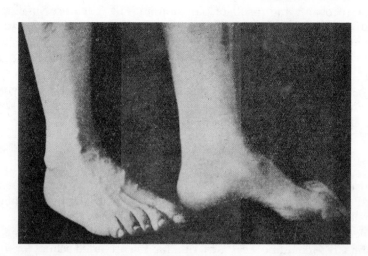

Figure 8. Foot, detail (Case 5). His shoe size was 39 (unusual for a man).

speech and intelligence could be considered normal. She had the same nasal deformity as her father (she had fallen on her nose), bilateral clubfoot, as well as very suspicious teeth [suspicious of congenital lues]. Her legs were pockmarked. There was marked *genu varum*. Her shoe size was 35 (quite small). Her gait had a wavering quality. When she stood she had the same difficulties as her father. This unsteadiness increased when she closed her eyes. Her hands were unequivocally weak, and hand movements were awkward. When she laced her shoes she held the lace between her thumb and the back of the proximal portion of her index finger (as do the patients with Charcot-Marie-Tooth disease). When she drank from a glass she was tremulous; she had great difficulty picking up coins from a table. Extremity tone and strength were preserved. *Her deep tendon and cutaneous abdominal reflexes were absent*, but sphincter function was preserved. The plantar reflex was flexor on the left and equivocal on the right. Standard cerebellar testing was normal, and the face was unremarkable except as noted above. A small corneal opacity was present on the right. The pupils were normal and equally reactive to light, and there was no nystagmus. Sensation was intact. There was thenar, hypothenar, and interosseus (especially on the left) atrophy.

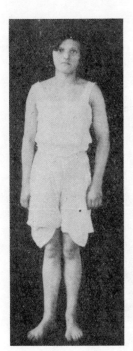

Figure 9.   Slender legs with clubfeet (Case 6).

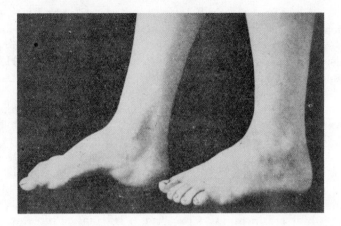

Figure 10.   Detail of the clubfeet (Case 6).

Summary: she was a seventeen-year-old who presented with difficulty walking, clubfoot, awkward hand movements, mild bilateral palmar atrophy, a markedly positive Romberg sign, absent cutaneous and
deep tendon reflexes, and a possible right extensor plantar response. No
nystagmus or other cerebellar signs were observed, and sensation was
intact.

CASE 7

Robert Bonn., was the nine-year-old third child of Case 5. He had the
facies of congenital syphilis—a large head and a saddle nose. He had a

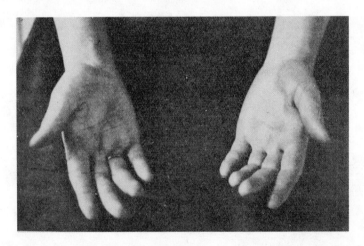

Figure 11.   Thenar and hypothenar atrophy (Case 6).

severe gait disorder, and he fell frequently. As result of these falls he refractured his right tibia, which had been broken before in a mishap with a bicyclist. His birth was normal at term. He was breast-fed, spoke at one year and walked at three years of age. He was considered to be very intelligent. He had had measles, mumps and gastrointestinal illnesses. On examination he appeared to be intelligent and quick to learn. He had normal speech and an unsteady gait. When he walked he seemed to throw his feet forward. Standing with his hands clasped together, he swayed and fell when he was pushed. The swaying increased when he closed his eyes. He could not stand on one leg and ran only with difficulty. At rest his legs gave way, as did those of other members of his family. His feet seemed of normal length. His left foot was slender and his right foot was rather flat—possibly a result of trauma. Muscle strength and tone were normal, but the deep tendon reflexes were absent. The cutaneous abdominal reflexes were preserved, and the plantar responses were equivocal on the right and flexor on the left. There were no cerebellar abnormalities, except for a mild intention tremor of the left arm. The face was unremarkable except as noted; the pupils contracted well, and there was no nystagmus. Although the child complained of foot cramps after walking, his sensory examination was normal (temperature testing was not performed).

The last three cases refused ophthalmolgic, electric, and serologic examination.

Summary: this nine-year-old child presented with a disturbance of gait and station, an equivocal left clubfoot, generalized tendon areflexia, and a mild left-sided intention tremor.

Thus, we have had the opportunity to analyze seven cases of a familial illness involving twenty individuals in four generations. In order of frequency, the features of this illness are: a. Disorder of station and gait; b. Generalized areflexia; c. Clubfoot. In addition, certain members show: d. Awkward hand movements; e. Palmar muscular atrophy (rare); f. Absent cutaneous abdominal reflexes with extension of toe (suggesting an extensor plantar response); g. Sphincter weakness (enuresis and stress incontinence). We will discuss the positive and negative features of this illness in detail.

POSITIVE FEATURES

Disorder of station and gait: The gait disturbance seems to be due to mild ataxia as well as cramps or pains associated with the foot deformities. The ataxic gait has an inebriated, steppage, swaying quality. The patient walks with his legs thrown forward, but the motions are not as brusque, nor do they have the great lurching to-and-fro quality seen in

SUMMARY TABLE

	Berthe Pli. 25 years Case 1	Simone P. 7½ years Case 2	Raymond 2 years Case 3	Julia U. 32 years Case 4	Mr. Bonne 38 years Case 5	Andrée B. 17 years Case 6	Robert B. 9 years Case 7
Gait	abnormal	abnormal	almost impossible	painful	normal	abnormal	very abnormal
Station	impossible on one foot +Romberg	impossible on one foot + Romberg	almost impossible	minimally impaired	+ Romberg	impossible on one leg + Romberg	impossible on one leg + Romberg
Finger movements	awkward	less awkward than Case 1	?	slightly awkward	normal	extremely awkward	normal
Vision and hearing	good	good	good	good, minor fundus malformations (congenital)	good	R. otitis, corneal opacity	good
Speech	normal	normal	normal	normal	normal	normal	normal
Intelligence	normal	normal	normal	normal	normal	normal illiterate	normal
Sphincters	enuresis to 12 years, stress incontinence	enuresis and stress incontinence	enuretic	—	—	—	—
Club foot	roughly	roughly	roughly				roughly

	1	2	3	4	5	6	7
Tendon reflexes	absent	absent	absent	absent	absent	absent	absent
Cutaneous reflexes	absent equivocal and in-constant extensor plantar	feeble extensor plantar	equivocal abdominals and plantars	absent abdominals plantars flexor	abdominals plantars flexor	absent abdominals absent (r) plantar doubtful	absent abdominals normal plantars equivocal on one side
Cerebellar signs	no	mild tremor	?	—	?	—	mild left intention tremor
Sensation	normal	normal	?	normal	?	normal	normal
Trophic changes	possible mild thenar atrophy	normal	normal	normal	normal	mild atrophy of palmar interossei, thenar and hypothenar	normal
Electrical responses	faradic and galvanic esp. in the small muscles of the hands and feet	identical to her mother (Case 1)	?	?	?	?	?
Nystagmus	no	mild nystagmoid jerks	—	—	—	—	—

cases of Friedreich's ataxia. Also, unlike Friedreich's ataxia, our patients become less ataxic as they grow older. Our most affected patient (Case 3) was also our youngest. Case 2 (age 7½), who showed only mild difficulty when examined, had been as disabled as her brother (Case 3) when she was younger. Their mother's difficulty showed the same pattern of evolution.

As we shall see later, the ataxia is most apparent on standing. Paradoxically, traditional tests of coordination do not reveal any abnormalities.

The episodic leg and foot cramps and pains occur after walking or standing. As in Case 4, these symptoms alone may be severe enough to make walking difficult or hesitant. These cramps may be associated with incoordination (Case 6).

The illness may present a range of abnormalities from ataxia without foot deformity (Case 3) to painful clubfoot without ataxia (Case 4), to clubfoot without gait disturbance (Case 5 is unique in this regard). The station difficulties reflect equilibrium problems as well as a tendency for the legs to quickly collapse. The disequilibrium is not completely explained by coordination difficulties. In the uncomplicated condition, when the patient is standing, disequilibrium shows itself as small-amplitude antero-posterior or transverse oscillations of the whole body (Cases 4 and 5). The unequivocal clubfoot and concomitant neurological symptoms seen in both patients may be responsible for the unsteadiness while standing and the inability to stand on one leg. However, these deformities would not explain the presence of Romberg's sign (increased unsteadiness with eyes closed) noted in most of our patients. It is also impossible to relate the patients' need to stand with legs spread and their titubation to the clubfoot deformity (a deformity clearly present in Case 6 but not in Case 3). One approach to the problem is to consider our patients' sudden lapses in leg control. These brusque, involuntary flexion movements of the legs sometimes associated with traumatic falls in our patients are also seen in tabetics. These episodic lapses seem to be of motor origin, are not provoked by pain, but may be preceded by activity (such as carrying a burden).

Generalized tendon areflexia: The second most constant symptom is complete absence of tendon reflexes in the upper (radial, brachial, and triceps) and lower (knee and ankle) extremities. Jendrassik's maneuver had no effect. In some patients the idiomuscular contractions in the posterior leg seemed feeble.

Clubfoot: A classic, bilateral clubfoot deformity was seen in four cases (Cases 1, 4, 5, and 6). In three others it was either unilateral or atypical. The classic deformity consists of antero-posterior compression, foreshortening, and widening of the foot (Case 4), sometimes associated with extension of the first phalanx of the great toe and flexion of the second phalanx without abnormalities of the remaining toes. In addition, the plantar arch, viewed from the lateral border of the foot, is exaggerated, and the foot seems to jut out dorsally. In Case 4 the deformity was so severe that the distal phalanges of the toes were on a level with the sole of the foot. X rays show abnormal size and position of the bones of the foot without abnormalities in their form or number. In less typical examples of the clubfoot there is (sometimes unilaterally) dorsal protrusion and excessively convex plantar arching without appreciable foreshortening. In addition, certain patients have slender lower legs, in contrast to the other calf (Case 5) and thigh muscles (Case 6), together with a *genu varum* (Case 6).

SECONDARY SYMPTOMS

In addition to the above three characteristic findings there are less constant ones listed here in order of frequency:

1. Toe extension (most often unilateral) in response to painful stimuli. In *no* case, however, was a clearly defined Babinski response present.
2. Frequent absence or diminution of the cutaneous abdominal reflexes.
3. Slight awkwardness of the hands during activities (sewing, peeling, buttoning, picking up coins) which involve finger movements. These activities were associated with a slight, atypical tremor in Case 1. Writing remains normal but is slow. In Case 2 it was associated with tremor and contraction of the digits. Marked weakness and movements usually associated with the Charcot-Marie-Tooth disease were present in Case 6. In several cases weakness could be demonstrated objectively in the hands or proximal lower extremities.
4. Atrophy and weakness of the thenar, hypothenar, and interosseus muscles were observed in one case. This combination of atrophy and weakness will be considered later when we discuss pathogenesis. The faradic and galvanic hypoexcitability of the muscles of the distal upper extremities is consistent with the theory of pathogenesis I will propose.
5. Sphincter dysfunction (enuresis and stress incontinence) were present in some of our patients.

NEGATIVE FEATURES

The illness is defined both by positive and negative findings. Our patients do not exhibit appreciable cerebellar dysfunction (with standard tests), objective or subjective sensory abnormalities, significant amyotrophy or scoliosis. Moreover, there is no evidence of cranial nerve dysfunction, nystagmus (with one mild exception), speech impairment, or intellectual decline.

EVOLUTION OF THE ILLNESS

The evolution of this illness is as mysterious as its symptoms. The child's first attempts to walk are delayed and difficult. As the foot deformities are probably congenital, it is probable that the major symptoms are also present from birth. This impression is supported by the fixed or even regressive nature of the neurological deficit. We are uncertain as to whether other, more seriously affected family members had a progressive form of this illness, since we were unable to examine them. Furthermore, we did not have exact information concerning previous generations. Our oldest patient was thirty-eight years of age. His deficit was so minimal that he would have been astounded to have been included among the afflicted family members. In fact he was remarkably robust and appeared practically normal. The other affected adults did not seem to have suffered from any progression of their disease since its onset. Some seemed to have improved!

FAMILIAL EVOLUTION

The precise mode of inheritance of this illness is unknown. The process affects and is transmited by both sexes. There is incomplete penetrance since certain patients have unaffected children, but we have been unable to prove that the disease is transmitted by otherwise healthy individuals.

DIAGNOSIS

In view of what we have already said about the illness, how is it to be classified, and what is its possible etiology?

DIFFERENTIAL DIAGNOSIS

The specific symptoms associated with the illness include a disorder of gait, clubfoot, and absent reflexes. These symptoms in combination with the familial character suggests a theoretical link to Friedreich's ataxia. However, the patients' symptoms and the mode of appearance and evolution of the illness distinguish it from Friedreich's ataxia. The latter is characterized by obvious and predominant cerebellar symptomatology, difficulty speaking, nystagmus, choreiform instability, club-foot, and spontaneous extension of the great toe. It appears most often in late childhood or adolescence and follows a progressive course.

By contrast, cerebellar symptoms were minimal in our patients and not related to the onset of the illness. As we shall mention later, even after very careful examination we were not able to make a definite statement regarding cerebellar symptoms. Our patients did not have choreiform instability, difficulty speaking, nystagmus, or scoliosis. If one disregards the fact that our patients become symptomatic first in early childhood, do not seem to progress, and do not exhibit tonic toe extension, they are linked to patients with Friedreich's ataxia by the presence of clubfoot and the absence of deep tendon reflexes.

If our cases are not typical of classic Friedreich's ataxia, could they be atypical forms of that illness? They might be attenuated, regressive, or possibly latent forms of Friedreich's ataxia. In truth, this hypothesis is not satisfying, nor does it resolve anything. No other published in-stances of *forme fruste* Friedreich's ataxia appear similar to ours. In this regard one fact is bothersome: Gardner* reported one family in which the mother suffered from spastic paraplegia, intention tremor, nystag-mus, clubfoot, etc.; three of the six children were affected, and three were considered "normal." All three "normal" children had absent knee jerks, one had scoliosis, and one had scoliosis and a clubfoot. Gardner considered that this reflected the multifaceted presentations of nervous-system illness. Thus, the general features (of these illnesses) permit their separation into large groups, while the secondary features separate the illnesses within these large groups. Our cases may repre-sent an intermediate or transitional form of familial illness linking Fried-reich's ataxia and Charcot-Marie-Tooth disease. Some of our cases seemed closer to the latter by virtue of awkward hand motions, amyo-trophic features, electrical abormalities, and the presence of clubfoot. In truth, this separation may be rather fanciful and should not replace the anatomo-clinical data.

Despite the lack of anatomic verification we feel that the clinical picture is so distinctive as to allow us to separate this illness from others and describe it in this report. Our ignorance of the cause and pathology of this illness leads us to several hypotheses.

HYPOTHESES CONCERNING THE NATURE OF THE ILLNESS

From an anatomo-physiologic point of view, how might we view the causal lesions in our patients? A lesion of the posterior columns is

---

*Gardner, "A Family in Which Some of the Signs of Friedreich's Ataxia Appeared Dis-cretely." *Brain*, 1906, p. 112.

suggested by the absence of deep tendon reflexes and the mild incoordination observed in all patients. We are aware that this is the clinical picture associated with cases of familial tabes (two brothers or sisters as reported by Londe or Crouzon). This incoordination could also be explained by a lesion of the cerebellar tracts as in Friedreich's ataxia.

The clinical picture leads only to hypotheses.

A posterior column rather than cerebellar tract lesion is suggested by the absence of dysmetria, true intention tremor, obvious cerebellar signs, and increased unsteadiness with eye closure.

However, the very mild pyramidal signs exhibited by some of our patients suggest an involvement of the lateral columns, such as is seen in Friedreich's ataxia.

Yet again, these signs may be due to lesions of the anterior horn cells. Such lesions would also explain the mild atrophic changes and above-mentioned electrical abnormalities. If one adds to these findings the involvement of the posterior columns, our cases resemble those with Charcot-Marie-Tooth disease.

The nature of the lesions in our patients eludes us. It would be easy to attribute this illness to hereditary syphilis, especially in view of the inadequate serologic examinations in our cases; but this would not explain the familial occurrence of the illness. This familial pattern is a general feature of the illness. None of our patients accepted a lumbar puncture, and only three had a serological examination. These serologies (two sisters and the child of one of them) were positive, which suggests an acquired illness rather than hereditary transmission. The criticisms are applicable to Cases 6 and 7, who had facial and dental deformities suggestive of hereditary syphilis. These two children did not have the same mother; and the father, who transmitted the familial illness, had somewhat suspect facies. As for other infections, none of our patients with the inherited illness became symptomatic after an acute infection. Moreover, we were unable to uncover any personal or genealogic fact which might explain the mysterious etiology of this malady. The problem of etiology is one which concerns all of the familial illnesses and, in a general way, reflects their hereditary nature.

CONCLUSIONS

1. We have described a unique familial illness (without pathologic verification) characterized by difficulty walking and standing, clubfoot, generalized tendon areflexia, and occasional mild clumsiness of the hands. Its clinical features permit us to separate it from the other familial illnesses.

2. We do not feel that this illness represents either an atypical form

of Friedreich's ataxia or an intermediate form of other familial diseases. It must be pointed out that this last statement is theoretical and does not lead to a definite classification. The two hypotheses complicate rather than elucidate, and raise the possibility of a unified pathogenesis for all the familial illnesses.

3. Even if future anatomic studies allow us to more clearly unite the various previously described forms of familial illness, the process we have described remains unique, in need of explanation, and worthy of our report. This report describes a separate and apparently new illness with common symptoms and a familial pattern, which makes it of some importance.

Even if this illness is ultimately proven to be an aberrant or transitional form of one of the already described familial maladies, the nature of the evolution, variety, and interrelationships of the familial illnesses will still represent a remarkable area for future research. Thus, we did not think that it was inappropriate to present this long, imperfect, and provisional description.

NARCOLEPSY

Introduction

William R. Shapiro, M.D.
Professor of Neurology
Cornell University Medical College

WESTPHAL (1) first described a narcoleptic sleep attack in 1877, but it was Gélineau, in 1890 (2), who defined narcolepsy as "an unusual, or at any rate little known, neurosis characterized by the recurrence at more or less frequent intervals of a sudden, transient but irresistible urge to sleep." Weir Mitchell (3) recorded what we now term sleep paralysis, and Lhermitte (4) commented both on hypnagogic hallucinations and on cataplexy, although Loewenfeld (5) probably described cataplectic attacks as early as 1902. Indeed, Gélineau's patient probably also had cataplexy. These four symptoms constitute the narcoleptic tetrad (6,7).

Narcolepsy consists of irresistible episodes of actual sleep occurring from a few to many times a day, between which episodes the patient may be alert or drowsy. Cataplexy is a sudden decrease or loss of muscle tone that may be generalized or confined to individual muscles. When mild it consists of a sense of weakness, a tendency to drop things, or of having one lower limb give way; when severe, the patient may fall in a heap. Such attacks generally last less than a minute and occur from once to 12–25 times in a twenty-four–hour period. They may be precipitated by heightened emotional tone—laughing, anger—but when severe they occur spontaneously or with any kind of movement. Sleep paralysis, like cataplexy, is also characterized by the inability to move, but occurs when the patient is either falling asleep or just coming out of a sleep spell. Hypnagogic hallucinations are vivid visual or auditory dreamlike states which occur while dozing or while being aroused. They are so vivid that patients may act out the dream state on awakening and are surprised to discover that they have been dreaming.

Twenty-five percent of narcoleptic patients only have sleep attacks while 70 percent have both narcolepsy and cataplexy (6,7). Approximately 12 percent of patients experience all four symptoms of the tetrad. The incidence in males is approximately equal to that in females. Although the disease commonly begins in the teens and twenties, the diagnosis is frequently delayed five to eight years because neither the patient nor his physician recognizes the nature of the attacks.

The pathogenesis of narcolepsy is unknown, but two theories have been proposed: Yoss and Daly (8) opined that narcolepsy represents one end of a continuous spectrum from full wakefulness to deep sleep. Narcoleptic patients are thought to have a genetically determined greater incidence of otherwise normal drowsiness (reduced vigilance), and the degree of sleepiness can be determined by pupillographic studies (9). The second theory of the pathogenesis of narcolepsy was advanced after the two different stages of sleep based on electroencephalographic (EEG) findings (slow-wave sleep and rapid-eye movement [REM] sleep) were recognized. Dement et al. (10) found that twenty of twenty-four patients with both narcolepsy and cataplexy had REM EEG patterns at the onset of sleep while seven of nine without cataplexy had non-REM sleep onset. The REM-onset sleep pattern contrasts with normal sleep which begins with non-REM sleep followed ninety minutes later by the first episode of REM. Hishikawa et al. (11) and Roth et al. (12) later demonstrated that narcoleptic patients without cataplexy may have non–REM-onset sleep attacks. REM sleep patterns are associated with inhibition of motor tone, a silent electromyogram (EMG), dreaming, and certain autonomic changes. The thesis that narcolepsy-cataplexy is associated with REM-onset sleep patterns explains cataplexy as the sudden loss of motor tone that occurs with REM. Hypnagogic hallucinations represent the dream component of the REM state, and sleep paralysis is also associated with loss of motor tone occurring during sleep.

Anatomic and pharmacologic studies suggest that certain brainstem structures represent the loci responsible for non-REM and REM sleep (13,14). Non-REM sleep is associated with serotonergic neurones lying in the midline raphe nuclei of the pons that project rostrally. REM sleep is associated with catecholaminergic and, perhaps, cholinergic neurones located more laterally in the region of the locus ceruleus. Amphetamines inhibit both non-REM and REM sleep, but only to a moderate degree (15), while tricyclic antidepressants profoundly inhibit REM sleep but do not influence non-REM sleep and have no effect on the sleep attacks of narcolepsy (16,17). It is the REM-inhibiting property of the antidepressants which makes them effective in treating cataplexy. That they do not prevent REM-onset sleep attacks may be explained by the fact that the brainstem contains mechanisms for both a phasic and a tonic component in the REM pattern. The phasic component consists of the desynchronized EEG patterns and rapid eye movements, the tonic component the marked inhibition of muscle activity and areflexia. The tricyclic antidepressants appear to suppress only the tonic components, apparently by inhibiting the caudal third of the locus ceruleus. The dissociation between the tonic and phasic components of REM sleep is demonstrable in cataplectic patients whose cataplexy and silent EMG occur before the EEG shows the desynchronization of REM sleep (18). Finally, recent demonstration that the antiserotonergic agent methysergide is mildly effective against narcoleptic sleep attacks suggests an effect on the non-REM serotonergic system (19). The narcoleptic disorder then may involve both the REM system (especially in patients who have associated cataplexy) and the non-REM system.

Treatment of narcolepsy began with Thomas Willis (20), who used caffeine as an agrypnotic. Ephedrine therapy, introduced by Doyle and Daniels in 1931, required doses approaching 300 mg per day (21). In 1935 Prinzmetal and Bloomberg (22) introduced the amphetamines as a specific treatment for narcolepsy. Modifications of the amphetamine derivatives were made by Prinzmetal and Alles (23) [dextroamphetamine] and by Eaton (24) [desoxyephedrine]. Dextroamphetamine sulfate in the form of sustained release capsules or tablets at doses of 15–50 mg per day are generally effective against the sleep attacks, especially in the first few years of use; tolerance develops, however, and the drugs become less effective. Methylphenidate was introduced by Daly and Yoss in 1956 (25) as a therapy for narcolepsy; tolerance develops more slowly than with the amphetamines, and it has a reduced excitatory potential. Methylphenidate must be administered on an empty stomach and can be used in doses up to 200 mg per day. It is the drug of choice in narcoleptic patients who are also hypertensive. Unfortunately, methylphenidate does not prevent cataplexy, and the amphetamines are only minimally effective. The first effective agent in the treatment of the ancillary cataplectic symptoms of narcolepsy was imipramine, introduced by Akimoto in 1960 (26). This drug completely blocked cataplexy but only at relatively high doses. Desmethylimipramine, introduced by Hishikawa in 1966 (27), was also effective. The most effective drug currently available to treat cataplexy is clomipramine, introduced in 1970 by Passouant (16) and confirmed by us (17). A number of other agents have been tested in the treatment of the narcoleptic tetrad including monamine oxidase inhibitors (28) and L-DOPA (29), but the side effects of these agents preclude their general use. Although narcolepsy is a benign disease, its course may be gradually progressive, the patient becoming refractory to therapy. Whether this constitutes progression of the disease or increasing tolerance to the medication produced by weight gain and other factors is not known.

Sleep is often a spirit of solace to troubled man, but in narcolepsy it is a demon, as Nietzsche wrote [quoted by Sours (6)]: "No small art is it to sleep; it is necessary for that purpose to keep awake all day."

REFERENCES

1. Westphal, C. "Eigentümliche [Krankheit] mit einschlafenverbundenen Anfällen." *Arch. Psychiatr* 7: 631–635, 1877.

2. Gélineau, J. B. E. "De la narcolepsie." *Gaz. Hop.* 55: 626–628, 1880.

3. Weir Mitchell, S. "Some disorders of sleep." In *Clinical Lessons on Nervous Diseases*. Philadelphia and New York: Lea Bros. & Co., 1897.

4. Lhermitte, J. Rapport du Congrès des Neurologistes et Aliénistes, Bruxelles, 1910. "Les maladies du sommeil et les narcolepsies." *Journal de Neurologie* 15: 1–17, 1910.

5. Loewenfeld, L: "Über Narcolepsie." *München. Med. Wschr.* 49: 1041, 1902.

6. Sours, J. A. "Narcolepsy and other disturbances in the sleep-waking rhythm: A study of 115 cases with review of the literature." *J. Nerv. Ment. Dis.* 137: 525–542, 1963.

7. Yoss, R. E. and Daly, D. D. "Criteria for the diagnosis of the narcoleptic syndrome." *Mayo Clin Proc.* 33: 320–328, 1957.

8. Yoss, R. E. and Daly, D. D. "On the treatment of narcolepsy." *Med. Clin. N. Amer.* 52: 781–787, 1968.

9. Yoss, R. E. "The inheritance of diurnal sleepiness as measured by pupillography." *Mayo Clin Proc* 45: 426–437, 1970.

10. Dement, W., Rechtschaffen, A., and Gulevich, G. "The nature of the narcoleptic sleep attack." *Neurology* 16: 18–33, 1966.

11. Hishikawa, Y., Nan'no, H., Tachibaba, M., et al. "The nature of sleep attacks and other symptoms of narcolepsy." *Electroenceph. Clin. Neurophysiol.* 24: 1–10, 1968.

12. Roth, B., Bruhova, S., and Lehovsky, M. "REM sleep and NREM sleep in narcolepsy and hypersomnia." *Electroenceph. Clin. Neurophysiol.* 26: 176–182, 1969.

13. Moruzzi, G. "The sleep-waking cycle." *Ergeb. Physiol.* 64: 1–165, 1972.

14. Jouvet, M. "The role of monamines and acetylcholine-containing neurons in the regulation of the sleep-waking cycle." *Ergeb. Physiol.* 64: 166–307, 1972.

15. Roth, B., Faber, J., Nevsimalova, S., and Tosovsky, J. "The influence of imipramine, dexphenmetrazine and amphetaminsulphate upon the clinical and polygraphic picture of narcolepsy-cataplexy." *Arch. Suisses de Neurol., Neurochir., Psychiat.* 108: 251–260, 1971.

16. Passouant, P., Baldy-Moulinier, M., and Aussillous, Ch. "Etat du mal cataplectique au cours d'une maladie de Gélineau; influence de la clomipramine." *Revue Neurologique* 123: 56–60, 1970.

17. Shapiro, W. R. "Treatment of cataplexy with clomipramine." *Arch. Neurol.* 32: 653–656, 1975.

18. Guilleminault, C., Wilson, R. A., and Dement, W. C. "A study on cataplexy." *Arch. Neurol.* 31: 255–261, 1974.

19. Wyler, A. R., Wilkus, R. J., and Troupin, A. S. "Methysergide (Sansert) in the treatment of narcolepsy." *Arch. Neurol.* 32: 265–268, 1975.

20. Willis, T. The London Practice of Physick: Or the Whole Practical Part of Physick Contained in the Works of Dr. Willis; Faithfully Made English, and Printed Together for the Publick Good. London: Thomas Bassett and William Crooke, 1685, Part 4, ch. 3; p. 397.

21. Doyle, J. B., and Daniels, L. E. "Narcolepsy: Results of treatment with ephedrine sulfate." *JAMA* 98: 542–545, 1932.

22. Prinzmetal, M., and Bloomberg, W. "The use of Benzedrine for the treatment of narcolepsy." *JAMA* 105: 2051–2054, 1935.

23. Prinzmetal, M., and Alles, G. A. "The central nervous system stimulant effects of dextroamphetamine sulfate." *Amer. J. Med. Sci.* 200: 665–673, 1940.

24. Eaton, L. M. "Treatment of narcolepsy with desoxyephedrine hydrochloride." *Mayo Clin Proc.* 18: 262–264, 1943.

25. Yoss, R. E., and Daly, D. D. "Treatment of narcolepsy with Ritalin." *Neurology* 9: 171–173, 1959.

26. Akimoto, H., Honda, Y., and Takahashi, Y. "Pharmacotherapy in narcolepsy." *Dis. Nerv. System* 21: 704–706, 1960.

27. Hishikawa, Y., Ida, H., Nakai, K., and Kaneko, Z. "Treatment of narcolepsy with imipramine (Tofranil) and desmethylimipramine (Pertofan)." *J. Neurol. Sci.* 3: 453–461, 1966.

28. Wyatt, R. J., et al. "Treatment of intractable narcolepsy with a monoamine oxidase inhibitor." *New Eng. J. Med.* 285: 987–991, 1971.

29. Gunne, L. M., Lidvall, H. F., and Widén, L. "Preliminary clinical trial with L-DOPA in Narcolepsy." *Psychopharmacologia* (Berl.) 19: 204–206, 1971.

On Narcolepsy

J. B. E. GÉLINEAU

I PROPOSE TO GIVE the name narcolepsy (from νάϱχωεις, stupor, and λαμβάνειν, to seize) to an unusual, or at any rate little known, neurosis characterized by the recurrence, at more or less frequent intervals, of a sudden, transient but irresistible urge to sleep. This name will bring to mind the double analogy between narcolepsy, somnolence, and catalepsy.

I thought at first that my observations (see below) were unique but later discovered in reading Dr. Delasiauve's *Journal de médicine mentale* (vol. 2, nos. 8 & 9, 1862) that Dr. Caffe published the princeps case of this sleep neurosis in his *Journal des connaissances médicales pratiques* (August 20, 1862). I relate Dr. Caffe's case with pleasure as indisputable proof of the existence of narcolepsy.

CASE 1

For more than a year, writes Dr. Caffe, I treated an employee of the Grand Cercle, 16 boulevard Montmartre, who was obliged to quit his job on account of an incessant, irresistible inclination to sleep. This forty-seven-year-old married man was tall and vigorous and had always been a model of sobriety. There was no history of previous illness. Heavy, half-closed eyelids signalled the onset of a sleep attack; attacks occurred while the patient was sitting, standing, lying down, or walking. He suffered from this somnolence—which was more or less irresistible de-

NOTE: Translated by D. A. Rottenberg and S. Fish from: Gélineau, J. B. E., "De la Narcolepsie," *Gazette des Hôpitaux* 53 (1880), 626–28 and 635–37.

pending upon his immediate circumstances—for more than four years. He awakened only to fall back asleep at once. The most extreme hunger pangs provided only a momentary distraction. He was lethargic and dull-witted, his face pallid and puffy, his attitude nonchalant; he remained portly and in good general health.

Various treatments were unsuccessful; taking the waters at Brides resulted in some amelioration of his condition but did not effect a cure.

Later, following upon a terrifying personal experience and a variety of illicit excesses (immoderate coitus, masturbation, and imbibition of alcoholic beverages) he suffered from hallucinations and a meningitic delirium, for which he was vigorously treated by Dr. Semelaigne.

CASE 2 (personal observation)

Mr. G., a thirty-eight-year-old cask merchant of a nervous-sanguine [sic] disposition, first attended my clinic on February 15, 1879.

There is no history of convulsions in childhood or, subsequently, of syphilis. G. has two children; the elder, thirteen years of age, always accompanies his father, and the younger is only a few months old. G.'s father was highly strung but not sickly; his mother died of cancer, his brother of a stomach ulcer. The patient drinks a moderate amount. Five years ago he suffered an attack of rheumatic fever and contracted ringworm of the scalp.

Three years ago during a rather heated argument over a money matter G. received a sharp blow from his adversary, to which he replied with a whip. He was subsequently apprehended by the superintendant of police and thrown into jail (which caused him considerable vexation).

Lastly, a short time later, a log fell on his head without, however, causing him much of a headache. (I was unable to elicit any tenderness or to detect any flattening worthy of note at the site of injury.)

A long symptom-free interval ensued, and it was not until two years later that G. began to experience drop attacks: his legs would suddenly give way when he burst out laughing or when he envisioned a profitable business transaction. When playing cards, if he was dealt a good hand he would succumb to a fit of weakness and be unable to move his arms; his head would droop, and he would fall asleep, only to awaken a moment later. Before long the slightest emotion—merely the sight of his winecasks—was sufficient to induce sleep. This urgent need to sleep became increasingly troublesome. At table his meals were interrupted four or five times by the desire to sleep: his lids would droop; his fork, knife or glass would fall from his hand; he would finish with difficulty—stammering in a whisper—the sentence which he had begun in a loud voice; his head would nod, and he would sleep. If he was sitting when stricken, he would rub his eyes in a vain attempt to ward off the urge to sleep; his hand would fall down lifeless; he would be overcome, slump forward, and sleep. If he was standing in the street when the urge to sleep overtook him, he would totter and stumble about like a drunkard; people would accuse him of being intoxicated and jeer at him. He would be unable to answer them. Their mockeries would bear him down, and he would fall, instinctively avoiding the horses and carriages that were passing by. When several people then formed a ring around him—which was always the case in Paris—he would hear (or imagine) them making charitable comments about his condition, and their amenities would exacerbate his weakness, paralyzing him and preventing him from regaining his feet.

If he experienced a strong emotion—painful or joyful—the need to sleep was even more imperious. Thus, if he concluded a profitable business transaction, caught sight of a friend, spoke to a stranger for the first time, or played a good hand at cards he would collapse and fall asleep immediately. If he went to the Botanical Garden and sat down near the monkey cage—the traditional rendezvous of the curious, nursemaids, soldiers, and wags—he would fall asleep watching the people laugh around him. An unmanageable horse, a passing carriage, the sight of a grotesquely dressed person prompting a smile—nothing more would be required to provoke an attack.

If he went to the theater he would fall asleep while entering it, merely at the thought of the pleasure he was about to experience. After taking his seat he would fall asleep again, and in order to arouse him his son would take to shaking and pinching him. But once the actors were on the stage his attacks would cease; he would follow the action with interest, and unless deeply moved by a touching scene he would remain awake during the entire performance.

Bad weather, especially the approach of a storm, would increase the frequency of his sleep attacks, which have numbered as many as two hundred in a single day.

The only way to arouse him was to shake him vigorously or to pinch him. Although he fell asleep less often when he was violently angry, a longer and deeper sleep would ensue when he recovered his temper. On awakening he walked straight and steadily until the next sleep attack overcame him a quarter of an hour later.

I shall always remember G.'s first visit to my clinic. He was led in and supported by his son, who had hold of his arm. He had scarcely entered my office and directed his eyes toward me when, overcome, his expression faded, his eyelids drooped, he staggered, stumbled, and fell, asleep, into a chair. His son spoke to him and shook him vigorously, whereupon he began to speak.

During sleep G.'s pulse, which is normally 66 to 68, drops immediately to 58 or 60. His pupils are miotic during wakefulness and somewhat less constricted during sleep. They constrict when the lids are raised and when a light is brought up close. The sleep attacks last from one to five minutes.

G. is otherwise in good health; his manner is calm and relaxed, and he eats well. His nocturnal sleep is unperturbed; he awakens only once during the night. He drinks coffee once a day and is not constipated. His sexual desires have greatly diminished. When I recalled that his wife had recently given birth he replied that the child was conceived when his affliction overtook him by surprise.

He belongs to a fraternal organization, and his membership card bears the diagnosis *morbus sacer* (epilepsy). He has been looked after at home and at the Salpêtrière. When he used to go to the Salpêtrière he would fall asleep several times: first at the front door, then in the waiting room and, finally, a third time, in front of the doctor whom he had come to consult. Potassium bromide, subcutaneous injections, hydrotherapy, electricity, and finally cauterizations of the neck were prescribed—all to no avail.

Asked to give a detailed account of the onset of a sleep attack, G. replied that he feels no pain at the moment of being stricken; he described a profound heaviness, a mental blankness, a sort of whirling around inside his head and a heavy weight on his forehead and behind his eyes. His thoughts grow dim and fade away, his lids droop. Hearing is unaffected; he remains conscious. Finally, his lids close completely, and he sleeps. All this occurs very rapidly so that the preliminary stage of physiologic sleep, which normally lasts five, ten or twenty minutes, lasts barely a few seconds in G.'s case.

If G. is asked to close his eyes while walking or talking (as one has an ataxic do), his voice becomes faint, and he falls asleep, sinking to the ground without extravagant movements. If he finds himself in a dark place such as a cellar, the urge to sleep is more insistent. When he walks down an incline or pushes a wheelbarrow he can hardly keep himself erect, whereas if he is harnessed to a cart he can pull it along without flagging or falling asleep—no doubt because his resolve is firmer under these circumstances.

He has never been incontinent of urine or feces during a sleep attack. On occasion I have chatted with him for more than half an hour without his falling asleep.

His memory is not in the least affected, and he is actively engaged in running his own business. Cognizant of the perils to which he is constantly exposed, he never ventures out unaccompanied. He has fewer attacks when he works alone; being fond of gossip he becomes animated in conversation and falls asleep.

The intermittent character of G.'s illness, its benign course, the frequency of his sleep attacks, and the absence of consecutive lesions suggest that we are dealing with a neurosis. But must it be assigned to one of the recognized subtypes, or does it merit a separate place within this group of illnesses, which is so important and already so large? That is the question which I propose to discuss.

First of all, can one see anything resembling epilepsy in G.'s illness? I think not. Certainly in both conditions the patient falls to the ground without being able to save himself. But the narcoleptic does not utter a harsh premonitory cry (the expression of profound terror); he does not blanch and blush in turn; he is not subject to tonic convulsions or clonic movements; he is aware of being pinched; he remains conscious of his surroundings; one can arouse him from sleep by shaking him; he is not at all lethargic when he awakens; and he immediately recovers his intellectual faculties, his power of sense-perception, and his strength and coordination. What is more, far from being oppressive, his repose seems indispensable and appears to refresh him. Finally, his memory is not impaired. Potassium bromide, that touchstone of anticonvulsant therapy, has no beneficial effect on G. whatever. Besides, what epileptic retains his memory and intelligence after one hundred or two hundred seizures a day for two years?

Dr. Semelaigne, however, seeks to relate G.'s illness to epilepsy. "One symptom," he writes, "has been more prominent than the others, but the concurrence of symptoms is nonetheless significant. Who knows but that such spells may occur for a long time before their true nature becomes apparent? Who knows whether or not they lead to drowsiness, dullness, memory loss, foolishness, intellectual impairment, or moral perversity? Between attacks, or when the attacks remit, intelligence and morality may be preserved. Such was the case with M. Doubtless his somnolence first attracted our attention, as it was his most prominent symptom, but he was also subject to daily faints, dizzy spells, and so-called sham fits. Attacks such as these are usually followed by drowsiness and not by stupor." As regards transient ischemic attacks, Dr. Semelaigne states that they are among the commonest complications of epilepsy. Lastly, he maintains that the acute meningitic delirium which complicated G.'s illness also falls within the "realm of the convulsive disorders."

I have reproduced my colleague's opinions in their entirety, but I find them most unconvincing. G., who has had daily drop attacks for more than four years, has never had a typical convulsive seizure! He falls, and he awakens immediately after an attack. He falls, but the ictus never hurls him, rigid, to the ground so as to occasion those injuries which are commonly sustained by epileptics. He falls, and he immediately recovers his senses and his intellect. His falls resemble those of a drunkard or of a sleeping child. His collapse results from and is *preceded* by sleep, whereas sleep *follows* the fall in an epileptic attack. I might add that Dr. Semelaigne does not allude to what, in my view, constitutes the cardinal feature of epilepsy (in its mildest as well as in its most severe forms), namely, memory loss—the inability to remember what has just happened. A patient who after a spell, a lapse, or a fall remembers what has happened to him or is aware of what is going on around him is not an epileptic.

Can G's illness be confused with kenophobia (τὸ χενὸν, empty; φοβέω, I fear), the fear of open spaces of Dr. Legrand du Saulle, the agoraphobia of the Germans? Not any longer. No doubt, while crossing a boulevard or a square G. is frightened, nervous, and hesitant; but the sight of an open space affects him less than the fear of being surprised by a carriage, a cart, or a horse. When an access of emotion brings his steps to a halt, sleep overpowers him and nails him to the spot. Besides, a kenophobe does not fall asleep. He frets, looks about, cries out, signals, calls, and hesitates if no one comes to take his hand. G.—anxious, troubled—does not fuss or look about at all; he falls asleep and collapses.

Neither can this illness be confused with vertigo accompanied by faintness, falling, and loss of consciousness. To begin with, there is no illusory movement of the environment; even when his eyes are half-shut G. perceives that his surroundings are stationary. When he totters—his eyes closed—it is because he wishes to stretch out and go to sleep. He does not try to catch hold of nearby objects as a vertiginous patient does; he gives up without a fight. For G., sleep is the rule; for the patient afflicted with vertigo, syncope is the exception. Finally, what a difference there is between G., sleeping peacefully, blissfully, his face glowing, and the patient plunged into syncope, livid, ice-cold, covered with a cold seat, and as pale as death!

Dr. Casse [sic] attributed this morbid state to a passive serous congestion of the brain and its meninges. But I must confess that I find it difficult to relate an intermittent symptom (recurrent sleep attacks) to such an anatomical lesion. The cerebral circulation hardly lends itself to the sudden fluxes and refluxes which must be invoked to explain the narcoleptic's recurrent sleep attacks. The concept of spasm provides a simpler explanation for the observed phenomena.

Can G.'s illness be related to any of the various degrees of morbid sleep—cataphora, sopor, stupor, coma, carus, lethargy—carefully distinguished by the ancients but seldom recognized nowadays? The form, duration, and the manifest unresponsiveness which characterize the last three immediately preclude any comparison.

One could, perhaps, compare G.'s affliction to cataphora; if one adheres to the meaning of the Greek words κατὰ (below) and φέρειν (to carry), a certain analogy between these two types of sleep can be discerned. But in cataphora the sleep, which is easily interrupted (as in G.'s case), resumes as soon as one stops talking to the patient. The sleep is continuous, has a fixed duration, and is not characterized by long intervals during which the patient thinks, acts, and works. Finally, cataphora would be unlikely to last for a period of years without ending in death or cure.

As for sopor or somnolence, an intermediate stage between cataphora and coma, the difference is even more striking. The patient, lying on his back, sleeps even more deeply, can be awakened only with difficulty, and presents clear-cut cerebral symptomatology—headache, vertigo, memory loss, and akinesia. But there is no evidence that G. suffers from a cerebral illness: he feels well, his memory is intact, he awakens easily, and, moreover, he is awake more than he is asleep.

As regards *sleeping sickness* (the sleeping dropsy of the English, the "somnosis" of Dr. Nicholas, the "hypnosis" of Dr. Dangaix), no confusion can possibly arise. To begin with, sleeping sickness is a disease of negroes living in the tropics and has not been observed to occur at temperate latitudes. However, since this is not a sufficient reason for rejecting the comparison, I will defer to Dr. Nicholas, who recently emphasized the progressive evolution of somnosis from drowsiness to death (*Transactions of the Academy of Science*, May 10, 1880). Somnosis, he writes, begins with somnolence, which is not at all different from normal sleepiness, and its course is characterized by progressively deeper and increasingly protracted sleep, from which, in the end, the patient can no longer be aroused. I might add that I invited my friend, Dr. Nicholas, to see G. in consultation, and that he, an expert in the field, immediately rejected any analogy between narcolepsy and sleeping sickness.

Moreover, neither Dr. Casse nor Dr. Semelaigne likened the illness of their patient, M., to the somnosis of the negroes. Dr. Semelaigne even went so far as to remark facetiously: "Let us leave sleeping sickness to the blacks, at least temporarily; the white race has afflictions enough without that particular one."

I considered comparing narcolepsy to *emotive delirium*, that peculiar form of neurosis described so well by Morel. The comparison was momentarily attractive, for all would agree that G. exhibits a conspicuous degree of emotivity and that this emotivity provokes his sleep attacks. But what a difference in the nature of the symptoms and the final outcome! It may be true that both illnesses result from the most trivial or the most bizarre causes, but in G.'s case each access is terminated by a sudden sleep attack, whereas the picture is far more complicated in the case of emotive delirium, which is characterized by sudden chills, pangs, palpitations, clouding of the senses, accelerations of the pulse, exaggerated ideas, and, ultimately, automania [sic]. G. has none of these symptoms. *He falls asleep without suffering;* the patient with emotive delirium trembles at the least provocation, is querulous, and *suffers without falling asleep.*

Nor do I believe that we can make a diagnosis of early, intermittent *ataxia* in the absence of lightning pains and jerky movements.

The weakness, the gait disability, and the aboulia which characterize G.'s illness also bring to mind the *neurasthenic form of spinal irritation.* But, on the one hand, the back pain, the fatigue, the sensations of compression and burning referred to the vertebral column are absent; and, on the other hand, G. does not manifest the slightest trace of melancholia or hypochondria which accompany irritable weakness and render this group of patients extremely wretched and peevish. Our man is a great conversationalist; he lacks neither strength nor energy; he never worries; and his limbs are strong except during attacks. So much for neurasthenia.

In view of the above I consider myself justified in separating narcolepsy from the other neuroses and in bringing it to the attention of my medical colleagues.

Let us recall the case of agoraphobia, confused for so long with vertigo; no sooner was agoraphobia set apart as a distinct clinical entity then it was recognized, overnight, by practitioners all over the world. Perhaps the same thing will happen to narcolepsy, which I regard as a neurotic illness characterized by somnolence and drop attacks or astasia. Has not the vernacular already acknowledged it after a fashion in the expression *"il tombe de sommeil,"* referring to a person who is exhausted from physical exertion and lucubration?

A few words about the cause, the role, and the necessity of physiologic sleep will help us, I believe, to understand the pathogenesis of narcolepsy.

Whether cerebral function is dependent upon a liquid or solid nutrient substance supplied by the gray matter or upon the movement of molecules within the fibers and ganglia of the brain, work or exercise will result in attrition, exhaustion, and loss of energy, and, consequently, in an absolute need for repair.

If cerebral activity varies in direct proportion to cerebral oxygen consumption (as is the case in other tissues), and if more oxygen is absorbed during wakefulness because cerebral blood flow increases, then the more active oxidation becomes, the greater the attrition of cerebral substance, the elimination of catabolites (especially phosphates), and the resultant cerebral exhaustion; and, also, the more urgent the need for a period of rest during which cerebral energy expenditure decreases and the elements of repair accumulate. Now what could be better than sleep to secure these pauses, these indispensable periods of repose and repair?

Having said this, I shall endeavor to explain the underlying cause of G.'s illness. I cannot believe that it resulted from his having been struck on the head by a falling timber and that the injury induced a recurring congestion of the surface of the hemispheres. Such an intermittent congestive process is no easier to explain than the intermittent functional disorder itself.

According to my view, G. is subject to the laws of two different kinds of sleep. Thus, like each of us (instinctively, in the early hours of the evening), he feels the need for rest after the fatigue of the day, and his sleep is then normal, physiologic sleep. But in the daytime it is otherwise; several times each hour he is forced to yield to a sudden, imperious, morbid urge to sleep.

Doubtless, owing to some idiosyncrasy, the quantity of oxygen accumulated in his nervous system is insufficient; or else oxygen is metabolized more rapidly than normal as a consequence of the frequency and intensity of his affective experiences. G.'s cerebral energy expenditure is, perhaps, greater than the next man's, his cerebral arterioles less numerous or of too narrow a caliber. Perhaps, in G.'s case, the elimination of catabolites, particularly phosphates, is too rapid.

Whatever the reason, in his state of relative impoverishment the slightest expenditure of energy, electricity, a storm, or an emotion exhausts his strength and robs him of his vitality. He becomes neuroparalyzed, or, to put it better, neurolyzed [sic], whence his frequent need to sleep (sleep being the principal restorer of the organism). This is also the opinion of Dr. Delasiauve, who writes in the first issue of his journal, "Following rapid depletions the nervous system must restore itself through immobility and rest."

If after hazarding the above explanation, borrowed from physiology, we seek to define the anatomical substrate of this neurosis, then we should place the lesion in the pons, falling back on the authority of Vulpian.* "The pons," writes Vulpian, "should be considered as the association center for emotional impulses; whether the excitant emanates from the brain or from without (and he gives several examples), strong emotional outbursts, dreams, and crying spells are all mediated in the pons. Under the influence of joy, gaiety, sadness, disappointment (as in G.'s case), and terror a certain proportion of the active elements of the pons are affected; the resultant excitation of motor fibers gives rise to a harmony of movement which varies according to the intensity of the stimulus." What a powerful argument in support of my cause! G.'s condition is thus attributable to overactivity of the pons, which goes into spasm, hyperfunctioning at the slightest provocation, and stimulates the other nervous centers. There ensues, on the one hand, a transient

*Lectures on the Physiology of the Nervous System, p. 549.

paralysis of the cerebrospinal axis, a suspension of nervous activity resulting in astasia or drop attacks, and, on the other hand, a momentary cerebral anemia which, in turn, induces sleep. These two symptoms—astasia and sleep—which constitute narcolepsy are precipitated in G.'s case by pontine apoplexy and cerebral shock.

In conclusion I must say a few words about treatment. Influenced at the outset by appearances and by the prior diagnosis of epilepsy—recognizing that affective experiences could precipitate G.'s sleep attacks and believing that vascular spasm could produce cerebral anemia, which is associated with sleep as well as with epilepsy—I prescribed picrotoxin. Picrotoxin prevents spasmodic contractions of the blood vessels by maintaining them in a state of relaxation. I added various bromides to diminish the irritability and reflex activity of the cerebrospinal axis.

I must admit that I did not obtain satisfactory results with this regimen, so I discontinued it. G. lost his vitality and slept more than ever.

Along these same lines, I advised him to inhale the vapors of amyl nitrate (poured onto a handkerchief) at the onset of a narcoleptic attack. Amyl nitrate has the effect of stimulating the cerebral as well as the visceral circulation and of increasing the caliber of blood vessels. It should be recalled that G.'s pulse is normally slow and that it drops even further during his attacks, giving rise to an empty feeling and a whirling sensation in his head. Thus, the use of this medication seemed indicated. It appeared to be effective for a few days, and G. flushed while breathing the vapors, but its use did not abort his attacks, so I discarded it, convinced that cerebral anemia did not contribute to the pathogenesis of his neurosis.

Next, I tried subcutaneous injections of apomorphine, touted in Germany for its efficacy in the convulsive disorders; administered in very small doses at first, and later to the point of nausea, it failed to produce any substantial improvement. Subsequently, I decided to employ symptomatic treatment, i.e., to combat the sleepiness directly. I maintained an issue in G.'s neck and prescribed caffeine valerianate and granules of caffeine. He improved slightly; but, wishing to obtain more marked results, I may, perhaps, have erred in abandoning this form of therapy in favor of another line of attack.

I prescribed strychnine arsenate in increasing doses until G.'s limbs began to shake. I employed this powerful agent in the hope of restoring body tone, combating weakness, and relieving G.'s constant neurolytic exhaustion. At the same time I ordered lukewarm revulsive douches to the vertebral column. I even had recourse to hypodermic injections of curare. In brief, I did my best to treat G. vigorously. I must admit in all humility, however, that these latter remedies scarcely afforded him a few hours respite from his sleep attacks, a few hours for sustained work in the morning and in the evening. In the end, we both realized that this limited success was not owing to our common efforts, and we parted ways, leaving the amelioration or cure of this troublesome neurosis to time and to nature.

Its refractoriness to treatment may be one of the distinguishing characteristics of this neurosis. In the treatment of M., Dr. Casse resorted to tea, coffee, quinine sulfate, iron compounds, purgatives, and baths in the Seine. A vesicatory was applied to M.'s neck—all without effect. As M.'s symptoms were aggravated by dyspepsia, heaviness in the head, and a gait disturbance, my colleague advised taking the waters at Brides. The strongly ionized mountain air and the action of the waters—within and without—restored M.'s appetite and strength; his skin took on a healthier color. Finally, after a season at Brides furthered by a trip to Switzerland, M. returned to Paris, much improved though not completely cured.

It appears from the above that the treatment of narcolepsy is unsatisfactory. In this respect narcolepsy resembles the other neuroses, which so often frustrate our therapeutic intervention. In any event, I am pleased to have been able to provide this first account of narcolepsy, which will undoubtedly stimulate further publications; I have already received from a physician in Lyons the report of a third case, which I intend to publish at a later date.

INFECTIOUS POLYNEURITIS

Introduction

P. Tsairis, M.D.
Assistant Professor of Neurology
Cornell University Medical College

THESE TWO PAPERS are important landmarks in the history of neurology. Landry's paper, written in 1859, is a description of the essential clinical features of a syndrome which he characterized as an acute ascending or "centripetal" paralysis; he clearly stated that sensation and motility could be equally affected. Following this report "Landry's paralysis" became a household word, which other neurologists have debated and elaborated over the last one hundred–plus years. In 1891 Quincke (1) introduced the technique of lumbar puncture which made possible the equally significant contribution in 1916 of Guillain, Barré, and Strohl, that is, the so-called associated albuminocytologic dissociation in the spinal fluid. Subsequently, the eponym "Guillain-Barré" came into vogue. The principal clinical features observed by Landry and the associated cerebrospinal fluid findings described by Guillain and his colleagues still hold and essentially define the syndrome as a specific nosological entity which can be readily differentiated from the more common chronic neuropathies. Every part of the nervous system except the cerebrum, cerebellum, and the first and second cranial nerves has been found to be involved occasionally, which has led to some confusion in establishing rigid diagnostic criteria. In 1938 Guillain tried to distinguish several forms of this syndrome. Subsequently, others proposed a variety of classifications, some of which are rather elaborate, but none of which has contributed very much to a further understanding of the pathogenesis. Major contributions have come from the pathologists and immunologists. The pathological identification of the disease was made by Walter in 1919 (2) and later by Haymaker and Kernohan (3). They reported that the peripheral nervous system was consistently affected; the primary lesion—presumed to be inflammatory—was located near the junction between anterior and posterior spinal roots and extended for a short distance proximally and, also, distally along the spinal nerve. Unfortunately, these authors did not have sufficient material to determine the nature and the total extent of the underlying pathological lesion in the peripheral nervous system. Later studies have revealed lymphocytic inflammatory lesions and myelin destruction without axonal degeneration throughout the peripheral nervous system; this has led logically to the consideration of an allergic, viral, or autoimmune mechanism for the disease (4, 5). It is interesting that Landry noted the onset of paralysis during convalescence from an acute illness in two of the ten cases that he reviewed, whereas in Guillain,Barré, and Strohl's cases there was no obvious antecedent illness. The disease has been associated with or preceded by almost every known illness, but no infectious agent has yet been isolated. Experimental studies have favored an immunological mechanism. In 1955 Waksman and Adams (6) pointed out the similarity as regards the clinical and pathological picture between this diesase and experimental allergic neuritis.

The course of the disease has been described as variable in duration. In most cases it lasts but a few months; however, at times a chronic remitting and/or progressive course may predominate. It seems possible, therefore, that the pathogenesis may be different in different cases. Since Landry's description of this presumably "fatal and pernicious illness," the prognosis is less ominous because of improved methods of general supportive care and, particularly, the use of assisted ventilation as early as possible when respiratory insufficiency develops. In summary, we have made a great deal of progress in understanding the pathology and pathogenesis of this syndrome since Landry and Guillain et al. laid the groundwork. No matter how one tries to identify and separate the various forms of this type of polyradiculoneuropathy, the detailed clinical aspects of the original cases and the associated cerebrospinal fluid changes still remain as hallmarks in establishing a diagnosis and providing a prognosis. If one is fond of eponyms, then Landry-Guillain-Barré-Strohl is the most appropriate descriptive term.

REFERENCES

1. Quincke, H. "Die Lumbarpunction des Hydrocephalus." Berlin, Klin. Wchnschr. 28: 929–933 (Sept. 21), 965–968 (Sept. 28), 1891.

2. Walter, F. K. "Zur Frage der Lokalization der Polyneuritis." Z. ges. Neurol. Psych. 44: 150–178, 1919.

3. Haymaker, W., and Kernohan, J. W. "The Landry-Guillain-Barré Syndrome: A clinicopathologic report of fifty fatal cases and a critique of the literature." Medicine 28: 59–141, 1949.

4. Asbury, A. K., et al. "The inflammatory lesion in idiopathic polyneuritis." Medicine 48: 173–215, 1969.

5. Wisniewski, H., et al. "Landry-Guillain-Barré Syndrome: A primary demyelinating disease." *Arch. Neurol.* 21: 269–276, 1969.

6. Waksman, B. H., and Adams, R. D. "Allergic Neuritis: An experimental disease of rabbits induced by the injection of peripheral nervous tissue and adjuvants." *J. Exper. Med.* 102: 213–235, 1955.

A Note On Acute Ascending Paralysis

O. LANDRY

PART I

I WOULD LIKE to focus attention on a rather rare and generally unknown illness which merits inclusion among the most remarkable afflictions in pathology.

In the "progressive diffuse" paralyses, the initially restricted area of paralysis gradually enlarges from its origin. This proximal propogation may be stepwise and orderly, as in the extenso-progressive ascending paralysis (ascending or centripetal paralysis), or intermittent and random (extenso-progressive intermittent paralysis). In the former, which is of some importance, the symptoms start in the distal extremities, progress proximally and cephalad, and become more intense with each area affected. The symptoms become generalized, producing a generalized paralysis which is quite distinct from syphilis.

I do not intend to present a description of this progressive diffuse paralysis (well described by Oliver of Angers, and Sandras) which characterizes many illnesses which have already been studied. However, it should be noted that, although almost always slowly evolving, it may also progress with extreme rapidity and be serious or even fatal. I would like to distinguish this latter variety by the name *acute ascending paralysis* or *centripetal paralysis*. This acute ascending paralysis shows features of malignant or pernicious illness by its insidious, ever worsening progression by the initial poorly defined symptoms and yet over-

NOTE: Translated by Fred H. Hochberg from: Landry, O., "Note sur la paralysie ascendante aigüe," *Gazette hebdomadaire*, July 29, 1859, 472–74; August 5, 1859, 486–88.

whelming effects, and by the absence of appreciable nerve lesions. From this point of view alone, the process merits special attention, even if it is not intrinsically interesting from every perspective.

I would like to present a case (noted in the service of M. Gubler at the Beaujon Hospital)which represents a complete and authentic example of this illness.

A Case Of Generalized Acute Ascending Paralysis Leading To Death With Autopsy Examination Failing To Reveal Lesions Of The Nervous System

The patient, Jean Baptiste Grellier was a forty-three-year old paver who was admitted to the Beaujon Hospital on June 1, 1859 (M. Gubler's service, Saint Louis Ward No. 22). The patient was small (1 meter 50), appearing weak, thin, pale, with light brown hair, grey eyes, and possessing unremarkable temperament.

The patient's sixty-eight-year old father was said to have been paralyzed during his last years, but his mother, brothers, and sisters had not had a similar illness. The patient had been sick in childhood. He said he had experienced a refractory intermittent fever from four to nine years of age, following which he remained deplorable, weak, and languid. He experienced a long bout of arthritis at the age of fifteen. From this time until 1858 he was well except for widely spaced disturbances, which he could not characterize. He denied venereal diseases except for gonorrhea, followed by painful swelling of the testicles without chancres or inguinal lymphadenopathy.

During the year 1858–1859, the patient experienced a series of almost continuous and increasingly severe illnesses. In July 1858, he developed a sudden chill, followed by fever, generalized malaise, and poorly described symptoms. He stayed in bed for several weeks without receiving specific therapy. His convalescence was short and complete. His appetite and strength returned promptly. Three months later, in November, he experienced another chill, this time accompanied by fever and pain in the left arm which migrated to all four extremities over the next several days. The joints were never red or swollen, and he could not state whether they were more painful than the soft tissues. The pains lasted continuously for three weeks, persisting as dull aches, and aggravated by the least movement. During this period, he was at times ambulatory. He subsequently felt better and returned to his work until March 16. He noted that his appetite was variable, his strength had not recovered, and he was easily fatigued and suffered from a vague generalized malaise.

In the beginning of January 1859, he developed oropharyngeal symptoms. These included swallowing difficulties, a mild continual cough and the sensation of having something stuck in his throat. He was afebrile and had minimal pain. These symptoms persisted, waxing and waning without ever becoming unbearable.

On March 16, the patient suddenly felt an intense chill and pleuritic pain while working, began to cough up sputum, and became febrile. He was diagnosed as having "pulmonary congestion" and was bled three times, following which emetics and topical agents to induce epidermal swelling [topical applications of cantharide which induced epidermal blebs were felt to be of diagnostic or therapeutic value] were applied to the left posterior thorax and the patient was instructed to restrict his dietary intake. He took no nourishment for eighteen days, following which he was allowed some bouillon. He slowly recovered and returned to work on May 9, still very weak and barely eating. His strength, far from improving, continued to diminish, and on May 15 he stopped working again. Feeling weaker, he returned and was admitted to the hospital on June 1.

From May 11 or 12, he felt formications in the tips of his fingers and toes. However, these sensations were minimal and he paid little attention to them. Although generally weak, he remained in control of all movements. His limbs functioned normally with the exception of the unaccustomed weakness that necessitated undue exertion. On June 1, he walked from Boulogne-sur-Seine to the Hospital Beaujon without difficulty. At that time he complained only of generalized weakness, and from his general appearance his complaints seemed somewhat exaggerated and difficult to believe to M. Gubler (who was suspicious of the story).

On June 13, the patient noted that his knees gave way frequently when he walked. On the following day, these flexions became more frequent, his feet seemed heavy and difficult to raise, as if glued to the ground. Several days before, the formications had involved his feet and had begun to gradually involve his legs, thighs, and arms. The sensations seemed to be moving upwards, as a band around the extremity. As they progressed, the caudal areas were left numbed as if by cold.

During the following days, walking became more and more difficult. He could no longer raise his legs, their movements now being slow and associated with dragging of the feet. During morning rounds on June 17, Grellier claimed he could no longer walk or hold himself upright. He stood up, held by two persons, who had to support him to prevent his legs from collapsing. When he tried to walk, his movements were slow and weak, but not abrupt or disorganized. He dragged his feet across the floor, being unable to lift them. When he lay down, he could not raise either of the lower extremities off the mattress and attempts to flex his thighs were painful. He could not turn onto his side as he could not move his legs across each other despite being able to rotate his trunk. Movements of the upper extremity were minimally involved. His grasp was sufficient to allow him to cling to helpers who might have abandoned him while walking; but he complained that his fingers were rigid and stiff, as if bound and compressed by twine—"all tied up." This sensation, apparent for several days, was also noted when he wiggled his toes, but the sensation only appeared during spontaneous movements and not with reflex movements. His joints were normal and the paralyzed areas were supple. In the upper extremity only the elevators of the arm were weakened. This deficit, worse on the right, made it impossible for him to raise and maintain his arm in a horizontal position.

There was no fever, no extremity or vertebral pain, headache, contracture or convulsive movements. Reflexes could not be elicited and sensation was only minimally impaired on the soles of the feet. Intellectual functions were intact. He had experienced diminished appetite without gastrointestinal tract difficulties. His general state was such that M. Gubler still feared that he was being deceived.

By June 20, the motor paralysis had increased in the previously involved areas and had affected formerly intact locations. The lower limbs were now almost completely paralyzed and the upper extremities could no longer be used, although their strength was not completely lost. The continually advancing formications were now felt around the thorax and at the base of the neck and Grellier now complained of slight respiratory difficulty—a sort of distressful constriction of the thorax. He spoke of an epigastric "barrier" which obstructed inspiration. On examination, his rib cage expanded as a passive wall, the individual intercostal movements were very limited, the epigastrium descended slightly during inspiration and rose during expiration. This was best seen when the patient lay on his back, but scarcely visible when he was seated. When Grellier made the effort to control it, his epigastrium moved normally during respiration. Slight dyspnea was present, his speech was halting in quality, and his cough was feeble. He complained that his tongue and jaw felt heavy and less mobile. Movements of eating were more difficult, food seemed harder to chew, and some dysphagia was present. His general condition had not changed from the preceding days.

On June 21, his clinical symptoms were more pronounced than previously. He continually sweated, appeared cachectic, and had a cough that produced a thick mucus. His pulse was rapid (85–90 beats per min.) but was thready and easily obliterated. His temperature was elevated, but was diminished in the distal portions of the limbs. Heart sounds were normal and his veins were not prominent. His appetite was fair, tongue normal (small, oval, and red) and gastrointestinal functions were undisturbed, with stool and urine unremarkable. His motor paralysis had now become generalized, but to varying degrees, and was most pronounced caudally. The distribution of the paralysis may be seen from the following details.

Lower extremities could only be minimally moved but not at all against gravity. Only the triceps surae (crural) contracted appreciably. There were no movements of the toes and feet and no contractions of the leg muscles with maximal effort. If his thigh was elevated, he could maintain his leg in extension for a short while. If the least force was exerted on this extended leg, it gave way, flexed and fell like a dead weight. With his leg supported (to lighten the weight of the limb) he was unable to flex his thigh. Adduction, abduction, extension, and rotation were completely absent. With effort, he could produce small adductor contractions which could be seen and felt by the examiner; but the glutei were silent. In summary, the paralysis was less complete in the anterior and internal thigh muscles than in those innervated by the sciatic nerve.

Upper extremity movements were limited in their range. Arm abduction and elevation were impossible. When his arm was placed at right angles to his shoulder, it fell without any opposition on his part. Contractions of the deltoid could be felt, but these were insufficient. Internal and external rotation of the arm was weak and incomplete. The remainder of the limb, except for distal areas, showed less complete paralysis. Finger abduction consisted only of a few oscillations; adduction and opposition of the thumb was almost nonexistent. His fingers were held semiflexed. Further flexion was slight and he could not grasp or hold objects placed in his hand. Extension of the fingers and wrists was impossible. Lateral and rotatory movements of the hands were restricted. On the left he could flex and extend the forearm—motions which could be impeded by the least resistance. The right forearm motions were weaker and more limited than the left.

Trunk, etc. Sitting was impossible. He fell forward or to the sides when not supported. Voluntary abdominal muscle contractions were feeble. The thoracic walls moved together in inspiration as a result of the isolated action of the cervical muscles. The widths of the intercostal spaces did not change in a physiologic manner. The patient could move his shoulder forward, backward, or upward provided there was no resistance on my part. The trapezius and pectoral muscles contracted well. When resisted minimally these muscles no longer moved. The serratus magnus did not move with any motion or with deep inspiration, and the scapula maintained its normal position. When he was placed in a sitting position, his head fell forward or to the side. He could raise it up again with effort.

The diaphragm was presumably paralyzed, as inspiration, especially if deep, caused the epigastrium to hollow only to raise again with expiration. He could bear down only for a short time, following which he became short of breath and exhausted.

As a result of the paralysis, the thorax filled incompletely and respiration was severely compromised by the defective diaphragmatic movements. Although the sternomastoid and scalene muscles contracted strongly, breathing was rapid, shallow and labored, marked by a very oppressive sensation and severe dyspnea. His speech was halting and the patient's strong voice intermittently became weak. Coughing lacked force. Expectoration was almost impossible.

The patient was dysphagic. His jaw was heavy, he chewed with difficulty and his tongue was less mobile and felt stiff and thick. He continually complained of paresthesias and stiffness in the cheeks. Although his speech was thick, all syllables were articulated and there was no tremor of the lips or tongue. Movements of the eyes and facial muscles were also not impaired.

He urinated and defecated spontaneously and never lost bladder sensation or voluntary voiding. Movements, which were not entirely lost, were soft, weak, slow, and limited, but without exception well-directed and coordinated. Tremors, involuntary contractions, and loss of muscular sensation, part of the picture of general paresis of the insane, were absent here. Muscular irritability was normal and the muscle mass did not appear atrophied. Finally, the nerve fibers retained their excitability to electrical stimulation.

Tendon retraction, muscle contracture, partial or generalized convulsions were not observed during the illness, nor were pathologic involuntary muscle contraction reflexes observed even with varied stimuli.

Sensation was much less affected than movement: pain and temperature sensation was normal, as was proprioception, which was preserved except in his feet and toes. Grellier was unaware of both movement and electrically induced contractions in these areas but was able to feel the intense, cramping pain, as well as the cutaneous pain associated with these stimuli. Elsewhere, proprioception was undiminished. Touch sensation, tested with objects of indifferent temperature, was no longer present on the sole or dorsum of the feet. These sensations improved over the inferior third of the leg and became better appreciated when tested in close proximity to the trunk. In the upper extremities, the sensory loss was complete in the fingertips and present up to the inferior third of the forearm. Touch was blunted over the posterolateral trunk. In these areas, Grellier could not tell the difference between simple touch and tapping of the skin, nor between touch of one's hand and a wool tuft brushed across the skin. Over the nonhypesthetic areas of the trunk he perceived heavy, but not light, touch (skimming the skin with a finger, feather, or pen).

The patient complained of torpor or fullness, especially distally in the paralyzed extremities, feelings which compared to a sensation of persistent intense cold. He stated that these areas always felt cold, indeed palpably cold, despite a cover, the warm temperature of the season and his rapid pulse (85–90). His feet, in particular, had a cadaveric temperature. Special sensation was normal.

Although naturally limited, the patient's intelligence had not deteriorated. He appeared more lucid, sharper, more appropriate, perhaps owing to lessening timidity. Moreover, his general condition was not alarming. His expression was calm, and at first sight, his dyspnea was scarcely noticeable. He was apprehensive about his state and at times seemed to have sad presentiments.

Treatment consisted of limb massages with volatile liniments (terebenthine, quinine) and electrical stimulation along with substantial nourishment (cutlets and Bordeaux wine). These approaches were in use for several days.

During the course of the day his symptoms became more aggravated. Towards 4 o'clock, dyspnea was extreme, his speech halting and weak, his face and neck became slightly cyanotic and were covered with a cold sweat. He complained of breathing difficulties and of a constricting sensation in the larynx.

At 5 o'clock, upon the insistence of the ward nurse, he decided to eat, but could not swallow. He then asked to sit up to facilitate respiration and swallowing, but after several moments, he became weak, asked for help, grew pale, and suddenly died, eight full days after the start of the paralysis.

Autopsy was performed on the evening of June 23 (good weather, 17°C) forty hours after death. Postmortem rigidity was marked, but the body was well-preserved, appearing as in life.

The skull and vertebral column were opened with care. The sinuses were engorged with blood as were the cortical and spinal meningeal veins, but there was no evidence of subarachnoid or subpial blood. There was very light serous fluid found, but no deposits or inflammation.

The cerebral convolutions and cerebellar lobes were normal in color and consistency. Some finely arborized plaques, which did not enter the grey matter, were seen on the mesial surface of the left hemisphere. At these points, as on the entire surface of the cerebral mass, the meninges were easily removed without tearing the subjacent tissue.

The most minute examination revealed no abnormality of the brain stem, cerebellum, or brain proper. The white and grey matter appeared normal. Petechiae, congestion, induration, softening or anemic change of the neuropil were not found. There was no trace of recent or old blood in the parenchyma or in the ventricles.

The spinal cord, likewise, was intact in its entirety and in all its elements. The nerve origins were well-formed. Several sections of the cord, taken at different levels, were submitted for microscopic examination by Messrs. Bourguignon, Gubler, Ch. Robin, and myself. These different examinations produced identical conclusions: the grey and white matter were entirely normal.

The muscles were deep red. Several microscopic specimens of the soleus appeared normal in character.

Very solid adhesions were present in the right thoracic cavity. The right lung appeared purplish wine-red and was engorged like a spleen throughout. Its tissue was harder and more friable than normal. However, several sections thrown into water floated. The largely intact left lung was similar to the right. In several places, the tissue was even more strongly discolored and appeared infiltrated with black pigment. Several calcific areas were seen in both lungs but nothing suggested fresh or softened tuberculous granulomas. The other organs were not examined.

In summary, we have presented a pitiful man of forty-three years of age, weakened by a series of acute illnesses, blood loss, and a prolonged restricted diet. During a slow and incomplete convalescence, he experienced gradually increasing generalized weakness without any sign of paralysis. Formications were initially limited to the toes and fingers and were not associated with impairment of movement or ambulation.

After a prodomal period of approximately six weeks characterized by these phenomena, the extremity paresthesias crept upwards, leaving numbness and paralysis behind. The latter, which especially affected ambulation, moved rapidly from the feet to the rest of the lower extremities, to the upper extremities, the trunk, the respiratory muscles, the tongue, etc. Movement was most impaired in the limbs, but micturition and defecation remained intact until the end. Muscle tone and irritability as well as nerve excitability were not altered. There were no contractures, convulsions, tremors, fibrillations, or pathologic muscle movements. The patient did not complain of pain in the extremities, vertebrae, or head, and tenderness was not present. Fever was absent and intelligence was unaffected.

Terminally, respiration became more and more difficult, signs of asphyxia appeared and the patient died suddenly, eight days after the onset of paralytic symptoms.

Autopsy did not reveal any lesion of the nervous system. We found only traces of pleurisy and recent pneumonia.

PART II

Thus, there exists a rapidly generalized paralysis which terminates with death in a few days. Autopsy examination provides no clue as to its origin, and its onset offers no hint of the proximity of its fatal outcome. On the contrary, observers have noted the contrast between the outcome of the disease and its benign initial appearance. This initial appearance is so benign that the observer often thinks that the patient has voluntarily exaggerated, or even simulated, his illness, so that even eight hours before death, there is little concern. The paralysis extends relentlessly from the lower to the upper extremities and from the limbs to the trunk, producing a quiet asphyxia when the respiratory muscles become involved. This insidious and rapid progression to an unexpected and fatal outcome suggests that the illness should be considered a malignant or pernicious disease.

I have observed four cases which were similar to the case described, and have uncovered five more from the literature, bringing the total to ten. I will limit myself to a brief presentation of the principal features of the group, rather than point out the differences in pattern of evolution, muscular irritability, etc., among the cases.

In this type of paralysis, sensation and movement can be equally involved. However, in general, movement is especially affected by gradual diminution of muscle strength and flaccidity of the limbs and loss of reflexes without tremor, contraction, localized or generalized convulsions, or pathologic muscle reflexes. In almost all cases, micturition and defecation remained intact, and there is no evidence of central neurologic symptoms—i.e. no pain along the vertebral column—occuring either spontaneously or as a result of compression, and there is no headache or delirium. Until the very end, intellectual faculties are completely preserved.

As in our patient, paralytic signs can be preceded by a slight generalized weakness, formications, and even fleeting cramps, or the onset can be sudden and unexpected. In each case, the paralysis rapidly advances from the lower to the upper extremities, with a constant tendency to become generalized. The first deficits always appear in the periphery of the limbs, most often in the lower extremities. From there they follow a progressively ascending course and invade the muscular system in an almost constant sequence: first, the muscles of the toes and feet, then the posterior muscles of the thigh and pelvis, and lastly, the anterior and medial muscles of the thigh; second, the muscles of the fingers of the hand and of the proximal arm at the shoulder, and the muscles between the forearm and the upper arm; third, the trunk muscles; fourth, the respiratory muscles, tongue, pharynx, and esophagus. The paralysis is then generalized, but is not as complete as it is in the extremities.

This phase of the illness is more or less rapid, occurring over eight days in M. Gubler's patient, and fifteen days in another case. More often, the process evolves over two or three days and sometimes over several hours.

When the paralysis has reached peak intensity, death by asphyxia is imminent. However, in eight of the ten cases, this fatal outcome was avoided by judicious intervention or a spontaneous arrest in the progression of the disease. Two of the ten cases died during this period.

An illness to which a fifth of the patients succumbs is without a doubt a grave process. It should be understood that in spite of the relatively favorable outcome of this illness, the danger is great and the prognosis remains uncertain. The patient remains in evident peril while the paralytic symptoms are rapidly ascending and his life may be endangered when his respiratory muscles are involved. As asphysia has been the most common cause of death, it is impossible to predict the extent of involvement and effectiveness of therapy in any single case.

The pattern of resolution of the paralysis reverses that of the development of the paralysis. The last invaded upper extremities are the first to recover; the area of resolution progresses from proximal to distal. Some patients may remit rapidly while others may enter a chronic state, from which they slowly improve. One patient who showed well-defined, frequent fluctuations between improvement and worsening over several months died during a seizure. A woman, reported by M. Cavare (of Toulouse), developed steady waves of paralysis—the illness ran its course in several hours.

I believe it is useless to dwell on the diagnostic features of acute ascending paralysis as no other disease state presents a similar constellation of signs.

The paucity of facts makes it impossible to study the etiology of this process, but the circumstances in which it develops can be noted.

In two instances, it developed during convalescence from an acute illness (our case description is one of these) which must play some role in the pathogenesis of the paralysis. The second subject developed the illness over five days while convalescing from a long bout of typhoid fever. The paralysis remitted spontaneously, and less than two weeks later he was entirely well.

In two instances, the acute ascending paralysis occurred against a background of menstrual difficulties. In one case, menses were retarded by a cold; leeches were applied to the vulva, and recovery was complete within seven days. In another case, suppression of menses during a moral crisis was followed by multiple neurologic symptoms and an acute ascending paralysis. The paralysis became generalized and life-threatening within three days. Remarkably, inhalation of chloroform and opium produced a sudden and marked improvement. After several remissions, the illness became chronic, resulting in death during an unexpected paroxysm.

In two additional cases, exposure to cold was associated with an acute and life-threatening illness which in one patient arrested spontaneously and in the other slowly advanced.

Paralysis leading to death in two days occurred in a woman convalescing from childbirth. Treatment consisted of bleeding and purges.

One patient presented during a syphilitic diathesis. The paralytic signs progressed more slowly and were less alarming than in the other cases, and rapidly disappeared following antisyphilitic treatment.

In the two remaining cases, there was no information as to the cause of the events. In one woman, the paralysis developed as steady paroxysms which responded to quinine sulfate (as I noted above).

As can be seen, the causes or circumstances under which the illness occurs are variable. The influences I have mentioned are remote causes. The direct cause of the distrubances remains to be determined.

The two autopsies performed prior to this writing have only furnished negative anatomic-pathologic data. However, Oliver (of Angers), who had a good knowledge of acute ascending paralysis, believed it was due to vascular congestion of the spinal cord. The symptoms do not suggest this is the case. It is known that the accumulation of a certain amount of blood in the veins of the nervous system, especially following asphyxia as in his patients, does not establish the nature of a disease. Indeed, this illness ought to be placed among the essential paralyses, i.e. those without an apparent lesion of the nervous system. I feel these facts are noteworthy. In this simple note, I would like to avoid considering the mode of production of ascending paralysis in general and of the acute form in particular.

On a syndrome of radiculoneuritis with hyperalbuminosis of the cerebrospinal fluid without a cellular reaction.

Remarks on the clinical characteristics and tracings of the tendon reflexes

G. GUILLAIN, J. A. BARRÉ, AND A. STROHL

WE WOULD LIKE to draw attention to a clinical syndrome observed in two patients that is characterized by motor difficulties, loss of the deep tendon reflexes with preservation of the cutaneous reflexes, paresthesias with slight impairment of objective sensation, muscle tenderness, slight alterations in nerve conduction and electromyographic patterns, and a remarkable increase in cerebrospinal fluid albumin in the absence of a cellular reaction (albumino-cytologic dissociation). This ostensibly infectious or toxic process appears to simultaneously involve nerve roots, peripheral nerves and muscles. It is distinct from the simple radiculopathies, pure polyneuropathies, and from the polymyositides. Experimental data derived from tracings of the latency and speed of the reflex response and muscular contraction indicate that the entire peripheral neuromuscular motor apparatus is involved. We particularly emphasize the increased cerebrospinal fluid albumin content without

NOTE: Translated by Fred H. Hochberg from: Guillain, G., Barré, J. A., and Strohl, A., "Sur un syndrome de radiculo-névrite avec hyperalbuminose du liquide céphalo-rachidien sans réaction cellulaire. Remarques sur les caractères cliniques et graphiques des réflexes tendineaux," *Bulletin Société Médicale des Hopitaux*, Paris, October 13, 1916, 1462–70.

309

cellular reaction, an observation which has not previously been reported.

CASE 1

D..., a twenty-five-year-old soldier of the...th cavalry, entered the Neurological Center of the Sixth Army on August 20, 1916, because of weakness of the upper and lower limbs. On about July 25, he first noted formication in the feet and weakness of the lower extremities, the latter forcing him to halt every 200 to 300 meters. During the following days, the formication spread to his upper extremities and lower face. Muscular weakness appeared in the upper limbs.

These signs and symptoms developed without apparent associated cause. He had had no recent infections (including sore throat and gastrointestinal disturbance) or fatigue. His past medical history was benign; he denied any syphilis or excessive alcohol intake.

When examined on August 25, he exhibited diffusely diminished muscle strength in the upper and lower limbs but without a total paralysis. This marked distal extremity weakness was especially obvious in the flexors and extensors of the toe, ankle, finger, and wrist.

The trunk muscles were weak. He could not rise from a lying position without using his hands for support. He was able to walk a few steps; some instability of upright posture was noted, and he was unable to stand on one foot.

There was no weakness of the facial muscles.

Electrophysiologic studies in the upper extremities showed normal faradic excitability and brisk jerk responses to galvanic excitation of all muscles. Polar inversion was not seen. Slight hypoexcitability of the common extensor of the fingers was detected. Faradic excitability in the lower extremities was slightly diminished, and galvanic excitability was diminished in the trunk of the sciatic and internal popliteal nerves, as well as in the semitendinosus muscle and the extensors of the fingers. Responses were sometimes slightly slowed. Polar inversion was seen in the external gastrocnemius but the degeneration reaction was very incomplete.

The deep tendon reflexes at the knee, ankle, and medial plantar surface, as tested with a percussion hammer, were abolished, as were those of the antebrachial radio- and cubito-pronator and olecranon areas.

The cutaneous plantar reflex induced frank flexion of the toes with distant contraction of the tensor fascialata. The cremasteric and cutaneous abdominal reflexes were normal. There were no defensive responses to pinching the sole of the foot or hyperflexion of the toes.

Neuromuscular excitability as elicited by the reflex hammer was preserved.

The patient constantly complained of formications just above the malleoli and just above the wrists. There was no deficit of objective sensation, except possibly for slightly hypesthetic touch, pain, and temperature sensation in the feet and hands. The muscles of the upper and lower limbs were painful to pressure.

The pupils, which were equal, reacted to light and to accommodation. There were sphincter difficulties. No fever, respiratory, or gastrointestinal signs were found, and the pulse was normal.

The urine, examined in the Army Bacteriologic and Chemical Laboratory, contained no sugar, albumin, or indoxyl, the chemical elements being in their normal proportions.

Lumbar puncture showed a clear cerebrospinal fluid under normal pressure; but with increased albumin (2.5 grams of albumin per liter) and without leukocytic reaction (two to four lymphocytes per field). The blood Wassermann reaction was negative. Pharyngeal and nasal mucosal cultures showed no diphtheritic bacilli.

Therapy consisted of absolute bed-rest, liniment massage of the upper and lower extremities, strychnine injections and oral salicylate of soda compounds.

On August 27, the lower extremity formications had diminished. On September 2, the muscular weakness had ameliorated and the foot formications had disappeared, although still present in the hands. The tendon reflexes were still absent. Another lumbar puncture showed, as previously, a marked increase in cerebrospinal fluid albumin without appreciable leukocyte reaction.

On September 19, the motor difficulties had very much improved. The patient was able to walk for an hour and stand on one foot. The paresthesias had completely disappeared in the inferior extremities, but persisted, although attenuated, in the hands. Tendon reflexes and withdrawal responses were still absent but cutaneous reflexes were normal. Neuromuscular excitability in the upper and lower limbs and in the face, elicited by reflex hammer, appeared normal.

The patient continued to improve and was sent to a convalescent center on September 30.

Case 2

D... , a thirty-five-year-old infantry soldier, was admitted to the Neurologic Center of the Sixth Army on September 5, 1916 with lower limb motor difficulties, which appeared under the following circumstances.

On August 28, after a march of fifteen kilometers, he experienced unusual fatigue, headache, and erratic pains in the upper and lower extremities. He lay down, but could not sleep, and shivered part of the night. The next morning, he walked with great difficulty to report to sick call, and was exempted from duty for the next four days. The weakness began in the lower extremities and subsequently involved the upper extremities. On the fourth day he decided to set out with his comrades at about 5:00 A.M. He dressed for the march, but fell backwards with his knapsack and could not get up again. He was taken to a first-aid station and then evacuated to the Army Neurological Center. These complaints developed without apparent cause: he had had no recent infectious illnesses, no symptoms of gastrointestinal intoxication or other disturbance. He very strongly denied having had syphilis.

On September 5, we found the patient able to make, with difficulty, little movements of flexion and extension of the toes, flexion of the leg on the thigh, and the thigh on the pelvis. The same difficulty was present with regard to movements of the upper extremities, where the difficulty was much more prominent peripherally. He held his head rotated to the left, and experienced difficulty in turning it to the right. He could open and close his mouth, but slowly and incompletely.

Electrophysiologic examination showed slight faradic hyperexcitability of the nerves and muscles. Excitability was slightly enhanced to galvanic stimulation, especially for the nerves of the upper extremity. There was no reaction of degeneration.

The knee jerks were very difficult to elicit because of increased muscular tone, but they seemed to be present. Ankle jerks and medial plantar responses could not be determined because of hypertonus and the impossibility of provoking a complete muscular movement. The cutaneous plantar reflexes showed frank flexion of the toes; the cremasteric and abdominal cutaneous reflexes were normal. No withdrawal response was seen, either by pinching the dorsum of the foot or hyperflexing the toes; but the patient perceived the sensations produced by these stimuli.

Neuromuscular excitability (tested with the reflex hammer) was preserved.

The patient complained of formications in the extremities. There was no impairment of objective sensation except possible touch, pain, and temperature hypesthesia in the feet and the hands. The muscles of the calf and forearm were tender on compression. The pupils were equal, reacted to light and to accommodation. The patient voided spontaneously. He felt the need to micturate but was unaware of urination. Fever, Kernig's sign, nausea or vomiting were not present. Urinalysis in the Army Bacteriologic and Chemical Laboratory showed no sugar, albumin, or indoxyl, and the chemical analysis was normal.

It should be noted that a cutaneous eruption had appeared three or four days earlier. This was erythematous and papulomacular in character and was localized principally to the upper part of the thorax and the lower part of the abdomen. In addition to the areas we have mentioned, eruptive lesions were disseminated over the rest of the thorax and the abdomen but not on the upper or lower extremities.

Lumbar puncture showed clear cerebrospinal fluid, not under increased pressure, with increased albumin content (more than 0.85 grams of albumin according to the rachialbuminmeter of Sicard) but without significant leukocyte reaction (three to four lymphocytes per field).

The symptoms found on the first exam remitted slightly. On September 20, distal extremity weakness was still present, all tendon reflexes except the left antibrachial were absent, the cutaneous reflexes were preserved, and muscular tenderness to pressure, as well as paresthesias in the extremities with slight hypesthesia persisted. Intermittent little myoclonic jerks were seen in the calf and thigh muscles. Another lumbar puncture revealed the same abnormalities seen on the antecedent examination, a clear fluid under normal pressure, containing markedly increased albumin without leukocytes (three to four lymphocytes per field).

The patient was evacuated to the rear on October 1....

These two cases are quite similar. Each developed a clinical syndrome without apparent cause, characterized by motor difficulties of all the muscles of the upper and lower extremities, but predominantly distally, by loss of deep tendon reflexes with preservation of cutaneous reflexes, by paresthesias with slight loss of objective sensation, by tenderness of the muscle bodies to pressure, and by minimal alterations in the electrophysiological reactions of the nerves and muscles, by a rather special abnormality of the cerebrospinal fluid characterized by increased cerebrospinal fluid albumin concentration without cellular reaction.

The significant rise in cerebrospinal fluid albumin concentration without cellular reaction seems to be an important peculiarity. This albumino-cytologic dissociation (Sicard and Foix) is seen most often in certain cases of medullary compression, in Pott's disease, and in certain instances of neurosyphilis, but it has not been reported, we believe, in the pure radiculopathies or polyneuropathies.

Notably, our second case developed muscle hypertonia in addition to paralysis. With the patient at rest, the muscle consistency was clearly greater than that of a healthy resting individual. The limbs maintained their full range of passive motion, but voluntary movements were limited and made with a certain stiffness and slowness. Tendon reflexes were difficult to elicit because the usual muscle responses were hindered by the continued contractions of their antagonists. In spite of these signs, also frequently found in meningitis, the patient could be seated, keeping his upper extremities almost completely extended. The slight knee flexion accompanying this maneuver could be overcome by insignificant pressure. Kernig's sign was not present in our patient: when the lower limbs were raised to form an almost right angle with the trunk they flexed as would those of a normal subject. *This state of hypertonicity has nothing in common with meningitis, but relates rather to a special state of muscular contractility which appears to depend on a peripheral nerve lesion. We have already stressed the fact that hypertonicity can be encountered in the course of certain peripheral neuritides and of incomplete nerve injuries, and specified on that occasion that contractures frequently observed in the course of certain facial palsies are not an exception among peripheral nerve lesions as had been classically believed.*

The syndrome observed in our two patients is due to simultaneous involvement of the nerve roots, peripheral nerves and muscles. The considerable increase in cerebrospinal fluid albumin indicates meningeal involvement, while the pattern of extremity muscle paralysis and the muscle pain in response to compression indicate the involvement of nerve and muscle. Besides, it seems to us that neurologists become too precise when they try to completely separate the polyneuritides and polymyositides. In a greater number of cases of infectious or toxic polyneuropathy, the intramuscular nerve endings and the muscle fibers themselves can be involved. In reality, the pathologic process is much more a polyneuromyositis than a pure polyneuritis.

In the case of our first patient, experimental research using myographic tracings enabled us to bring out certain new features in the study of reflexes and muscular contractility. Such tracings can give us important data for the interpretation of symptoms and lesions.

In the first case, although the tendon reflexes (by clinical examination) appeared to have been lost throughout the course of the illness the tracing of the distension of the quadriceps femoris and gastrocnemius muscles following percussion of the tendons or muscle bodies displayed interesting features. Thus, from the onset of the illness, the knee jerk showed a contraction following a mechanical blow (Fig. 1). This contraction, notably weaker than that obtained in a normal subject, appeared after a latency of 0.056 seconds, but was *not* followed by a second contraction of greater amplitude and duration that represents the true "reflex" response in a normal tracing. Scarcely 0.152 seconds after the beginning of excitation, we noted a very slight upward deflection of the curve, indicating the vestige of the reflex contraction. The knee jerk was thus almost completely reduced to an idio-muscular contraction up to the end of the illness. During this period, percussion of the quadriceps provoked a good muscular contraction with a latency of 0.051 seconds followed by a second contraction having all the characteristics of a response of reflex origin and appearing 0.150 seconds after the onset of excitation. The muscle, which only weakly and incompletely responded to mechanical excitation of its tendon (transmitted by propagation to the muscular fibers), demonstrated, when it was struck directly, a double

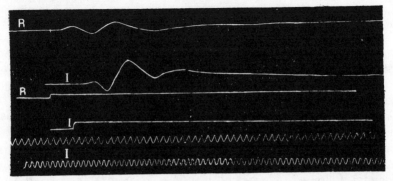

Figure 1. R.R.R. Myogram of the quadriceps femoris during patellar reflex. The signal of Desprez indicates the percussive stimulus and indicates the time in fractions of 1/100 second. I.I.I. The same tracing for direct percussion of the quadriceps femorus, recorded on August 21, 1916. Of note is the almost total absence of "reflex" contraction following patellar percussion in comparison to its clear preservation in response to direct percussion.

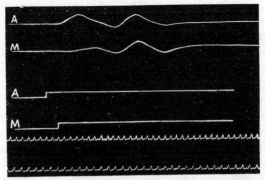

Figure 2. A. Myogram of the internal gastrocnemius during the Achilles reflex. M. The same during the medial-plantar reflex, recorded on August 21, 1916. The first evaluation in record A is a mechanical jerk, the second is a "muscular" contraction which is absent during the Achilles reflex but weakly visible during the medial-plantar reflex.

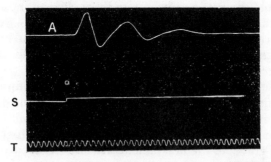

Figure 3. A. Myogram of the external gastrocnemius during the Achilles reflex, recorded September 15, 1916. The reflex shows three characteristic elevations. The "muscular" contraction and especially the "reflex" contraction are weaker than normal.

315

contraction which was almost normal. The muscle seems to be mechanically hypoexcitable except to sudden blows to the muscle body itself.

The ankle jerk was similarly altered and reduced, leaving only its mechanical response. The latter (Fig. 2), of very low amplitude, appeared after an extremely long latent period of around 0.110 seconds. It was not followed by reflex contraction. In contrast to the knee jerk, these changes partially resolved and already on September 5 (Fig. 3), we detected a higher-amplitude muscular jerk, more brisk, more rapid (0.035 seconds), followed by a second response (recognizable as a reflex) appearing after a latency of 0.140 seconds. The neuromuscular response of the gastrocnemius followed a similar course and gradually resumed a more normal shape.

It is interesting to note that, at the start of the illness, when percussion of the Achilles and gastrocnemius tendons elicited only a muscular response, study of the medial plantar reflex, even at this time, showed a second contraction which was weak, but clearly a reflex, with a latency of 0.144 seconds.

In summary, while the clinical exam permitted only the demonstration that tendon reflexes were lost, detailed analysis of the myographic curves indicated which elements of the reflex were altered, and led us to the following observations: First, the reflex segment of the myographic curve is either absent, or when it persists, extremely reduced in amplitude with a markedly slow inscription. Its considerable latency, almost double the normal, demonstrates the profound and predominant alteration of nerve conduction of the central part of the reflex. Furthermore, the muscular response appears equally modified, diminished in height, and slowed and delayed in appearance, which leads one to think that the muscular element has been equally affected by the toxic process. Finally, comparison of the curves obtained after percussion of the patella and Achilles tendons shows a different evolution for the two reflexes. While the first had been rapidly abolished and had not reappeared by the patient's discharge from hospital, the second, which seemed clinically absent, had begun to approach normal by myography. *This emphasizes the fact that the graphic method is a more precise indicator of the state of the tendon reflex than is the reflex hammer.*

The pathogenesis of this radiculoneuropathic syndrome cannot be precisely defined. Although an infection or toxic insult should be considered, we have found no supporting evidence for either. Judged by the evolution of the disease in our two patients, the prognosis does not appear to be grave, as the first patient was almost cured and the second on the road to recovery when discharged from the army.